ECTOPARASITIC DISEASES

ECTOPARASITIC DISEASES

JAMES H. DIAZ

Environmental and Occupational Health Sciences,
School of Public Health, Louisiana State
University/LSU Health, New Orleans, Louisiana,
United States

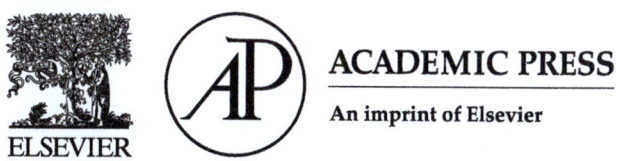

ELSEVIER

ACADEMIC PRESS

An imprint of Elsevier

ISBN: 978-0-443-26724-6

For information on all Academic Press publications visit our website at https://www.elsevier.com/books-and-journals

Publisher: Stacy Masucci
Acquisitions Editor: Kattie Washington
Editorial Project Manager: Deepak Vohra
Production Project Manager: Vishnu T. Jiji
Cover Designer: Greg Harris

Typeset by TNQ Technologies

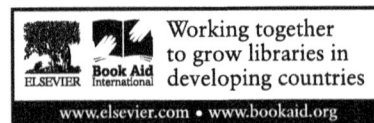

Contents

About the author   xi
Foreword   xiii
Preface   xv

1. Introduction to ectoparasitic diseases   1

Definitions   1
Taxonomy   1
Epidemiology   2
Pathophysiology   2
Infectious disease transmission   3
Conclusions   3
References   8

2. Pediculosis (lice)   9

Definitions   9
Epidemiology   12
Diagnosis   14
Clinical manifestations and differential diagnosis   19
Therapy   20
Prevention   25
References   26

3. Trombidiosis (larval chigger mites)   27

Definitions and taxonomy   27
Life cycle   28
Regional distribution and ecology   29
Feeding behavior   30
Clinical manifestations   31
Treatment   32
Complications   33
Prevention and control   33
References   33
Further reading   33

4. Scrub typhus (larval typhus mites)   **35**

Introduction   35
Taxonomy   35
Arthropod vectors   35
Ecology   36
Epidemiology   37
The microbiology and pathophysiology of rickettsial infectious diseases   40
Clinical manifestations of scrub typhus   41
Laboratory diagnosis   42
Treatment   43
Empirical treatment with doxycycline in patients with undifferentiated non-malaria
fever with eschar   44
Prevention and control of scrub typhus   44
Rickettsialpox and scrub typhus as widely distributed and neglected mite-transmitted
infectious diseases   45
References   45
Further reading   46

5. Scabies (scabies mites)   **47**

Definitions   47
Epidemiology   47
Transmission   49
Clinical manifestations   49
Diagnosis   55
Therapy   56
Prevention and control   60
Conclusions   61
References   61

6. Rickettsialpox (rat mites)   **65**

Reservoirs and vectors   65
Life cycle and feeding behavior   65
Epidemiology   66
Clinical manifestations   66
Differential diagnosis   68
Laboratory diagnosis   68
Therapy   69
Prevention and control   69
References   69

7. Animal (zoonotic) and insect mites   **71**

   Animal (zoonotic) mites   71
   Domestic animal-transmitted cheyletiellosis   71
   Domestic animal scabies in humans (Scabietic mange)   75
   Zoonotic acariasis: Definitions   76
   Rat, bat, and snake mite bites   78
   Insect (itch) mites   81
   References   86

8. Plant, food, dust, and follicle mites and allergies   **87**

   Plant, food, and food storage mites   87
   Dust mites and dust mite allergies   92
   Follicle mites   96
   References   100

9. Myiasis, murine typhus, tungiasis, and plague (flies and fleas)   **103**

   Myiasis   103
   Flea infestations   109
   Murine typhus   112
   Tungiasis   113
   Plague   117
   References   124

10. Tick-transmitted bacterial diseases   **127**

   Introduction   127
   Vector behavior   127
   Biology and taxonomy   127
   Epidemiology   129
   Borrelioses   133
   Rickettsioses   143
   Tularemia   152
   Anaplasmosis and the ehrlichioses   155
   Prevention and control of tickborne diseases   160
   References   161

11. Babesiosis   **165**

   History   165
   Vectors, reservoirs, and regional distributions   165
   Microbiology   165

Epidemiology 166
Clinical manifestations 169
Laboratory Diagnosis 170
Therapy 171
Prevention and control 171
References 172

12. Tick-transmitted viral diseases 173

Introduction 173
Epidemiology 173
Tickborne viral encephalitides 177
Hemorrhagic fever viruses 180
Coltiviruses 181
References 182

13. The tick sialome, tick-transmitted coinfections, and tick paralysis 185

The tick sialome 185
Tick-transmitted coinfections 186
Tick paralysis 187
The differential diagnosis of tick paralysis 191
References 194

14. Red meat allergies after tick bites 197

Introduction 197
Epidemiology 197
Geographic distribution 198
Immunology 199
Risk factors 204
Clinical manifestations 206
Diagnosis 206
Treatment 207
Prevention and control 207
Conclusions 208
References 209

15. True bugs (Order Hemiptera) as ectoparasites: Bedbugs 213

Introduction and taxonomy 213
Biology and life cycle 213
Bed bug behavior 214
Epidemiology 216
Clinical manifestations 216

Detection and diagnosis 218
Management 219
Control and prevention 219
Conclusions 220
References 220

16. Insect repellents, insecticides, and vector control **221**

Introduction 221
Definitions 221
Why use insect repellents? 221
The history of insect repellents 222
Selecting the best insect repellents 222
Chemical versus plant-based insect repellents: Which are the best? 222
Insect repellent use in children and during pregnancy 231
Insect repellents and sunscreens 232
Area and barrier chemical insect repellents 232
Nonchemical measures for the management, control, and prevention of arthropod-borne
infectious diseases 233
Conclusions 233
References 234
Further reading 236

17. Delusional ectoparasitosis (Morgellons disease) **237**

Introduction 237
History and disease definitions 239
Epidemiology 239
Clinical behavioral manifestations 241
Differential diagnosis 241
Treatment 244
Conclusions 246
References 247

18. Conclusions **249**

Introduction 249
Bartonella quintana — A reemerging pathogen 249
Babesiosis — Increasing regional prevalence 249
Rhipicephalus sanguineus — A new and unanticipated vector 250
Conclusions 251
References 251

Index 253

About the author

James H. Diaz, MD, MPH & TM, Dr PH, FACMT, FASTMH, is a Professor of Public Health and Preventive Medicine at the LSU School of Public Health in New Orleans, LA. He is board certified in general preventive medicine and public health, occupational and environmental medicine, and medical toxicology and is a Fellow of the American Society of Tropical Medicine and Hygiene and the American College of Preventive Medicine.

Dr. Diaz's current academic and clinical research interests include the following: (1) occupational and environmental toxicology; (2) infectious diseases, poisonings, and injuries in international travelers; (3) emerging environmentally associated diseases and poisonings, particularly food-borne, water-borne, and vector-borne infectious diseases and poisonings; and (4) the impact of climate change on infectious disease outbreaks and natural disasters and their public health outcomes. Dr. Diaz has published 5 textbooks and over 350 original articles and chapters in scientific journals and textbooks.

Foreword

First encounters with ectoparasites

Growing up, the sounds of mosquitoes near my ears and the checking of my dog for ticks were a trade-off for spending the summer in a woodsy area. I never thought of it as an introduction to the realm of ectoparasites. However, when I got to college, the life cycles of parasites grabbed my interest and that begat my education in epidemiology and public health. However, when my father, living in eastern Long Island, was bitten by a deer tick, my journey changed from being an academic interested in ectoparasites to a son witnessing the sequela of a tick-borne illness.

A new textbook

This personal interaction with ectoparasites deepened my appreciation for the subject matter explored in this new textbook by Professor James Diaz. It highlighted the real-world implications of the intricate relationships between hosts and parasites and the challenges faced in mitigating the impact of these interactions on human and animal health.

International travel and ectoparasites

Working with international health organizations, I also had the opportunity to travel to many countries, particularly those where arthropod-associated diseases are still significant causes of morbidity and mortality. There, I was reminded of the intricate balance between humans and ectoparasites. The vibrant ecosystems of these regions introduced me to a diverse array of external ectoparasites, each with its unique story and ecological role.

Climate change and ectoparasites

Furthermore, our warming climate, increased coastal flooding, and the expansion of human activity into previously wild areas increase the risk of exposure. As we delve into the pages of this textbook, let us draw inspiration from our real-world encounters that underscore the significance of ectoparasitology on local and global populations.

Recommendations

Through my encounter with ectoparasites, I came to appreciate the importance of the knowledge contained within these pages. This text provides a theoretical foundation and resonates with the practical experiences of those who have encountered these external freeloaders in their natural habitats. I hope that, just as my personal experience enriched my understanding, Dr. Diaz's comprehensive textbook on ectoparasites will leave a lasting impression on all who embark on their journey into this fascinating field.

Edward J. Trapido, MSPH, ScM, ScD, FACE
Interim Dean
Associate Dean of Research
Professor of Epidemiology
LSU School of Public Health
New Orleans, Louisiana

Preface

Ectoparasites infest the skin and its appendages, such as the hair and sebaceous glands, and most external orifices, especially the ears, nares, and orbits, and can cause systemic infections, such as Lyme disease, scrub typhus, and plague. Over the past two decades, there have been several reports of significant outbreaks of ectoparasitic diseases, principally myiasis, scabies, tungiasis, scrub typhus, and tick-borne infections and coinfections both in indigenous populations and in travelers returning from developing nations and even exclusive temperate and tropical zone resorts.

About the new text

The new text, *Ectoparasitic Diseases*, covers the neglected topic of arthropod ectoparasites, their diversity, and the conditions caused or vectored by them. This text provides information in a single reference on the full array of ways in which lice, mites, flies, fleas, and ticks can be parasites, vectors of parasitic infections, allergens, commensals, or the cause of psychological issues. This text also covers the diagnosis, treatment, and prevention of ectoparasitic conditions caused by arthropods of medical importance, such as the Oriental rat flea, *Xenopsylla cheopis*, which transmits plague. No other text has ever addressed the topic of ectoparasitic diseases exclusively and has only treated ectoparasitic diseases with a few chapters inserted in the text, comprising a small percentage of the chapters (Table 1.1).

Some key features of ectoparasitic diseases

- Identifies the types of ectoparasites and differentiates between the infections transmitted by ectoparasites from ectoparasitic infestations and allergies.
- Provides information on diagnoses, treatments, prevention, and control strategies.
- Examines the psychological and socio-economic impact of infections, infestations, health disparities, and ectoparasite-associated conditions, allergies, and predisposing risk factors.
- Addresses topics not covered in other texts on parasitic diseases, such as the ones given in the following paragraphs.

Tick paralysis

Tick paralysis is a rare, regional, and seasonal cause of acute ataxia and ascending paralysis with an incubation period of 4—7 days after female tick attachment, mating, and blood-

Table 1.1 Existing textbooks of medical parasitology/parasitic diseases.

Authors	Titles	Editions	Publishers	Chapters	Ectoparasitic disease chapters
Markell EK, John DT, Krotoski WA	*Markell and Voge's Medical Parasitology*	8th	Saunders	16	1
Neva FA, Brown HW	*Basic Clinical Parasitology*	6th	Appleton and Lange	19	3
Peters W, Pasvol G	*Atlas of Tropical Medicine and Parasitology*	6th	Mosby	10	1
Despommier DD, Gwadz RW, Hotez PJ, Knirsch CA	*Parasitic Diseases*	4th	Apple Trees	11	2
Bogitsh BJ, Cheng TC	*Human Parasitology*	2nd	Academic Press	18	1

feeding. Although 43 species of ticks have been implicated in tick paralysis cases worldwide, most cases occur in the United States, the Canadian Pacific Northwest, and Australia. In the US Pacific Northwest, tick paralysis is caused by the American dog tick (*Dermacentor variabilis*) or the Rocky Mountain wood tick (*D. andersoni*) during April through June, when *Dermacentor* ticks emerge from hibernation to mate and seek blood meals. The mechanism of neurotoxic paralysis in *Dermacentor* tick paralysis is unknown. Neuroelectrophysiologic studies have suggested that the sodium flux across axonal membranes is blocked at the nodes of Ranvier, leaving neuromuscular transmission unimpeded.

Host immune responses to tick-transmitted salivary substances

The combinations of bioactive compounds in the tick salivary complex or sialome act synergistically to secure the initial and sustained tick attachment, permit immediate and prolonged blood-feeding, disarm host humoral and cellular immunity, and assure pathogen transmission. Investigators have now identified many immunomodulatory compounds in the tick sialome that are family-specific, and even species-specific, as a result of the different tick blood-feeding behaviors. Ixodid or hard ticks attach firmly to the host and feed for days with a greater likelihood of transmitting pathogens than argasid or soft ticks which attach to hosts repeatedly to blood-feed for minutes to hours.

Host immune responses and red meat allergies after tick bites (alpha-gal syndrome)

Like tick paralysis, tick bite—induced red meat allergy, also known as the alpha-gal syndrome, is a rare, noninfectious, poorly understood phenomenon. The sensitizing food-borne allergen following tick bites, most commonly by the lone star tick, *Amblyomma americanum*, in the United States, is galactose-alpha-1, 3-galactose (alpha-gal), an oligosaccharide constituent of all types of red meat (beef, lamb, pork, horse, and game meat) that structurally resembles the human blood group antigen B. All life stages of ticks feed on warm-blooded mammals and absorb alpha-gal sugars from their animal hosts. During human blood-feeding, lone star ticks inject small amounts of alpha-gal into bite wounds in addition to many other salivary chemicals in their sialomes, such as anticoagulants and local anesthetics. Repeated lone star tick bites over time may predispose certain individuals to IgE-mediated allergic responses, including anaphylaxis on reexposure to alpha-gal antigens in red meat, dairy products, drugs and foods containing animal-derived gelatin, and during cetuximab chemotherapy, a monoclonal antibody produced in mouse cell lines.

Insect repellents and insecticides

The most effective applications of insect repellents are a combination of the topical repellents, either N-diethyl-3-methylbenzamide (formerly N,N-diethyl-m-toluamide or DEET) or picaridin, and insecticidal permethrin-impregnated or other synthetic pyrethroid-impregnated clothing layered over topically treated skin. The insecticide-treated clothing will provide contact-level insecticidal effects and provide better, longer lasting protection against malaria-transmitting mosquitoes, mites, and ticks than that of topical DEET or picaridin alone. In special cases, where environmental exposures to disease-transmitting ticks, biting midges, mites, sandflies, or blackflies are anticipated, topical insect repellents containing IR3535, picaridin, or oil of lemon eucalyptus (p-menthane-3,8-diol or PMD) offer better topical protection than topical DEET alone.

Target audience for ectoparasitic diseases

The target audience for *Ectoparasitic Diseases* includes masters and doctoral-level graduate students, researchers, academics, infectious disease specialists and fellows, tropical medicine specialists and fellows, general internists, physicians practicing in tropical and temperate regions, veterinarians, animal handlers and groomers, dermatologists, cosmetologists, and professionals in related industries.

CHAPTER 1

Introduction to ectoparasitic diseases

Definitions

Ectoparasites infest the skin and its appendages, such as the hair and sebaceous glands, and external orifices, especially the ears, nares, and orbits. Ectoparasites may be obligatory parasites, programmed to feed on human hosts to complete their life cycles, or facultative parasites, preferring to feed on nonhuman hosts, infesting humans only as accidental or dead-end hosts. Over the past 2 decades, there have been reports of significant outbreaks of ectoparasitic diseases, principally myiasis, scabies, and tungiasis, both in indigenous populations and in travelers returning from developing nations and even from exclusive tropical beach resorts.

Many common ectoparasites, such as head lice and scabies mites, are also developing increasing resistance to medical therapies, including the safest topical insecticides (Meinking et al., 2002; Hodgdon et al., 2010). Other ectoparasites, such as the New World human botfly, *Dermatobia hominis,* and the jigger or chigoe flea, *Tunga penetrans,* are resistant to systemic and topical antiparasitics and can be treated only surgically.

Ectoparasitic diseases have reemerged as unusual, but not uncommon, infectious diseases worldwide, especially in high-risk populations. High-risk indigenous populations of ectoparasite-endemic tropical nations often have recurrent ectoparasitic infestations and superinfestations that can result in severe disfigurement from facial cavitary myiasis or permanent disability from tungiasis-associated autoamputations of toes and feet.

Taxonomy

The phylum Arthropoda is the largest phylum of the animal kingdom and includes the classes Insecta and Arachnida. All of the medically important ectoparasites, including fleas, flies, lice, mites, and ticks, belong to the phylum Arthropoda. Arthropods have chitinous exoskeletons, segmented bodies, and jointed appendages.

Fleas, flies, and lice are six-legged members of the class Insecta, which also includes the mosquitoes and true bugs (order Hemiptera). Mites, including chigger mites and scabies mites, and ticks are the eight-legged members of the class Arachnida, subclass Acari. The arthropod ectoparasites of medical importance are stratified by their taxonomic classes and distinguishing external anatomic characteristics in Table 1.1.

Ectoparasitic Diseases
ISBN 978-0-443-26724-6,
https://doi.org/10.1016/B978-0-443-26724-6.00001-1

Table 1.1 Taxonomy of arthropods (phylum arthropoda) of major medical importance.

	Common name	Number of legs and body segments, other identifying anatomic features
Phylum arthopoda, class insecta		
Order Diptera, family Culicidae	Mosquitoes	Six, three, wings
Order Diptera	Flies[a]	Six, three, wings
Order Hemiptera	True bugs (e.g., bedbugs, reduviid bugs)	Six, three, ± wings
Order Hymenoptera	Ants, bees, wasps	Six, three, ± wings
Order Phthiraptera	Lice[a]	Six, three, no wings
Order Siphonaptera	Fleas[a]	Six, three, no wings
Phylum arthropoda, class arachnida		
Subclass Acari	Mites and ticks[a]	Eight, one globose body, no distinct heads[b], no wings
Order Araneae	Spiders	Eight, two, no wings
Order Scorpiones	Scorpions	Eight, two, abdomens with terminal stingers

[a]The arthropod ectoparasites of major medical importance by taxonomic order and distinctive anatomic features.
[b]Mouthparts visible dorsally only in ixodid (hard) ticks.
Adapted from Diaz, J.H., 2019. Section on ectoparasitic diseases. Chapter 291. Introduction to ectoparasitic diseases. In: Bennett, J.E., Dolin, R., Blaser, M.J. (Eds.), *Mandell, Douglas and Bennett's Principles and Practice of Infectious Diseases*, Ninth Edition. Elsevier, Philadelphia. Elsevier Publication.

Epidemiology

Ectoparasitic diseases share many of the general characteristics of emerging infectious diseases. Commonly shared characteristics of ectoparasitoses and emerging infectious diseases include the following: (1) Origination as zoonoses, disease establishment dependent on arthropod vector competency and endemicity; (2) introduction into new, naïve host populations; (3) infection by endemic agents given selective advantages by changing civil, ecologic, or socioeconomic conditions; and (4) recent movement from rural to urban endemic areas, often following refugee resettlements or migrating human host populations seeking better economic opportunities (Marano et al., 2007).

Pathophysiology

The arthropod ectoparasites can threaten human health directly by burrowing into and feeding, dwelling, and reproducing in human skin and orifices (mites, fleas, flies), or by blood or tissue fluid feeding (fleas, lice, mites, ticks). Tissue fluids are composed of liquid combinations of serum, lymph, and epithelial cells dissolving in the lytic secretions of feeding arthropods. With rare exceptions, mites are primarily tissue fluid-feeders as compared with ticks, which are blood-feeders.

Infectious disease transmission

The arthropod ectoparasites (fleas, mites, ticks) can also threaten human health indirectly by transmission of infectious disease. They can transmit and even cotransmit a variety of infectious diseases (viral, bacterial, and protozoan) during blood and tissue liquid feeding. Many species of gravid ticks are capable of injecting paralytic toxins (tick paralysis) during their prolonged blood meals. Unlike other ectoparasites, ticks can be infective as males and females at birth (by transovarial pathogen transmission) and throughout all stages of their life cycles (by transstadial pathogen transmission).

Life cycles

The similar stages in the life cycles of commonly encountered human ectoparasites are compared in Table 1.2. The most commonly encountered arthropod ectoparasites, excluding ticks, and the major clinical manifestations of their infestations are featured in Table 1.3. The tick-borne pathogens and the clinical manifestations of their infections are featured in Chapter 9–11.

Conclusions

Recent epidemiologic evidence now supports the endemicity of several ectoparasitic diseases and their arthropod vectors and their human and animal reservoir hosts throughout the developing world and in many parts of the developed world, including Europe and the United States (Table 1.4). Ectoparasitic diseases have also reemerged in regions where they were once effectively controlled.

Ectoparasitic diseases will continue to be present in the developed world for several reasons, including: (1) The globalization of trade and commerce with ectoparasites and their human and animal hosts traveling worldwide on humans, airplanes, and ships; (2) mass movements of populations from rural to urban areas and from developing to developed nations; (3) the worldwide legitimate and illegal trade of exotic animals and animal hides and skins; (4) the accidental and intentional introduction of exotic animal species into new regions with supportive ecosystems; (5) the increasing frequency of pyrethroid-resistant strains of ectoparasites, especially head lice and scabies mites; and (6) the growing populations of susceptible, and often immunocompromised, human hosts living in long-term care facilities and in crowded and impoverished periurban communities (Marano et al., 2007).

Table 1.2 Similar stages of the life cycles of common human ectoparasites.

Order or subclass (common names)	Phthiraptera (lice)	Acari family sarcoptidae (mites)	Diptera (flies)	Siphonoptera (fleas)	Acari family ixodidae (hard ticks)
Examples (common names)	*Pediculus humanus capitis* (Head louse)	*Sarcoptes scabiei* (Scabies or itch mite)	*Dermatobia hominis* (human botfly)	*Tunga penetrans* (chigoe or jigger flea)	*Ixodes scapularis* (Black-legged deer tick)
Eggs (only viable eggs on hosts indicate infection)	Viable egg (nit) Diagnostic stage	Viable egg Diagnostic stage	Human botflies latch onto mosquitoes and other flying insects in mid-flight and attach their eggs. When the insect lands on human skin and bites, the eggs burrow into the bite wound and develop into larvae. Diagnostic stage	Female jigger flea laying eggs in wound. Diagnostic stage	Female deer tick-laying eggs in environment and away from hosts. Nondiagnostic
Larval or developmental stages (nymphs or instars)	Viable nymphs (2 stages) Diagnostic stage	Viable nymph Diagnostic stage	Viable larva Diagnostic stage	Viable larva Diagnostic stage	Viable nymph Diagnostic stage
Female adults	Gravid female head louse with eggs. Infective stage	Gravid female scabies mite with egg. Infective stage	Female Human Botfly Vector	Female Chigoe or jigger Flea Vector	Female Black-legged Deer Tick Infective stage

Adapted from Diaz, J.H., 2019 Section on ectoparasitic diseases. Chapter 291. Introduction to ectoparasitic diseases. In: Bennett, J.E., Dolin, R., Blaser, M.J. (Eds.), Mandell, Douglas and Bennett's Principles and Practice of Infectious Diseases, Ninth Edition. Elsevier, Philadelphia. Elsevier Publication.

Table 1.3 Common arthropod ectoparasites (excluding ticks) and clinical manifestations of ectoparasitoses.

Representative species of infesting arthropods	Common names of infesting arthropods	Geographic distributions	Major clinical manifestations of ectoparasitoses
Class insecta, order phthiraptera, suborder anoplura lice			
Pediculus humanus corporis	Body louse	Worldwide	Pediculosis corporis
Pediculus humanus capitis	Head louse	Worldwide	Pediculosis capitis, trench fever (*Bartonella quintana*)
Phthirus pubis	Crab (pubic) louse	Worldwide	Pediculosis pubis (phthiriasis)
Order diptera flies			
Family Calliphoridae	Screwworms		
Auchmeromyia senegalensis	Congo floor-maggot fly	Sub-Saharan Africa, Cape Verde Islands	Larvae are nocturnal blood feeders, no myiasis (tissue invasion); wound (cutaneous) myiasis
Callitroga Americana	American screwworm	North and Central America	Cavitary (invasive) myiasis
Chrysomyia bezziana	Old World screwworm	Tropical Africa, Asia, Indonesia	Cavitary (invasive) myiasis
Cochliomyia hominivorax	New World screwworm	Central and South America	Furuncular myiasis
Cordylobia anthropophaga	Tumbu (mango) fly	Africa	Furuncular myiasis
Family oestridae	Botflies		
Cuterebra spp.	Rodent botfly	North and Central America	Furuncular myiasis
Dermatobia hominis	Human botfly	Central and South America	Furuncular myiasis
Order siphonaptera fleas			
Ctenocephalides spp.	Cat (*C. felis*) and dog fleas (*C. canis*)	Worldwide	Bite groupings (mechanical vectors of dog and rat tapeworms, less efficient bubonic plague vectors)

Continued

Table 1.3 Common arthropod ectoparasites (excluding ticks) and clinical manifestations of ectoparasitoses.—cont'd

Representative species of infesting arthropods	Common names of infesting arthropods	Geographic distributions	Major clinical manifestations of ectoparasitoses
Pulex irritans	Human flea	Worldwide	Bite groupings (efficient plague vector in Chilean Andes)
Tunga penetrans	Chigoe (jigger) flea	Central and South America, Africa Europe, Asia	Tungiasis
Xenopsylla cheopis	Oriental rat flea	Africa, Americas	Most efficient bubonic plague vector

Class arachnida spiders, mites, ticks subclass acari mites and ticks

Sarcoptes scabiei	Itch (scabies) mite	Worldwide	Scabies, crusted (Norwegian) scabies
Eutrombicula alfreddugesi	Common chigger (redbug chigger)	Worldwide	Chiggers
Leptotrombidium akamushi	Japanese-Asian rodent chigger	Japan, India, Australia	Potential scrub typhus (Tsutsugamushi disease) vector
Leptotrombidium deliensis	Indian-Asian rodent chigger	Eurasia-Eastern Asia, Southeast Asia, India, Australia, Indo-Pacific Islands	Potential scrub typhus (Tsutsugamushi disease) vector

Adapted from Diaz, J.H., 2019. Section on ectoparasitic diseases. Chapter 291. Introduction to ectoparasitic diseases. In: Bennett, J.E., Dolin, R., Blaser, M.J. (Eds.), Mandell, Douglas and Bennett's Principles and Practice of Infectious Diseases, Ninth Edition. Elsevier, Philadelphia. Elsevier Publication.

Table 1.4 Selected infectious diseases transmitted by arthropods.

Infectious disease	Vector
Anaplasmosis (human granulocytotropic)	Hard ticks
Arbovirus diseases (including yellow fever, dengue fever, encephalitis)	Mosquitoes and ticks
Babesiosis	Hard ticks
Boutonneuse fever (tick bite fever; *Rickettsia conorii*)	Hard ticks

Table 1.4 Selected infectious diseases transmitted by arthropods.—cont'd

Infectious disease	Vector
Cat scratch disease, cat scratch fever (*Bartonella henselae*)	Cat fleas
Chagas disease (American trypanosomiasis)	Triatomine (kissing) bugs
Colorado tick fever	Hard ticks
Ehrlichiosis, monocytotropic (*Ehrlichia chaffeensis*) and granulocytic (*Ehrlichia ewingii*)	Hard ticks
Endemic relapsing fever (*Borrelia duttonii*)	Soft ticks
Epidemic relapsing fever (*Borrelia recurrentis*)	Human body lice
Epidemic typhus (*Rickettsia prowazekii*)	Human body lice
Filariasis (*Wuchereria bancrofti, Brugia malayi*)	Mosquitoes
Leishmaniasis (*Leishmania* spp.)	*Lutzomyia* sand fly in the Americas, phlebotomine flies elsewhere
Loiasis (*Loa loa*)	Tabanid flies
Lyme disease (*Borrelia burgdorferi*)	Hard ticks
Malaria (*Plasmodium* spp.)	Mosquitoes
Murine typhus (*Rickettsia mooseri*)	Rat fleas, lice
Onchocerciasis (*Onchocerca volvulus*)	Black flies
Plague (*Yersinia pestis*)	Rat fleas
Q fever (*Coxiella burnetii*)	Hard ticks, fleas
Rickettsial pox (*Rickettsia akari*)	Mouse mites
Rocky Mountain spotted fever (*Rickettsia rickettsii*)	Hard ticks
Scrub typhus (*Orientia tsutsugamushi*)	Larval mites (chiggers)
Trench fever (*Bartonella quintana*)	Body lice, potentially head lice
African trypanosomiasis, African sleeping sickness	*Glossina* (tsetse) flies
West Nile fever	Mosquitoes

Adapted from Diaz, J.H., 2019. Section on ectoparasitic diseases. Chapter 291. Introduction to ectoparasitic diseases. In: Bennett, J.E., Dolin, R., Blaser, M.J. (Eds.), Mandell, Douglas and Bennett's Principles and Practice of Infectious Diseases, Ninth Edition. Elsevier, Philadelphia. Elsevier Publication.

Socioeconomic and behavioral factors

The isolation of the trench-fever pathogen, *Bartonella quintana*, in head lice from homeless persons in the United States exemplifies how socioeconomic factors, human behavioral trends, and vector adaptations can support ectoparasite persistence with significant public health consequences (Bonilla et al., 2009). Formerly felt to be susceptible to the safest pyrethroid pesticides and incapable of transmitting infectious diseases, head lice have now acquired the capability to harbor *B. quintana* and potentially to transmit trench fever to new naïve host populations (Bonilla et al., 2009). In 2015, investigators reported a new clade of African body and head lice infected by both *B. quintana* and *Yersinia pestis* indicating that body and head lice could possibly represent new arthropod vectors for plague (Drali et al., 2015).

The eradication of pyrethroid-resistant head lice infestations in homeless persons in crowded shelters and children in schools will require the use of more powerful pesticides with increased potential for adverse effects, such as carbaryl, lindane, and malathion; or the use of new, safer alternatives, such as oral and topical ivermectin-containing pediculicides (Meinking et al., 2002; Hodgdon et al., 2010).

References

Bonilla, D.L., Kabeya, H., Henn, J., Kramer, V.L., Kosoy, M.Y., 2009. *Bartonella quintana* in body lice and head lice from homeless persons, San Francisco, California, USA. Emerging Infectious Diseases 15 (6), 912–915. https://doi.org/10.3201/eid1506.090054.

Drali, R., Shako, J.C., Davoust, B., Diatta, G., Raoult, D., 2015. A new clade of African body and head lice infected by *Bartonella quintana* and *Yersinia pestis*—Democratic Republic of the Congo. The American Journal of Tropical Medicine and Hygiene 93 (5), 990–993. https://doi.org/10.4269/ajtmh.14-0686.

Hodgdon, H.E., Yoon, K.S., Previte, D.J., Kim, H.J., Aboelghar, G.E., Lee, S.H., Marshall Clark, J., 2010. Determination of knockdown resistance allele frequencies in global human head louse populations using the serial invasive signal amplification reaction. Pest Management Science 66 (9), 1031–1040. https://doi.org/10.1002/ps.1979.

Marano, N., Arguin, P.M., Pappaioanou, M., 2007. Impact of globalization and animal trade on infectious disease ecology. Emerging Infectious Diseases 13 (12), 1807–1809. https://doi.org/10.3201/eid1312.071276.

Meinking, T.L., Serrano, L., Hard, B., Entzel, P., Lemard, G., Rivera, E., Villar, M.E., 2002. Comparative in vitro pediculicidal efficacy of treatments in a resistant head lice population in the United States. Archives of Dermatology 138 (2). https://doi.org/10.1001/archderm.138.2.220.

CHAPTER 2

Pediculosis (lice)

Definitions

Pediculosis is the term for three distinct human infestations with two species of blood-sucking lice of the insect order Phthiraptera, suborder Anoplura: (1) *Pediculus humanus* and (2) *Phthirus pubis.* Sometime after early humans began to wear clothes, initially made from animal skins, *P. humanus* evolved into two clinically distinct ectoparasitic variants, *P. humanus* var. *corporis,* the body louse (Fig. 2.1), and *P. humanus* var. *capitis,* the head louse (Fig. 2.2) (Whitfield et al., 1999). Although morphologically indistinct, these human louse variants do not interbreed, prefer unique anatomic niches on human hosts, and are now considered separate and distinct species (Whitfield, 2003; Whitfield et al., 1999). Although not initially suspected of transmitting infectious diseases such as body lice, head lice may be infected with *Bartonella quintana* and *Yersinia pestis* and may be capable of transmitting both trench fever and plague (Drali et al., 2015b; Downs et al., 1999).

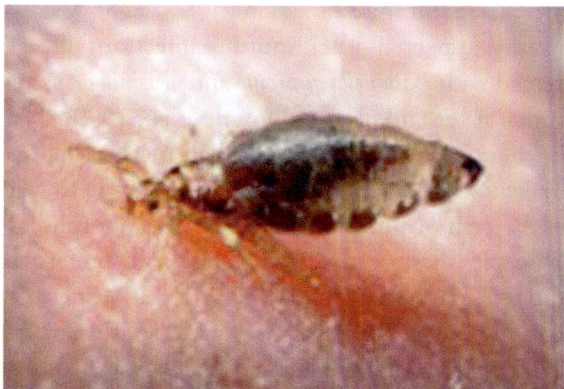

Figure 2.1 Dorsal view of a female body louse, ***Pediculus humanus*** var. ***corporis.*** Dorsal view of a female body louse, *Pediculus humanus* var. *corporis.* Note the eggs within the abdominal segment, which assist in identifying the female body louse. Unlike pubic lice, body lice can transmit several bacterial diseases including: (1) relapsing fever caused by *Borrelia recurrentis,* (2) trench fever caused by *Bartonella quintana,* and (3) epidemic typhus caused by *Rickettsia prowazekii.* Homeless, immunocompromised, and refugee populations are at greatest risk for body lice infestations and epidemics of body louse–borne bacterial diseases. *(From Centers for Disease Control and Prevention [CDC], Atlanta, GA. CDC Public Health Image Library, image 9204.)*

Ectoparasitic Diseases
ISBN 978-0-443-26724-6,
https://doi.org/10.1016/B978-0-443-26724-6.00002-3

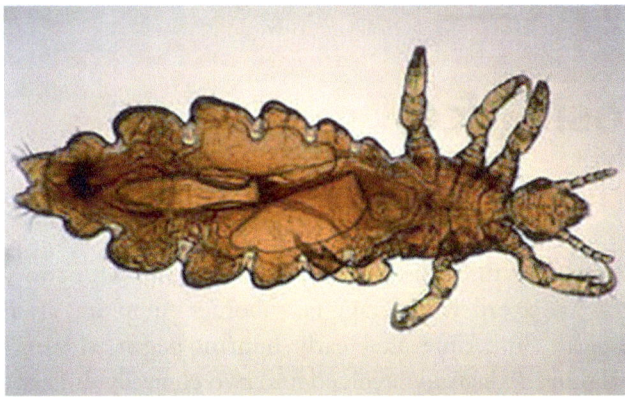

Figure 2.2 Dorsal view of a female head louse, **Pediculus humanus** var. **capitis,** containing eggs or nits. Dorsal view of a female head louse, *Pediculus humanus* var. *capitis,* containing eggs or nits. Note the eggs within the abdominal segment, which assist in identifying the female head louse. Although not initially suspected of transmitting infectious diseases such as body lice, head lice may be infected with *Bartonella quintana* and *Yersinia pestis* and may be capable of transmitting both trench fever and plague (Drali et al., 2015a,b). *(From Centers for Disease Control and Prevention [CDC], Atlanta, GA. CDC Public Health Image Library, image 377.)*

Unlike pubic lice, body lice can transmit several bacterial diseases including: (1) Relapsing fever caused by *Borrelia recurrentis*, (2) trench fever caused by *Bartonella quintana*, and (3) epidemic typhus caused by *Rickettsia prowazekii*. Homeless, immunocompromised, and refugee populations are at greatest risk for body lice infestations and epidemics of body louse—borne bacterial diseases.

Although not initially suspected of transmitting infectious diseases such as body lice, head lice may be infected with *Bartonella quintana* and *Yersinia pestis* and may be capable of transmitting both trench fever and plague (Downs et al., 1999).

Head lice *(P. humanus capitis)* leave their hair shaft nests for blood meals on the scalp, and body lice *(P. humanus corporis)* leave their clothes' seams nests for blood meals on the body. *Phthirus pubis,* the crab or pubic louse (Fig. 2.3), is morphologically distinct from the two *P. humanus* species, has a crab-shaped body, and prefers to dwell in the hair-bearing areas of the pubic and inguinal areas, but may also infest the hairy areas of the axillae, nipples, chest, abdomen, and even eyelashes (phthiriasis palpebrarum). Pubic lice remain relatively stationary, anchored to the bases of hair shafts while blood feeding, unless mating or egg-laying.

Phthirus pubis, the crab or pubic louse, is morphologically distinct from the two *P. humanus* species, has a crab-shaped body, and prefers to dwell in the hair-bearing areas of the pubic and inguinal areas, but may also infest the hairy areas of the axillae, nipples, chest, abdomen, and even eyelashes (phthiriasis palpebrarum). Pubic lice remain relatively stationary, anchored to the bases of hair shafts while blood feeding, unless mating or egg-laying.

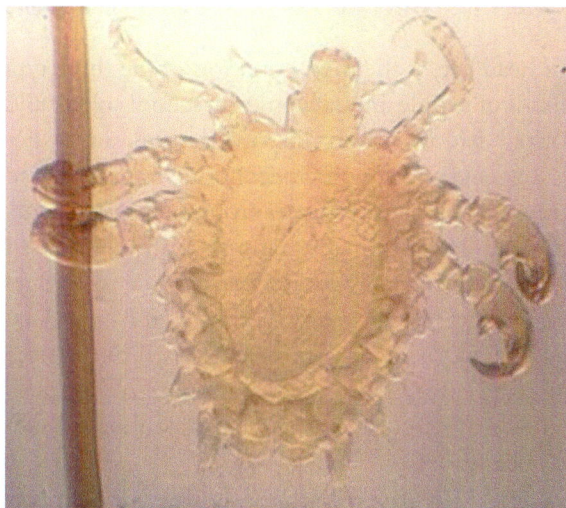

Figure 2.3 Enlarged ventral image of a pubic or crab louse, *Phthirus pubis. Phthirus pubis,* the crab or pubic louse, is morphologically distinct from the two *P. humanus* species, has a crab-shaped body, and prefers to dwell in the hair-bearing areas of the pubic and inguinal areas, but may also infest the hairy areas of the axillae, nipples, chest, abdomen, and even eyelashes (phthiriasis palpebrarum). Pubic lice remain relatively stationary, anchored to the bases of hair shafts while blood feeding, unless mating or egg-laying. *(From Centers for Disease Control and Prevention [CDC], Atlanta, GA. CDC Public Health Image Library, image 4077.)*

Lice are among the oldest ectoparasites of man and are distributed into six separate mitochondrial clades (A, B, C, D, E, and F) based on their geographic origins (Whitfield, 2003). Clades A and B are the most widely distributed clades worldwide, while the other clades are restricted in geographic distributions. Recently, a mitochondrial clade D of head and body lice infected with both *B. quintana* and *Y.pestis* was discovered in lice-infected persons living in plague-endemic areas of the Democratic Republic of the Congo (Drali et al., 2015a,b).

Since the analysis of ancient DNA from Old World archeological sites is often compromised by low concentrations in poor specimens, the DNA from ancient head louse eggs or nits detected by reverse transcriptase—polymerase chain reaction (RT-PCR) has recently proven to be valuable in mapping the migration patterns of ancient humans and the spread of their louse-borne infectious diseases such as epidemic typhus, relapsing fever, and trench fever (Whitfield, 2003).

Epidemiology

Pediculosis capitis, or head lice, is the most common of the three types of human pediculoses, afflicting millions of people annually, mostly school-aged children, in both developing and industrialized nations. Body lice infestations, or pediculosis corporis, are associated with poor hygiene and low socioeconomic status and occur primarily in the indigent, institutionalized, homeless, refugees from civil unrest, and the immunocompromised. Body and head lice are usually transmitted by direct body or head-to-head contact and, much less commonly by indirect contact with fomites, such as bedding, clothing, towels, and headgear, such as hats, combs, and hair brushes.

Pubic lice infestations, or phthiriasis pubis, are caused by *P. pubis,* the pubic or crab louse. Pubic lice are more often transmitted during sexual contacts rather than fomite contacts and often coexist with crusted (Norwegian) scabies, genital scabies, and other sexually transmitted diseases.

Unlike pubic lice, body lice can transmit several bacterial diseases. Homeless, immunocompromised, and refugee populations are at greatest risk for body lice infestations and have amplified epidemics of body louse–borne bacterial diseases including: (1) Relapsing fever caused by *Borrelia recurrentis,* (2) trench fever caused by *Bartonella quintana,* and (3) epidemic typhus caused by *Rickettsia prowazekii.* Body lice have been recognized as infectious organisms of high importance, not only in displaced populations in evacuee and refugee camps but also in immunocompromised subjects, particularly homeless individuals with the acquired immunodeficiency syndrome (AIDS).

In a retrospective epidemiological analysis of body infestations in homeless persons in Marseille, France, over 18 years (2000–17), investigators reported a 12.2% prevalence of body lice in 2288 persons living in homeless shelters. In a nested multivariate analysis of comorbidities and demographics, the investigators identified the following significant risk factors for pediculosis corporis in homeless persons: (1) age $\geq$50 years ($P = .022$) (Ly et al., 2017), (2) duration of residence in France of $\geq$5 years ($P = .001$), (3) frequent alcohol use ($P < .0001$), and (4) tobacco smoking ($P = .001$) (Drali et al., 2015a).

Although other investigations have reported higher prevalence of body lice in homeless persons, this study was the first to identify several independent risk factors for body lice (Bonilla et al., 2014; Drali et al., 2015a; Ly et al., 2017). Prior investigations in homeless persons sleeping in public areas in Paris identified additional significant risk factors for body lice including prior history of public lice, begging, and not using municipal showers (Ly et al., 2017; Whitfield et al., 1999). In a survey of homeless persons in San Francisco, California, risk factors significantly associated with body lice included male gender, African American race, and sleeping outdoors (Arnaud et al., 2016; Bonilla et al., 2014).

Human immunodeficiency virus (HIV) infection in the homeless may be an additional risk factor for louse-borne infectious diseases. In a study of 382 HIV-positive patients with fever in San Francisco, Koehler et al. found that 18% were positive for *Bartonella* spp. (Bonilla et al., 2014; Koehler et al., 2003).

Rickettsia prowazekii, the causative agent of epidemic typhus, is frequently isolated from body lice in homeless persons and displaced refugees. Louse-borne *R. prowazekii* caused regional epidemics of typhus during World War I and, more recently, in refugee camps. Although body lice have not been clearly implicated in the transmission of *R. typhi*, the causative agent of murine or endemic typhus, a retrospective immunological analysis of pathogens detected in body lice collected from 153 homeless persons in Bogota, Colombia, who had an 11.7% point prevalence of lice infestation, identified seroprevalences of 19% for *B. quintana* and 56% for typhus group rickettsiae in collected lice (Faccini-Martínez et al., 2017; Koehler et al., 2003). Since *R. prowazekii* was not detected in collected body lice, *R. typhi* was assumed to be the predominant typhus group rickettsiae in this investigation (Koehler et al., 2003). Although not confirmed, these data suggest that body lice in homeless persons can transmit *R. typhi* as well as other rickettsiae (Koehler et al., 2003).

B. quintana has now been isolated in head lice as well as body lice from homeless persons in the United States, establishing the potential for transmission of trench fever by blood-feeding head lice in addition to body lice (Arnaud et al., 2016; Downs et al., 1999). During a 2011 outbreak of relapsing fever in Ethiopia, investigators demonstrated *B. recurrentis* DNA by quantitative real-time polymerase chain reaction (RTqPCR) in 23% of head lice from patients with positive blood smears, establishing the potential for transmission of relapsing fever by head lice in addition to body lice (Faccini-Martínez et al., 2017; Tasher et al., 2017). As noted, the DNA from ancient head louse eggs or nits detected by quantitative polymerase chain reaction (qPCR) has now proven to be valuable in mapping the migration patterns of ancient humans and the spread of their louse-borne infectious diseases such as relapsing fever (Whitfield, 2003).

Bartonella quintana can also cause culture-negative endocarditis in adults and has now been identified as a cause of endocarditis in children (Boutellis et al., 2013). In a case series reported from Ethiopia, investigators described five cases of endocarditis, primarily of the aortic valve (n = 4), in children 7—16 years of age with preexisting congenital or rheumatic valvular heart defects with four cases caused by *B. quintana* and one case caused by a *Bartonella* of unknown species (Boutellis et al., 2013; Tasher et al., 2017). Despite no direct evidence for body lice by history or physical examination, they remained a likely source for the *B. quintana* infections (Boutellis et al., 2013).

In addition to serving as vectors for epidemic typhus (*R. prowazekii*), trench fever (*B. quintana*), and relapsing fever (*B. recurrentis*), body lice have now been suspected in the transmission of another pathogen, *Yersinia pestis*, the causative agent of plague. In 2010, Drali et al. collected body and head lice from 37 infested individuals in plague-hyperendemic areas of the Democratic Republic of the Congo (Drali et al., 2015b). Using multiplex PCR to rapidly differentiate head and body lice, the investigators detected evidence of *B. quintana* in 33.5% of body lice and 19% of head lice and *Y. pestis* in one head louse that was PCR-negative for other pathogens and two body lice that were PCR-positive for *B. quintana* (Drali et al., 2015b). Although these results will require independent confirmation, plague may possibly be added to the list of pathogens that can potentially be transmitted by body and head lice (Drali et al., 2015b).

Diagnosis

Lice infestations are diagnosed by demonstrating live adult lice, nymphs, and viable eggs, or nits, in their precise human ecologic niches. Adult lice are flattened dorsoventrally and are 1 mm (pubic lice) to 3 mm (head and body lice) in length, have three pairs of legs ending in powerful claws that can grip hair shafts, and exhibit a reddish-brown hue after blood feeding (see Figs. 2.2 and 2.3, and Table 2.1). Females can live on their hosts for up to 3 months, lay up to 300 nits in a lifetime, and die within 24 hours when separated from hosts (see Fig. 2.2). Nits are oval, less than 1 mm in diameter, and grayish white (Fig. 2.4); they fluoresce in ultraviolet or Wood's light when viable. Nits are deposited on hair shafts at the skin surface and hatch nymphs within 6—10 days (see Fig. 2.4). Nymphs resemble miniature adults and grow to adulthood within about 10 days. Empty egg cases remain attached to hair shafts after hatching and are not diagnostic of active infection. Head lice and their viable nits are often attached to hairs close to the scalp, especially in occipital and postauricular locations. Body lice infest clothing and, when not blood-feeding, may be found along with their nymphs and eggs or nits residing in alignment with the inner seams of clothing (Fig. 2.5). Pubic lice and their nits may be found in the pubic, perianal, and inguinal areas, in axillary and chest hair, and even in the eyelashes (phthiriasis palpebrarum) (Fig. 2.6). The life cycles, pathogenesis, and clinical manifestations of the three types of human louse infestations are shown in Table 2.1.

Today, "no-nit policies" in schools have been modified. As noted, nonviable nits on hair shafts are simply empty egg cases without a red eye spot and do not indicate active louse infestation. Dermoscopy can clearly distinguish viable nits from hatched, empty nits and pseudo-nits immediately and reliably and offers a more sensitive screening tool for head lice infestations than visual inspection alone.

Despite the fact that body lice reside in clothing, often along seams and not on the body, like head lice, pediculosis corporis infestation is often much more symptomatic than pediculosis capitis and causes severe pruritus with extensive self-inflicted excoriations.

Infestation with pediculosis pubis (phthiriasis), or crab lice is less symptomatic compared with pediculosis capitis. These organisms affect all hair-bearing regions, most commonly the pubic and perianal areas, but also the upper eyelashes and the hairy areas of the axillae, chest, nipples, and abdomen. More extensive infestations usually occur in males with more body hair—bearing areas than females.

Table 2.1 The life cycles, pathogenesis, and clinical manifestations of pediculosis corporis, pediculosis capitis, and phthiriasis pubis.

Ectoparasitic infestations	Pediculosis corporis	Pediculosis capitis	Pediculosis (phthiriasis) pubis
Common names of ectoparasitic infections	*Pediculus humanus corporis* Body lice, gravid female with eggs. Source: Same as Fig. 2.1.	*Pediculus humanus capitis* Head lice, gravid female with eggs. Source: Same as Fig. 2.2.	*Pthirus pubis* Pubic lice, gravid female with egg. Source: Same as Fig. 2.3.
Egg laying by gravid females	Gravid females live up to 30 days and lay eggs (nits) at the base of body hair shafts within 6 mm of skin and on the seams of clothing.	Human hosts typically harbor only 10–12 head lice. Gravid females live up to 30 days and lay 5–10 eggs (nits) per day at the base of single hair shafts on the scalp, especially behind and above the ears and on the back of the neck. Typically, 1–2 eggs are laid on a single hair shaft.	Gravid females live 3 –4 weeks and lay 150 –200 eggs (nits) which are smaller than those of body and head lice. Several eggs are laid in a row on a single hair shaft primarily in the public and perineal regions, but may also be laid on coarse hairs in other hair-bearing places such as the axilla, chest, mustache, beard, and eyelashes (phthiriasis palpebrarum).
Egg hatching on human hair shafts	Eggs hatch within 6–9 days releasing nymphs which resemble small adults.	Eggs hatch within 8–12 days releasing nymphs which resemble small adults. Since hair grows 0.4 mm per day, the distance between the scalp and the furthest egg on a hair shaft provides an estimate of the duration of infestation.	Eggs hatch within 7 days releasing nymphs which resemble small adults.

Continued

Table 2.1 The life cycles, pathogenesis, and clinical manifestations of pediculosis corporis, pediculosis capitis, and phthiriasis pubis.—cont'd

Ectoparasitic infestations	Pediculosis corporis	Pediculosis capitis	Pediculosis (phthiriasis) pubis
Developmental (nymph or instar) stages in humans	Nymphs mature on clothing after 3 molts and mature into adults within 3 days of hatching. Nymphs must feed immediately on hatching.	Nymphs mature after 3 molts and become adults within 3 days of hatching. Nymphs must feed immediately on hatching. Nits that are more than 1 cm from the scalp have likely failed to release their nymphs and are considered nonviable.	Nymphs mature after 3 molts and mature into adults within 10–17 days of hatching. Nymphs must feed immediately on hatching.
Human-to-human transmission	Transmitted by close bodily contact and contact with infested clothing. Viable eggs can survive up to 4 weeks in discarded clothing. Adults will leave seams and hair shafts several times per day to blood feed. Adults can only survive 1–2 days away from human hosts.	Transmitted by close bodily contact more so than by contact with fomites such as combs, hair brushes, scarfs, caps, and hats. Viable eggs can survive up to 10 days in the environment. Adults can only survive 1–2 days away from the human scalp.	Transmitted by close bodily contact, most often by sexual contact. Much less frequent transmission by fomites, such as infested, discarded underclothing and bed linens. Public lice can only survive on fomites for 24 hours. Adults can only survive 2 days away from human hosts.
Feeding behaviors of nymphs and adults and the pathogenesis of clinical manifestations.	Although nymphs blood feed only at night, adults blood feed throughout the day and night, especially on soft, moist, folded skin covered by tight clothing or elastic bands. Nymphs	Nymphs and adults leave hair shafts and feed on blood from the scalp 2–6 times per day causing discomfort and pruritus confined to	Nymphs and adults blood feed 4–5 times per day mostly at night. Nymphs and adults of both sexes feed by piercing the skin

	and adults of both sexes feed by piercing the skin and sucking blood every 2–3 hours. Light infestations may only cause moderate itching over infested areas exacerbated by sensitization to louse saliva. Symptoms are often increased in recurrent infections due to prior saliva sensitization.	the head. Nymphs and adults of both sexes feed by piercing the skin and sucking blood every 2–3 hours. Light infestations may only cause moderate itching of the scalp exacerbated by sensitization to louse saliva. Symptoms are often increased in recurrent infections due to prior saliva sensitization.	and sucking blood every 2–3 hours. Light infestations may only cause moderate itching of infested areas exacerbated by sensitization to louse saliva. Symptoms are often increased in recurrent infections due to prior saliva sensitization.
Infectious disease transmission capability and causative pathogens	Epidemic typhus (*Rickettsia prowazekii*), Relapsing fever (*Borrelia recurrentis*), Trench fever (*Bartonella quintana*), Suspected: Endemic (murine) typhus (*R. typhi*), and plague (*Yersina pestis*).(2)	Cannot typically transmit infectious diseases.Suspected: *B. quintana* and *Y. pestis*.(2)	Cannot typically transmit infectious diseases.Persons with phthiriasis should also be evaluated for other sexually transmitted infectious diseases, including syphilis and HIV/AIDS.

Adapted from Diaz, J.H, 2014. Section on Ectoparasitic Diseases. Chapter 293. Lice (Pediculosis). In Bennett, J.E., Dolin, R., Blaser, M.J. (Eds.), Eight Edition, Elsevier, Philadelphia, pp. 3246–3249. Elsevier publication.

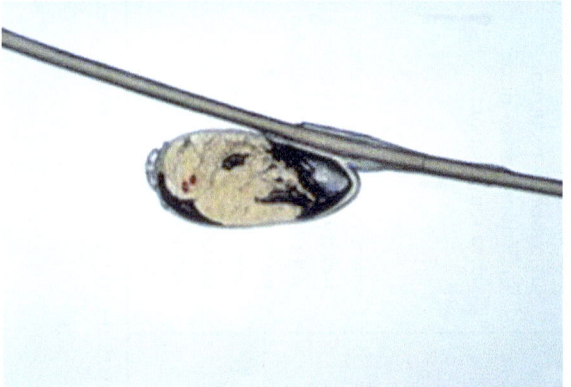

Figure 2.4 The unhatched nit or egg of the head louse, ***Pediculus humanus*** var. ***capitis,*** attached to a hair shaft. The unhatched nit or egg of the head louse, *Pediculus humanus* var. *capitis,* attached to a hair shaft. Note the red eye spots of the developing nymph embryo, identifying the nit as infectious. Today, "no-nit policies" in schools have been modified. As noted, nonviable nits on hair shafts are simply empty egg cases without a red eye spot and do not indicate active louse infestation. Dermoscopy can clearly distinguish viable nits from hatched, empty nits and pseudo-nits immediately and reliably and offers a more sensitive screening tool for head lice infestations than visual inspection alone. *(From Centers for Disease Control and Prevention [CDC], Atlanta, GA. CDC Public Health Image Library, image 378.)*

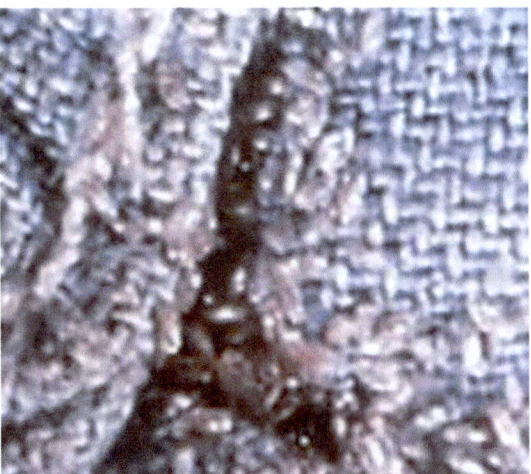

Figure 2.5 Live eggs from the body louse, ***Pediculus humanus*** var. ***corporis,*** lining the seams of clothing. Live eggs from the body louse, *Pediculus humanus* var. *corporis,* lining the seams of clothing. Despite the fact that body lice reside in clothing, often along seams and not on the body, such as head lice, pediculosis corporis infestation is often much more symptomatic than pediculosis capitis and causes severe pruritus with extensive self-inflicted excoriations. *(From Centers for Disease Control and Prevention [CDC], Atlanta, GA. CDC Public Health Image Library, image 5270.)*

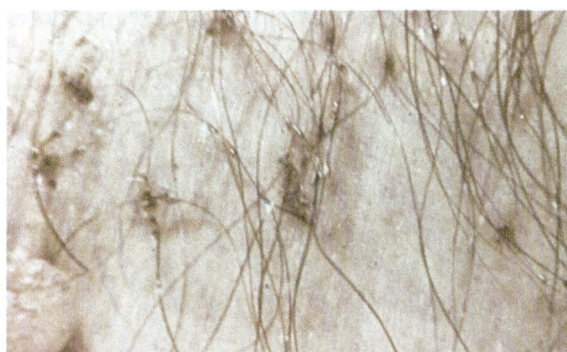

Figure 2.6 Erythematous lesions seen in the pubic region of a patient in response to the bites of blood-feeding crab or pubic louse, ***Phthirus pubis.*** Erythematous lesions seen in the pubic region of a patient in response to the bites of blood-feeding crab or pubic louse, Phthirus pubis. Infestation with pediculosis pubis (phthiriasis), or crab lice is less symptomatic compared with pediculosis capitis. These organisms affect all hair-bearing regions, most commonly the pubic and perianal areas, but also the upper eyelashes and the hairy areas of the axillae, chest, nipples, and abdomen. More extensive infestations usually occur in males with more body hair—bearing areas than females. *(From Centers for Disease Control and Prevention [CDC], Atlanta, GA. CDC Public Health Image Library, image 4078.)*

Clinical manifestations and differential diagnosis

Head lice

The clinical manifestations of pediculosis capitis range from asymptomatic infestations to severe pruritus, with self-inflicted, often secondarily infected, excoriations with impetigo and postoccipital lymphadenopathy. The differential diagnosis of pediculosis capitis includes eczema, lichen simplex chronicus, dandruff, seborrheic dermatitis, and bacterial impetigo.

Body lice

Despite the fact that body lice reside in clothing, often along seams and not on the body, such as head lice, pediculosis corporis infestation is often much more symptomatic than pediculosis capitis and causes severe pruritus with extensive self-inflicted excoriations (see Fig. 2.5). The sites of blood feeding are often present as erythematous macules, papules, or areas of papular urticaria with a central hemorrhagic punctum. The differential diagnosis includes eczematous dermatitis, lichen simplex chronicus, and scabies.

Crab lice (pediculosis pubis or phthiriasis pubis)

Infestation with pediculosis pubis (phthiriasis) or crab lice is less symptomatic compared with pediculosis capitis. These organisms affect all hair-bearing regions, most commonly the pubic and perianal areas, but also the upper eyelashes and the hairy areas of the axillae, chest, nipples, and abdomen. More extensive infestations usually occur in males with more body hair—

bearing areas than females. Pubic lice may appear as 1—2-mm brownish-gray specks in infested hairy areas, where they remain stationary for days with claws gripping hair shafts and mouth parts embedded in the skin (see Fig. 2.3). The average life span for *Phthirus pubis* is 17 days for females and 22 days for males. Females deposit grayish-white eggs or nits at the skin-hair junctions. The egg incubation period is 7—8 days, and the life cycle from egg to adult is 22—27 days. Clinical manifestations include papular urticaria and self-inflicted, often infected, excoriations at blood-feeding sites and regional, usually inguinal, lymphadenopathy (see Fig. 2.6).

Pathognomonic findings may include maculae ceruleae *(taches bleues)*, bluish-gray irregularly shaped macules, 0.5—1 cm in diameter, scattered over the lower abdominal wall, buttocks, and upper thighs. Maculae ceruleae may be caused by subcutaneous tissue staining from heme pigments in excreta altered by louse saliva and digestion. The differential diagnosis of crab lice includes eczematous dermatitis, seborrheic dermatitis, tinea cruris, folliculitis, molluscum contagiosum, and scabies, which frequently coexists with phthiriasis and may also be sexually transmitted.

Therapy

Both *Pediculus humanus* species (head and body lice) and *Phthirus pubis* (the crab or pubic louse) now have high levels of resistance worldwide to the safest topical pediculicides, specifically the natural pyrethrins and synthetic pyrethroids (permethrin, phenothrin) (Meinking et al., 2002; Downs et al., 1999; Tasher et al., 2017). In addition, resistance to lindane, an organochlorine insecticide, and malathion, an organophosphate insecticide, both alone and combined with pyrethroids, has been reported in the United Kingdom and elsewhere (Tasher et al., 2017).

In a randomized comparison of wet combing versus 0.5% malathion shampoos for head lice in the United Kingdom, Roberts et al. reported a 78% cure rate for malathion shampoo versus 38% for wet combing (Downs et al., 1999; Roberts et al., 2000). In an in vitro pediculicidal efficacy comparison of five pediculicides available in the United States, Meinking et al. reported: (1) significant differences in the pediculicidal efficacies of the five pesticides tested; (2) malathion was the only tested pesticide that had not become less effective as a pediculicide; (3) therapeutic effectiveness ranged from 0.5% malathion (best), undiluted natural pyrethrins with piperonyl butoxide, 1% permethrin, diluted natural pyrethrins with piperonyl butoxide, to 1% lindane; and (4) some head lice in the United States had become resistant to most pediculicides (Meinking et al., 2002; Roberts et al., 2000).

The increasing resistance of head lice to the pyrethrins and pyrethroids has led to the increasing use of more toxic pesticides, specifically lindane, malathion, and carbaryl (not approved by the Food and Drug Administration [FDA] in the United States) in treating pyrethroid-resistant pediculosis capitis worldwide (Downs et al., 1999; Meinking et al., 2002).

Lindane is being inappropriately overprescribed, especially for recurrent infestations with lindane-resistant head lice (Diaz, 2008; Meinking et al., 2002). Lindane is an organochlorine insecticide that bioaccumulates in adipose and nerve tissue; overapplication or, if ingested, can cause seizures, especially in children (Meinking et al., 2002). Although malathion, an organophosphate pesticide, has the greatest therapeutic efficacy against head lice in the United States, it is an irreversible acetylcholinesterase inhibitor that can cause a cholinergic toxidrome and fatal neuromuscular paralysis after overapplication or ingestion (Downs et al., 1999; Meinking et al., 2002). Carbaryl, a carbamate pesticide, highly effective against both head lice and scabies, is being increasingly prescribed for pediculosis capitis, especially in the United Kingdom and Europe (Downs et al., 1999; Meinking et al., 2002). Carbaryl is a reversible acetylcholinesterase inhibitor that is closely related to the organophosphate pesticides that can also cause a cholinergic (muscarinic and nicotinic) toxidrome after overapplication or ingestion (Meinking et al., 2002).

Unfortunately, all of the topical pesticides used to treat ectoparasitic infections share the same characteristics as the three most commonly ingested childhood poisons: prescribed or over-the-counter (OTC) medications; household products; and pesticides (Meinking et al., 2002). As the prevalence of pesticide-resistant ectoparasite infestations increases, alternative pesticides more toxic than pyrethrins and pyrethroids will be prescribed; medications will continue to be administered in households; and thus, household accidental overapplication or ingestion of these more toxic pesticide formulations may increase unless there is enhanced public health education measures (Diaz, 2008; Meinking et al., 2002).

Therapy for pediculosis capitis

Therapy for pediculosis capitis should include two topical or systemic treatments with pediculicides, 7—10 days apart, and removal of all viable nits by carefully combing wet hair. Olive oil, petroleum jelly, and Hair Clean 1-2-3 are preferred hair-wetting agents, and plastic combs are preferred over metal combs (Roberts et al., 2000). Unfortunately, the ideal pediculicide with 100% killing activity against lice and nits does not exist. Table 2.2 presents the most commonly used pediculicides for lice infestations. As noted, drug resistance is increasing against the safest pediculicides, the pyrethrins and synthetic pyrethroids, and even against lindane and malathion, an effective ovicidal insecticide with 95% efficacy against viable nits (Tasher et al., 2017; Roberts et al., 2000; Meinking et al., 2002).

Topical ivermectin lotion 0.5% has now been FDA-approved for sale over the counter for the treatment of head lice in patients 6 months of age and older. Ivermectin is a fermentation product of a soil-dwelling actinomycete, *Streptomyces avermitilis*.

Table 2.2 Recommended pediculicide treatments for pediculosis capitis.

Pediculicides	Trade names	Therapeutic efficacies	Safety profiles	Contraindications
0.33% pyrethrins + 4% piperonyl butoxide shampoo	A-200 (OTC) RID (OTC)	95% ovicidal; no residual activity; increasing drug resistance	Excellent	Chrysanthemum and daisy (plant family Compositae) allergies possible contraindications
1%–5% permethrin cream rinse	Acticin (OTC) (Rx) Nix (OTC)	2-wk residual activity; increasing drug resistance	Excellent	Prior allergic reactions
0.5% malathion lotion, 1% malathion shampoo	Ovide (Rx)	95% ovicidal; rapid (5 minutes) killing; good residual activity; increasing drug resistance, but not in the United States	Flammable 78% isopropyl alcohol vehicle stings eyes, skin, mucosa; potential for scalp fire and burn risks if using a hair dryer or curling/flat iron when wet after applying; increasing drug resistance; organophosphate poisoning risks with overapplication and ingestion	Infants and children <6 mo of age; pregnancy; breast-feeding
1% lindane lotion and shampoo	Generic (Rx)	95% ovicidal; no residual activity; increasing drug resistance	Potential for CNS toxicity from organochlorine poisoning, usually manifesting as seizures, with overapplication and ingestion	Preexisting seizure disorder; infants and children <6 mo of age; pregnancy; breast-feeding; not recommended for use due to toxicity. No longer available in the US since 2022.

0.9% Spinosad suspension	Natroba (Rx)	New to market; no reports of resistance; not ovicidal	Excellent	Infants and children age 4 yr and younger; presumed safe in pregnancy based on animal studies
5% benzyl alcohol lotion	Ulesfia (Rx)	No resistance reported; not ovicidal	Excellent	Infants and children age 6 mo and younger; presumed safe in pregnancy based on animal studies
0.5% ivermectin lotion	Sklice (Rx)	No resistance; single 10-minute application, not ovicidal but nymphs die when they emerge from nits	Excellent	Infants and children age 6 months and younger; safety in pregnancy uncertain
Ivermectin, 200–400 µg/kg single PO dose, repeated in 7–10 days	Stromectol (Rx); not ovicidal; second dose recommended	Excellent	Excellent, but not in widespread use; nausea and vomiting possible; take on empty stomach with water only	Safety in pregnancy uncertain; not recommended for children weighing <5 kg; not FDA approved for pediculosis in United States

CNS, central nervous system; *FDA*, U.S. Food and Drug Administration; *OTC*, over-the-counter availability; *Rx*, available by prescription only.
Carbaryl (Sevin), a carbamate pesticide, is not currently approved or available as a human topical preparation for use for pediculosis in the United States. Carbaryl is prescribed for pediculosis in Europe and elsewhere. Ectoparasite resistance to carbaryl has not been reported.

Adapted from Diaz, J.H., 2014. Section on Ectoparasitic Diseases. Chapter 293. Lice (Pediculosis). In Bennett, J.E., Dolin, R., Blaser, M.J. (Eds.), Eight Edition, Elsevier, Philadelphia, pp. 3246–3249. Elsevier publication. Diaz, J.H., 2014.Section on Ectoparasitic Diseases. Chapter 293. Lice (Pediculosis). In Bennett, J.E., Dolin, R., Blaser, M.J. (Eds.), *Mandell, Douglas and Bennett's Principles and Practice of Infectious Diseases*, Eight Edition, Elsevier, Philadelphia, pp. 3246–3249. Elsevier publication. Updated reference: Drugs for head lice. 2024. The Medical Letter on Drugs and Therapeutics 66 (1704), 89–91.

Ivermectin binds to glutamate-gated chloride channels in lice and other ectoparasites causing paralysis and death. Although ivermectin 0.5% lotion is not directly ovicidal like other pediculicides, the nymphs that hatch from ivermectin-treated eggs will die within 48 hours, making retreatment at 7–10 days unnecessary.

A randomized controlled trial has shown that a single oral dose of ivermectin, 400 µg/kg of body weight, and repeated at 7 days, established higher louse-free rates by day 15 (97.1%) than two applications of 0.5% malathion lotion (89.8%) in patients with pyrethroid-resistant head lice infestations (Chosidow et al., 2010; Diaz, 2008; Pariser et al., 2012). In 2012, the FDA approved the use of topical single application of 0.5% ivermectin lotion for head lice infestations based on the results of two multisite, randomized, double-blind studies (Chosidow et al., 2010).

In these studies, investigators compared a single application of one tube of 0.5% ivermectin lotion with vehicle control for the elimination of head lice infestations without nit combing in patients ≥6 months of age (Chosidow et al., 2010). A total of 765 patients completed the studies. In the intention-to-treat population, significantly more patients receiving topical ivermectin than patients receiving topical vehicle control were louse-free on day 2 (94.9% vs. 31.3%), on day 8 (85.2% vs. 20.8%), and on day 15 (73.8% vs. 17.6%) ($P < .001$ for each comparison) (Chosidow et al., 2010). The severity and frequency of adverse events were not significantly different in the two groups (Chosidow et al., 2010). The investigators concluded that a single, 10-minute, at-home application of ivermectin was more effective than vehicle control in eliminating head-louse infestations at 1, 7, and 14 days after treatment (Chosidow et al., 2010).

Resistance of head lice to ivermectin is rare (Pariser et al., 2012). Adverse reactions to ivermectin lotion are uncommon, but were reported in less than 1% of patients enrolled in clinical trials (Pariser et al., 2012). Reported adverse reactions included eye irritation, ocular hyperemia, conjunctivitis, dandruff, dry skin, and burning sensations.

Today, both oral ivermectin and topical ivermectin lotion for head lice offer convenient, single-dose treatments that kill nymphs when they emerge from nits and can be reserved for drug-resistant head lice cases to limit the potential for ivermectin resistance. Unfortunately, these newer treatments are more expensive than the topical pesticides, and access to them is limited to nonexistent in many low-income settings where louse-borne infestations are hyperendemic.

Therapy for body lice

Management includes initial bathing with soap and water, followed by two topical or systemic treatments with pediculicides, 7–10 days apart (Table 2.1). Topical medications should be applied to clean affected areas, allowed to dry, and not rinsed for 8 (malathion) to 24 (pyrethrins, pyrethroids) hours.

Prevention

Prevention strategies for head lice include combinations of sanitizing the environment and, more importantly, eliminating all human reservoirs of carriage of head lice in households, apartments, housing complexes, homeless shelters, classrooms, and schools. Some common preventive interventions include: (1) Avoiding contact with potentially contaminated items, such as hats, head sets, clothing, towels, combs, brushes, bedding, and upholstery; (2) soaking all combs and brushes in isopropyl alcohol or 2% Lysol solution; (3) sanitizing the household environment by high heat-cycle washing and drying of all bedding, clothing, and headwear; and (4) inspecting high-risk schoolchildren for active head lice, viable nits, and nymphs.

Today, "no-nit policies" in schools have been modified. As noted, nonviable nits on hair shafts are simply empty egg cases and do not indicate active louse infestation (Table 2.1). Dermoscopy can clearly distinguish viable nits from hatched, empty nits and pseudo-nits immediately and reliably and offers a more sensitive screening tool for head lice infestations than visual inspection alone (Chosidow et al., 2010).

Prevention and control strategies for pediculosis corporis should include:

1. Hot-cycle washing and drying of all clothing and bedding
2. Clothing and body delousing with 1% permethrin dusting powder, especially in outbreak situations with potential for bacterial disease transmission
3. Institution of basic personal hygiene and sanitation measures, including showering, body washing, and frequent clean clothing changes

Bathing and immersion of clothing in water heated to at least 60°C over a charcoal, wood, or propane gas fire to kill body lice are both time-consuming and costly for many people, especially in low income regions, such as in the Horn of Africa, where louse-borne relapsing fever (LBRF) caused by *B. recurrentis* is a hyperendemic and frequent cause of healthcare visits (Pariser et al., 2012).

In a review of several simpler methods to control LBRF in Ethiopia, investigators recommended holding infected clothes away from human hosts in plastic shopping bags for 10 days to starve adult and nymphal body lice to death and prevent eggs from hatching. Several experiments in vitro have supported this strategy since adults must feed regularly every few days and nymphs must feed immediately upon maturation (Pariser et al., 2012).

Prevention strategies for pubic lice are similar to the prevention strategies for body lice and should include:

1. Hot-cycle washing and drying of all clothing and bedding
2. Institution of basic personal hygiene and sanitation measures
3. Treatment of sexual contacts with active infestations
4. Examination and laboratory testing of patients and their sexual contacts for other sexually transmitted diseases, especially crusted scabies and AIDS.

References

Arnaud, A., Chosidow, O., Détrez, M.-A., Bitar, D., Huber, F., Foulet, F., Le Strat, Y., Vandentorren, S., 2016. Prevalences of scabies and pediculosis corporis among homeless people in the Paris region: results from two randomized cross-sectional surveys (HYTPEAC study). British Journal of Dermatology 174 (1), 104—112. https://doi.org/10.1111/bjd.14226.

Bonilla, D.L., Cole-Porse, C., Kjemtrup, A., Osikowicz, L., Kosoy, M., 2014. Risk factors for human lice and bartonellosis among the homeless, San Francisco, California, USA. Emerging Infectious Diseases 20 (10), 1645—1651. https://doi.org/10.3201/eid2010.131655.

Boutellis, A., Mediannikov, O., Bilcha, K.D., Ali, J., Campelo, D., Barker, S.C., Raoult, D., 2013. Borrelia recurrentis in head lice, Ethiopia. Emerging Infectious Diseases 19 (5), 796—798. https://doi.org/10.3201/eid1905.121480.

Chosidow, O., Giraudeau, B., Cottrell, J., Izri, A., Hofmann, R., Mann, S.G., Burgess, I., 2010. Oral ivermectin versus malathion lotion for difficult-to-treat head lice. New England Journal of Medicine 362 (10), 896—905. https://doi.org/10.1056/nejmoa0905471.

Diaz, J.H., 2008. Increasing pesticide-resistant ectoparasitic infections may increase pesticide poisoning risks in children. Journal of the Louisiana State Medical Society: Official Organ of the Louisiana State Medical Society 160 (4), 210—220.

Downs, A.M.R., Stafford, K.A., Harvey, I., Coles, G.C., 1999. Evidence for double resistance to permethrin and malathion in head lice. British Journal of Dermatology 141 (3), 508—511. https://doi.org/10.1046/j.1365-2133.1999.03046.x.

Drali, R., Shako, J.C., Davoust, B., Diatta, G., Raoult, D., 2015a. A new clade of african body and head lice infected by bartonella quintana and yersinia pestis-democratic republic of the Congo. The American Journal of Tropical Medicine and Hygiene 93 (5), 990—993. https://doi.org/10.4269/ajtmh.14-0686.

Drali, R., Mumcuoglu, K.Y., Yesilyurt, G., Raoult, D., 2015b. Studies of ancient lice reveal unsuspected past migrations of vectors. The American Journal of Tropical Medicine and Hygiene 93 (3), 623—625. https://doi.org/10.4269/ajtmh.14-0552.

Faccini-Martínez, Á.A., Márquez, A.C., Bravo-Estupiñan, D.M., Calixto, O.-J., López-Castillo, C.A., Botero-García, C.A., Hidalgo, M., Cuervo, C., 2017. Bartonella quintana and typhus group rickettsiae exposure among homeless persons, Bogotá, Colombia. Emerging Infectious Diseases 23 (11), 1876—1879. https://doi.org/10.3201/eid2311.170341.

Koehler, J.E., Sanchez, M.A., Tye, S., Garrido-Rowland, C.S., Chen, F.M., Maurer, T., Cooper, J.L., Olson, J.G., Reingold, A.L., Hadley, W.K., Regnery, R.R., Tappero, J.W., 2003. Prevalence of Bartonella infection among human immunodeficiency virus-infected patients with fever. Clinical Infectious Diseases 37 (4), 559—566. https://doi.org/10.1086/375586.

Ly, T.D.A., Touré, Y., Calloix, C., Badiaga, S., Raoult, D., Tissot-Dupont, H., Brouqui, P., Gautret, P., 2017. Changing demographics and prevalence of body lice among homeless persons, Marseille, France. Emerging Infectious Diseases 23 (11), 1894—1897. https://doi.org/10.3201/eid2311.170516.

Meinking, T.L., Serrano, L., Hard, B., Entzel, P., Lemard, G., Rivera, E., Villar, M.E., 2002. Comparative in vitro pediculicidal efficacy of treatments in a resistant head lice population in the United States. Archives of Dermatology 138 (2), 220—224. https://doi.org/10.1001/archderm.138.2.220.

Pariser, D.M., Meinking, T.L., Bell, M., Ryan, W.G., 2012. Topical 0.5% ivermectin lotion for treatment of head lice. New England Journal of Medicine 367 (18), 1687—1693. https://doi.org/10.1056/nejmoa1200107.

Roberts, R.J., Casey, D., Morgan, D.A., Petrovic, M., 2000. Comparison of wet combing with malathion for treatment of head lice in the UK: a pragmatic randomised controlled trial. The Lancet 356 (9229), 540—544. https://doi.org/10.1016/s0140-6736(00)02578-2.

Tasher, D., Raucher-Sternfeld, A., Tamir, A., Giladi, M., Somekh, E., 2017. Bartonella quintana, an unrecognized cause of infective endocarditis in children in Ethiopia. Emerging Infectious Diseases 23 (8), 1246—1252. https://doi.org/10.3201/eid2308.161037.

Whitfield, J., 2003. Lice genes date first human clothes. Nature. https://doi.org/10.1038/news030818-7.

Whitfield, J., Drali, R., Mumcuoglu, K.Y., Yesilyurt, G., Raoult, D., Drali, R., Shako, J.-C., Davoust, B., 1999. Presence of scabies and pediculosis corporis among homeless persons in the Paris region: results from two randomized cross-sectional surveys (HYTPEAC Study). Ethiopia Emerging Infectious Diseases 93 (3), 304—310. https://doi.org/10.1038/news030818-7.

CHAPTER 3

Trombidiosis (larval chigger mites)

The remaining genera of larval trombiculid mites can cause chigger bites, but do not transmit scrub typhus or other infectious diseases. "*Chiggers*" is also a colloquial American term for trombidiosis describing the intensely pruritic clusters of erythematous welts resulting from bites by larval chigger mites.

Definitions and taxonomy

There are over 700 species of chigger mites (Family Trombiculidae) in the world, but only about 20 species cause trombidiosis or transmit scrub typhus (McClain et al., 2009). In the United States, the term "*chiggers*" includes immune reactions to bites by the six-legged larval stage of the American trombiculid mite, *Eutrombicula alfreddugesi* (Fig. 3.1) (McClain et al., 2009). Other local names for larval trombiculid mites in the United States include jiggers, harvest mites, red bugs, red mites, harvest lice, and mower's

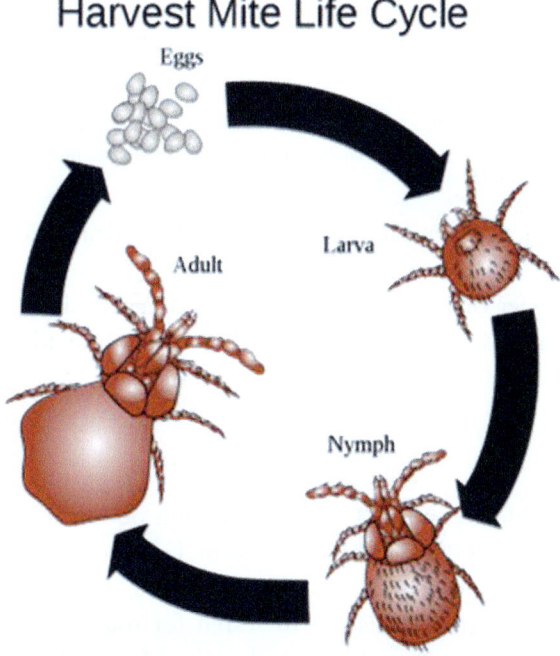

Figure 3.1 The life cycle of the American chigger or harvest mite, ***Eutrombicula alfreddugesi.*** *(Wikipedia. Public domain, No copyright permission required. This is the life cycle of the American chigger mite from egg to adult.)*

Ectoparasitic Diseases
ISBN 978-0-443-26724-6
https://doi.org/10.1016/B978-0-443-26724-6.00003-5

Table 3.1 Representative larval trombiculid mites (Family Trombiculidae) causing chiggers.

Latinnames	Commonnames	Animal reservoirs for nymphs and adults	Geographic distributions	Skinconditions
Eutrombicula alfreddugesi	American chigger mite, red bug, red mite, harvest lice, mower's mite	Birds, rodents, insects, and small mammals	Americas	American chiggers, trombidiosis
Eutrombicula hirsti	Australian scrub itch mite, tea tree itch mite	Birds, rodents, insects, insectivores, small mammals	Australia	Australian chiggers, Australian scrub itch
Eutrombicula sarcina	Asian chigger mite	Birds, insects, rodents, and small mammals	Asia, Australia	AsianChiggers, non-typhus chiggers, trombidiosis
Neotrombicula autumnalis	European harvest mite, European autumn mite	Birds, insects, rodents, and small mammals	Europe, Scandinavia	EuropeanChiggers, trombidiosis
Trombidium holosericeum	Red spider mite, velvet mite	Birds, insects, rodents, and small mammals	Asia, Europe, North Africa, Scandinavia	Chiggers, trombidiosis

Adapted from Diaz, J.H., 2023. *Mite-Human Encounters: Nuisances, Vectors, Parasites, Allergens, and Commensals.* Elsevier, Cambridge, MA. Elsevier publication. No permission required.

mites. Other indigenous species of trombiculid larval mites cause trombidiosis worldwide (Table 3.1).

The life cycle of the American chigger or harvest mite begins with eggs laid by a gravid female that hatch into larvae, which develop into nymphs that mature into adult males or females.

Life cycle

The eight-legged adult female chigger mite lays up to 40 eggs per month on leaf litter, ground cover, and grasses (McClain et al., 2009). The eggs hatch in 1–2 weeks and, following short prelarval dormant phases, release reddish-colored, mobile, six-legged larvae which climb up to 30 cm on plants and vegetation to search for rodent hosts (Fig. 3.2) (McClain et al., 2009). Once the larvae find a host, they feed for 2–4 days

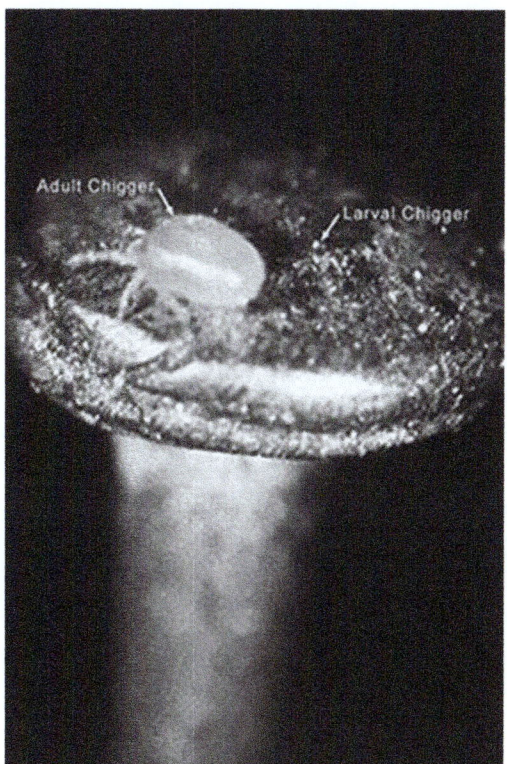

Figure 3.2 Adult and larval American chigger mites, ***Eutrombicula alfreddugesi***, on the head of a pin. *(Adult and larval chigger mites are barely visible to the unaided eye and both are so small that they can fit together on the head of a pin. CDC. Public domain.)*

before dropping off and developing into free-ranging nymphs and adults that feed only on insects (McClain et al., 2009). Adult red chigger mites are less than 1 mm in length, barely visible without magnification, and usually unnoticed even when biting humans or feeding on zoonotic hosts (See Fig. 3.2).

Adult and larval American chigger mites are so small that both can sit together on the head of a pin.

Regional distribution and ecology

Chigger mites are found in greatest abundance in the southeastern and south central United States where environmental conditions support egg-laying and maturation and provide a range of rodent and insect hosts (McClain et al., 2009). The best seasonal and environmental conditions to support larval feeding and maturation are achieved during summer and early fall, with temperatures between 10°C (50°F.) and 32°C (90°F.) and a relative humidity around 80% (McClain et al., 2009).

Feeding behavior

Chigger mites do not burrow beneath the skin to feed like scabies mites do. They crawl on the skin to find a suitable area for feeding where the skin is soft, warm, and moist, particularly where clothing is tight and compresses the skin restricting mite movement. Preferred areas include under waistbands, underwear bands, collars, cuffs, and socks. When ready to bite and feed, chiggers will attach their mouthparts at a skin pore or at the base of a hair shaft to initiate a unique manner of feeding on tissue juices using their specialized stylostomes (See Fig. 3.3) (Hase et al., 1978). Unlike ticks, chiggers are tissue juice feeders, not blood feeders. Tissue juices are composed of edema fluid, lymph, and dissolved epithelial cells (Hase et al., 1978).

A trombiculid mite larva feeds by first attaching to human skin and then penetrating the skin with a hollow, straw-like stylostome that can suck dissolved tissue juice from the host.

Larvae pierce the skin with sharp chelicera and inject tissue-dissolving saliva to create a pool of tissue juices for feeding. The tissue-dissolving components of the saliva of trombiculid mite larvae have not been identified. The repeated injection of mite saliva containing tissue and epithelial cell−dissolving lytic enzymes into the

Figure 3.3 The feeding position of a trombiculid mite larva on the skin of a human host. Diagram depicting the feeding position of a trombiculid mite larva with a hollow, straw-like stylostome penetrating deeper under the host's skin and permitting the siphoning of fresh tissue juices dissolved by salivary enzymes. *(CDC and Wikipedia. Public domain. Available at: https://en.wikipedia.org/wiki/Trombiculidae#/media/File:Chigger_bite.svg.)*

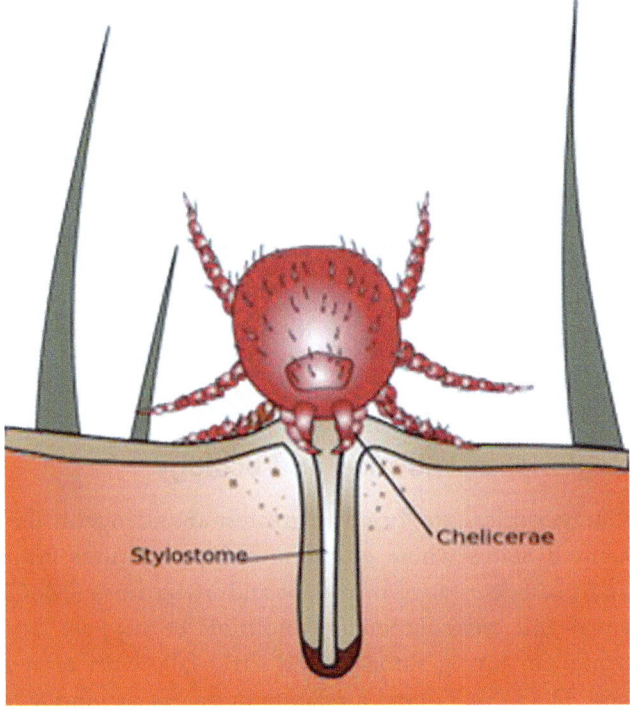

bite wound induces a host humoral immune response that assists in the extension of a long straw-like hollow tube or siphon, known as a stylostome (Hase et al., 1978). The humoral immune response to stylostome penetration is most likely initiated by Th2 T-cells that soften the skin, stimulate B-cells to release IgM antibodies, and trigger the scratch-itch reflex as in other types of pruritic insect bites. As the host's surrounding tissues harden in a fibrotic reaction to the deeper penetrating stylostome, the mite's mouthparts are firmly anchored to the bite wound for prolonged, uninterrupted feeding (Hase et al., 1978).

Clinical manifestations

Initially painless, chigger bites become symptomatic within 3—6 hours. They often cluster in patterns and progress through a sequence of stages from macules to papules, to papulo-vesicles, to urticarial wheals, and later to draining pustules (Fig. 3.4) (McClain et al., 2009). The lesions become intensely pruritic as they progress and accumulate in areas where clothing impedes mite movement in a downward direction, such as under

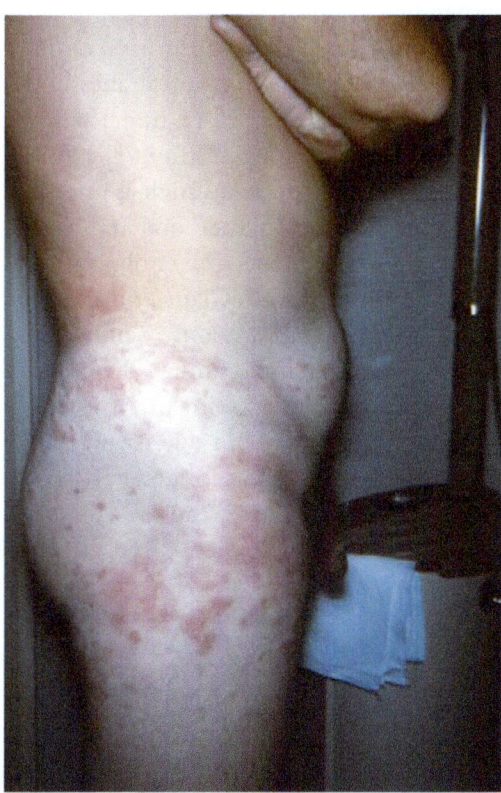

Figure 3.4 The rash caused by multiple larval chigger mite bites is intensely pruritic and usually confined to regions covered by underclothing or socks. An intensely pruritic papulovesicular rash caused by chigger mite bites and characterized by draining pustules confined to a circumferential area around the waist, hips, and genitals usually covered by underwear. *(CDC. Public domain. United States Centers for Disease Control and Prevention, Atlanta, GA. Public Health Image Library (PHIL). Image Number 20202. Available at =phil.cdc.gov/Details.aspx?pid=20202.)*

belts, waistbands, sleeves, socks, and underwear elastic waist and thigh bands. As a result, these groupings may exhibit a circumferential pattern around wrists, knees, waists, thighs, ankles, toes, male genitalia, and under the elastic bands of under garments (McClain et al., 2009).

The rash caused by multiple chigger mite bites is intensely pruritic, characterized by draining pustules, and usually confined to body areas covered by underclothing.

Patients who have previously experienced chigger bites or have developed significant immune responses to past chigger bites often suffer from severe local bite site reactions to subsequent chigger bites. These reactions include bullae and weeping pustules and may be misdiagnosed with scabies or bullous pemphigus (Fig. 3.4) (McClain et al., 2009). A hypersensitivity reaction known as the "*summer penile syndrome*" has been described in prepubertal males, usually summertime campers, with multiple circumferential penile and scrotal chigger bites causing significant penile and scrotal edema with intense pain and pruritus (Smith et al., 1998).

Treatment

The treatment of chigger bites is nonspecific, supportive, and symptomatic including topical applications of local anesthetics, antiseptics, antipruritics, antihistamines, cooling counterirritants, and corticosteroids. Effective topical anesthetics applied in ointments, creams, foams, or incorporated into or placed under patches include lidocaine, prilocaine, benzocaine, and pramocaine (McClain et al., 2009). Effective topical antibiotic ointments for low-grade skin infections such as impetigo include 2% mupirocin or bacitracin. Effective antipruritics include oral and parenteral antihistamines, such as diphenhydramine and hydroxyzine, and cooling topical counterirritants, such as calamine, camphor, and menthol (McClain et al., 2009). Topical diphenhydramine should not be used because it can cause sensitization with subsequent allergic reactions to topical or oral diphenhydramine. Temporary occlusion of bite sites by occlusive plastics, collodion, liquid skin, or clear finger nail polish has been reported to increase itching, erythema, and edema (McClain et al., 2009). If it is necessary to use an occlusive dressing for prolonged corticosteroid application, these symptoms can be alleviated by covering the dressing with plastic bags filled with ice and inserting a cloth barrier between the ice and the dressing to prevent frostbite (McClain et al., 2009).

In rare cases, intralesional corticosteroids and excision of bite lesions have provided permanent relief when topical and oral treatments have failed to control itching (Elston, 2006). Low concentrations of corticosteroids between 2.5 and 5.0 mg/mL are recommended for intralesional injections to avoid fat atrophy with permanent skin dimpling (McClain et al., 2009; Elston, 2006).

Complications

Chigger bites may be secondarily infected with common skin contaminants.

Prevention and control

All mite species have developed very close associations with their supporting ecosystems and preferred zoonotic reservoirs referred to as mite islands. Mite islands typically border cleared land and scrub brush. Environmental requirements include warm soil temperatures with high humidity to support grassy vegetation frequently visited by rodents. Humans stumbling onto or camping within mite islands are at significantly greater risks for multiple larval chigger bites.

Preventive strategies for chigger bites include avoidance of high risk mite island areas of grassland during the late summer and early autumn in endemic areas and the application of synthetic pyrethroid insecticides, such as permethrin, on clothing, shoes, tents, tarps, hammocks, and sleeping bags. In addition to permethrin-impregnated or sprayed clothing and bedding, other personal protective measures should include the topical applications of 10%−30% N, N-diethyl-meta-toluamide (DEET, also known as N, N-diethyl-3-methyl-benzamide) or 10%−20% picaridin (also known as icaridin) to skin surfaces, especially in high risk bite areas around the wrists, elbows, waists, knees, and ankles. Combination preparations of insect repellents and sunscreens are not recommended because sunscreens require more frequent applications than insect repellents and may potentiate insect repellant toxicity, especially in children.

References

Elston, D.M., 2006. What's eating you? Chiggers. Cutis 77 (6), 350−352.
Hase, T., Roberts, L.W., Hildebrandt, P.K., Cavanaugh, D.C., 1978. Stylostome Formation by Leptotrombidium mites (Acari: Trombiculidae). The Journal of Parasitology 64 (4), 712−718. https://doi.org/10.2307/3279967.
McClain, D., Dana, A.N., Goldenberg, G., 2009. Mite infestations. Dermatologic Therapy 22 (4), 327−346. https://doi.org/10.1111/j.1529-8019.2009.01245.x.
Smith, G.A., Sharma, V., Knapp, J.F., Shields, B.J., 1998. The summer penile syndrome: seasonal acute hypersensitivity reaction caused by chigger bites on the penis. Pediatric Emergency Care 14 (2), 116−118. https://doi.org/10.1097/00006565-199804000-00007.

Further reading

Liu, C., Bayer, A., Cosgrove, S.E., Daum, R.S., Fridkin, S.K., Gorwitz, R.J., et al., 2011. Clinical practice guidelines by the Infectious Diseases Society of America for the treatment of methicillin-resistant *Staphylococcus aureus* infections in adults and children. Clinical Infectious Diseases 52 (3), 18−55.

CHAPTER 4

Scrub typhus (larval typhus mites)

Introduction

Mites, including chigger and scabies mites, are among the smallest arthropods, being most barely visible without magnification. Only about 20 species of the more than 3000 species of chigger, animal, plant, and scabies mites are of any medical importance, and most of these are simply biting nuisances that do not transmit infectious diseases (McClain et al., 2009). Mites are closely related to ticks but not as prodigious at blood-feeding. They do not transmit as broad a range of infectious microbial diseases to humans as ticks. The most serious diseases transmitted by mites are scrub typhus and rickettsialpox. The most common mite affecting humans, *Sarcoptes scabiei* var. *hominis*, causes scabies and is considered separately in Chapter 5.

Taxonomy

The family Rickettsiaceae contains two genera: (1) the genus *Rickettsia* subdivided into the spotted fever group of more than 20 species, including *R. akari*, the causative pathogen of rickettsialpox, and the typhus group with two species, *R. prowazekii* and *R. typhi*, the causative pathogens of epidemic and murine (endemic) typhus, respectively; and (2) the scrub typhus-causing genus *Orientia*, which contains only one recognized species, *Orientia tsutsugamushi* (originally *Rickettsia tsutsugamushi*).

Although initially classified among the *Rickettsia*, *O. tsutsugamushi* has now been reclassified into a separate genus (McClain et al., 2009). This reclassification was based on molecular evidence that the pathogen's cell wall differed significantly from that of the Rickettsiaceae both structurally and in its component proteins. Unlike North American "chiggers," scrub typhus is a serious and potentially fatal zoonotic infectious disease caused by bites from *O. tsutsugamushi*-infected *Leptotrombidium* species chigger larvae.

Arthropod vectors

Among the trombiculid chiggers (Family Trombiculidae), including the scrub typhus—transmitting *Leptotrombidium* species, only the larvae are human and animal scrub typhus transmitters (Fig. 4.1) (McClain et al., 2009). Originally considered vectors of a rodent zoonosis, scrub typhus chiggers are the main environmental reservoirs and the only

Ectoparasitic Diseases
ISBN 978-0-443-26724-6
https://doi.org/10.1016/B978-0-443-26724-6.00004-7

Figure 4.1 *Leptotrombidium* species chigger larvae, the vector of scrub typhus in endemic areas. Only the larval form of the Asian chigger mite can transmit scrub typhus in endemic areas. The larger chigger nymphs and adults are free-living and feed on small insects and their eggs. *(Wikipedia.)*

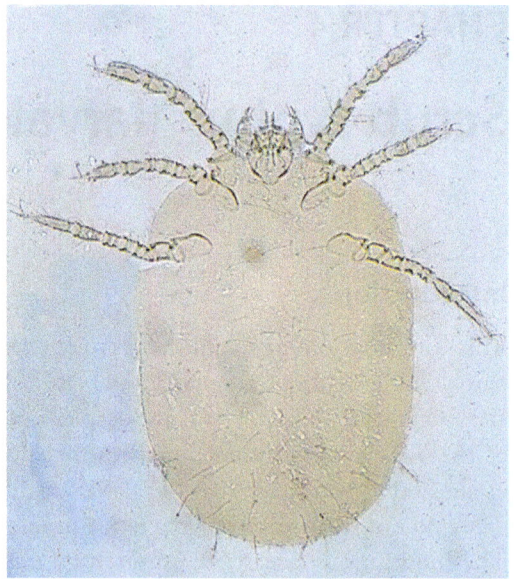

arthropod vectors of *O. tsutsugamushi* in endemic regions, with much smaller secondary bacterial reservoirs in wild rodents.

Once infected by feeding on humans with scrub typhus, gravid females will pass the infection by transovarian transmission to their progeny and to new hosts (McClain et al., 2009). The larger chigger nymphs and adults are free-living and feed on insects, birds, and, especially, rodents. A female mite will lay one to five eggs a day on leaf litter during seasonal cycles in temperate areas and year-round in tropical areas. The eggshells will split in less than a week revealing a six-legged nymph that remains in its shell for about a week before exiting to quest tick-like on higher vegetation for passing hosts. After three nymph states, two of which are infective (protonymph and deutonymph), larvae mature into adults over a period of 3—4 weeks ready for mating. The entire life cycle occurs over 40—75 days, but can be prolonged by colder and drier environmental conditions. *O. tsutsugamushi* infection is maintained throughout the generations of developmental stages of chigger mites by transstadial transmission.

Ecology

All mite species develop close generational associations with their ecosystems and zoonotic reservoirs, often referred to as mite islands. Mite islands usually border cleared land and scrub bush and have several habitat requirements, including grassy vegetation with warm soil temperatures and high humidity, frequently visiting rodent hosts for larvae to feed on, and sufficient small insect fauna to feed nymphs and reproducing adults. Humans stumbling onto mite islands are at significantly higher risk for multiple larval chigger bites or trombidiosis worldwide or scrub typhus in the endemic regions of Asia and Northern Australia.

Epidemiology

Larval feeding and disease transmission

Among the trombiculid chiggers (Trombiculidae), including the scrub typhus—transmitting *Leptotrombidium* species, only the larvae are human and animal ectoparasites (McClain et al., 2009). The larger chigger nymphs and adults are free-living and feed on small insects and their eggs. All trombiculid larvae exhibit a unique method of feeding on their human hosts and transmitting salivary secretions, which may contain *O. tsutsugamushi* in endemic regions (See Image 3.3 from Chapter 3: Trombidiosis (Larval Chigger Mites)). When larval mites have selected a human host, they will congregate where the skin is soft, warm, and moist, particularly where clothing is tight against the skin, such as under waistbands, undergarment elastic bands, and socks. Initially painless, chigger bites cluster in these regions on the genitalia, perineum, thighs, buttocks, waist, and ankles and become symptomatic in 3—6 hours (See Image 3.4 from Chapter 3: Trombidiosis (Larval Chigger Mites)). Larvae pierce the skin with sharp mouthparts and inject tissue-dissolving saliva to create a pool of lymph, other body fluids, and dissolved epithelial cells to feed on.

Noninfectious chigger bites

All of the noninfectious chigger larvae can cause trombidiosis or trombiculiasis (trombiculidiasis), with the American chigger mite *(Eutrombicula alfreddugesi)* being the most common culprit in the United States; the European harvest mite, *Neotrombicula autumnalis,* the most common in Europe; and the Asian chigger, *Eutrombicula sarcina,* the most common in Asia (McClain et al., 2009).

In Asia and Northern Australia, similar clusters of larval mite bites may be referred to as *"scrub itch,"* especially in Australia, where the scrub itch mite, *Trombicula hirsti,* commonly cause trombidiosis. Among the scrub typhus—carrying *Leptotrombidium* larval chigger mites, *Leptotrombidium deliense,* the Asian rodent chigger, is a principal vector throughout eastern Asia and Northern Australia.

Immune responses

The repeated injection of mite saliva into the bite wound induces a host immune reaction that forms a straw-like hollow tube, known as a hypostome or stylostome, which extends downward into the host's skin, anchoring the mite firmly (See Image 3.3 from Chapter 3: Trombidiosis (Larval Chigger Mites)) (McClain et al., 2009). Some trombiculid larvae remain attached to and feeding on human hosts for up to a month, but the larval vectors of scrub typhus feed only for 2–10 days before dropping to the ground engorged and ready to mature into free-ranging nymphs.

The most common antigen used to detect serum immunoglobin responses (IgM and IgG) to *O. tsutsugamushi* infection is the 56 kDa-type-specific antigen, which displays significant antigenic variation among many different strains of the pathogen throughout Asia (Rodkvamtook et al., 2013). Investigation of a scrub typhus outbreak among soldiers and residents living near a military installation in Thailand in 2013 identified seven genogroups and three genotypes in a genetic sequence analysis of the *O. tsutsugamushi* strains collected from infected chiggers and rodents (Rodkvamtook et al., 2013). The phylogenetic trees also indicated that *O. tsutsugamushi* strains isolated from chiggers differed from those obtained from rodents, confirming high genetic variability in a very localized scrub typhus outbreak (Rodkvamtook et al., 2013).

In addition to the genetic variability in the causative strains of scrub typhus and the variability in immunoglobulin responses, the cytokine responses to scrub typhus cases are also complex and variable (Eisermann et al., 2020). In a study of cytokine responses to 11 cases of imported scrub typhus in Germany between 2020 and 2018, investigators demonstrated simultaneously upregulated Th1, Th 2, and Th 17 cytokine responses (Eisermann et al., 2020). The complex variation in immune responses to *O. tsutsugamushi* antigens from many genetic strains in scrub typhus-infected mites has precluded the development of effective vaccines for scrub typhus (Eisermann et al., 2020).

Geographic distribution

As a result of experiences with scrub typhus among US troops in the Pacific during World War II and later during wars in Korea, Vietnam, and Afghanistan, scrub typhus was originally considered a regional zoonosis confined to the "Tsutsugamushi Triangle," which extended from Pakistan in the west to the Pacific coast of Russia in the east to northern Australia in the south (Fig. 4.2) (Weitzel et al., 2016).

In 2006, additional cases of scrub typhus were detected in the Middle East caused by a new species, *Orientia chuto*, and in Chile caused by *O. tsutsugamushi* (Weitzel et al., 2016). Although the zoonotic reservoirs and larval mite vectors of scrub typhus outside of the tsutsugamushi triangle remain unidentified, there is now a wider global distribution of the disease than initially assumed.

Seasonal transmission

In the temperate regions of Asia, there is a definite scrub typhus seasonal transmission cycle determined by peaking temperatures and humidity during weeks of marked seasonal

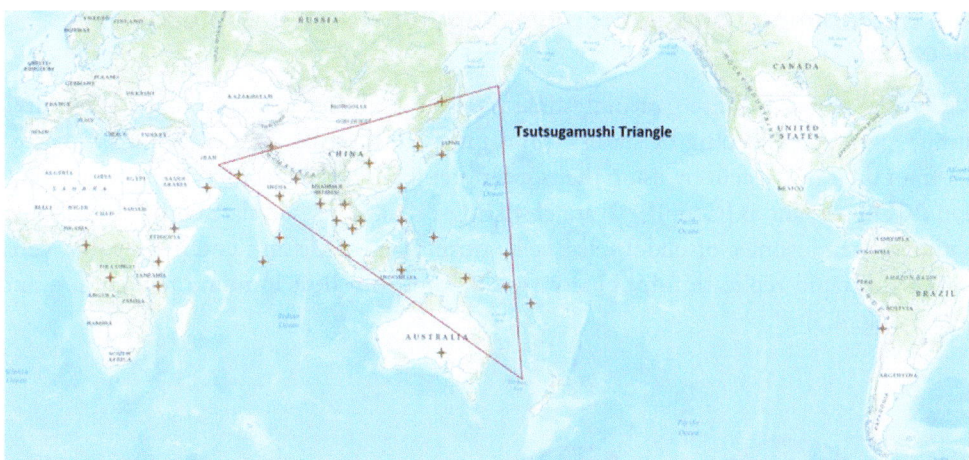

Figure 4.2 The Tsutsugamushi Triangle. *(Wikipedia. Public domain. No copyright permission required. Original Wikipedia Source: Xu, G., Walker, D.H., Jupiter, D., Melby, P.C., Arcari, C.M., 2017. A review of the global epidemiology of scrub typhus. PLoS Negl. Trop. Dis. 11(11), e0006062. https://doi.org/10.1371/journal.pntd.0006062)*

change in late spring to early summer and again in late fall to early winter. In the tropics, scrub typhus transmission occurs year-round.

Risk factors

In a hospital-based matched case—control studies during scrub typhus season (October—December 2015), investigators identified major environmental, occupational, and demographic risk factors for clinical scrub typhus in Bhutan (Zangpo et al., 2023). The major risk factor was farming and harvesting cardamom (odds ratio [OR]1519; $P < .0001$). Cardamom, *Elettaria cardamomum*, is a perennial herb related to ginger that produces seeds used as popular spices and in teas and herbal supplements throughout Bhutan, Nepal, and India (Zangpo et al., 2023). The investigators concluded that the cardamom fields were highly infested seasonally during harvest time with larval scrub typhus mites (Zangpo et al., 2023). Other significant risk factors for scrub typhus included childhood age under 18 ($P = .001$) or elderly age over 65 years ($P = .007$), living in traditional housing with an outside toilet (OR 472; $P = .002$), frequently (>10 times) sitting or sleeping on grass (OR 16; $P = .016$), clearing brush fulltime (OR 4.71; $P = .005$), and owning a goat (OR 37; $P = .002$) (Zangpo et al., 2023). Females had a significantly lower risk of contracting clinical scrub typhus than men (OR 0.19; $P = .01$) which the investigators attributed to less frequent involvement in outdoor activities during scrub typhus season (Zangpo et al., 2023).

The microbiology and pathophysiology of rickettsial infectious diseases

Rickettsiae thrive in mite gastrointestinal tracts and salivary glands and are transmitted during tissue juice feeding by scrub typhus mites. Rickettsiae gain entry into the cytoplasm of their host's cells by using their outer membrane proteins (outer membrane protein A [OmpA] and B [OmpB]) to attach to host cells and to stimulate endocytosis. Once within the endosomes of endothelial cells, rickettsiae escape and enter the white cell's cytosol for rapid replication by binary fission, safe from host immune recognition and attack (Fig. 4.3).

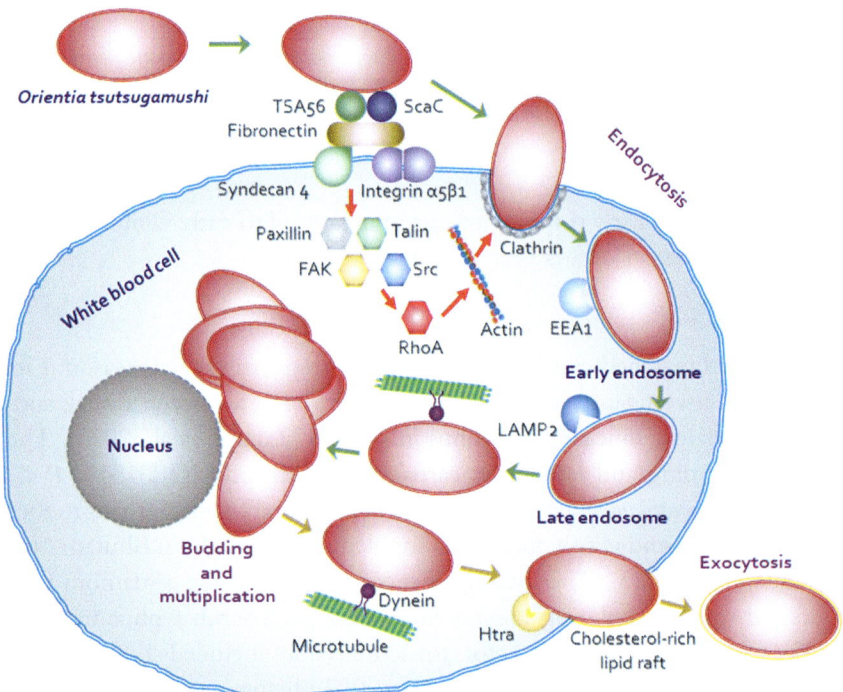

Figure 4.3 *Orientia tsutsugamushi* uses its outer membrane proteins to stimulate endocytosis for entry into the host cell. Endosomes engulf the rickettsiae protecting them from intracellular attack. Rickettsiae escape the endosomes for multiplication in the cytosol, and leave the cell by exocytosis. *EEA1*, early endosome antigen 1; *FAK*, focal adhesion kinase; *HTRA*, serine protease HTRA1 enzyme; *LAMP2*, Lysosomal associated membrane protein 2; *RHOA*, Ras Homolog family Member A; *TSA 56*, 56 kDa type specific antigen. *(Wikipedia. Public domain.)*

Clinical manifestations of scrub typhus

Once injected into the host, rickettsiae are initially distributed regionally through lymphatics with some species including *Orientia* causing regional lymphadenopathy, typically proximal to the bite site eschars. Within 2—14 days (mean, 7 days), rickettsiae are disseminated hematogenously to vascular endothelial lining cells and other cells of target organs and systems, including the gastrointestinal tract, central nervous system (CNS), lungs, liver, kidneys, and myocardium (McClain et al., 2009).

After *O. tsutsugamushi*—infected *Leptotrombidium* chigger bites, an 8—10-day incubation period precedes the onset of classic clinical manifestations of scrub typhus with bite eschar, regional lymphadenopathy, conjunctival injection, central nervous system (CNS) manifestations (e.g., headache, confusion, delirium, hearing loss), and centrifugal rash (Figs. 4.4 and 4.5) (McClain et al., 2009).

In a systematic review and metaanalysis of 458 published articles on the geographical distributions and clinical manifestations of scrub typhus cases, investigators found an overall eschar prevalence of 58.0% with greatest prevalence in East Asia (78.7%), followed by Oceania (52.2%) and Southeast Asia (41.4%), and with the lowest prevalence in South Asia (32.8%) (Yoo et al., 2022). The frequency of eschar distribution was greatest in the inguinal area (28.5%) followed by the anterior body area (28.0%) and lower extremities (22.0%) (Yoo et al., 2022). The upper extremities (8.9%), back (6.6%), and head and neck (6.1%) had low frequencies of lymphadenopathy (Yoo et al., 2022).

The most common CNS manifestations of scrub typhus are meningitis and meningoencephalitis (Lee et al., 2017). In a retrospective analysis of 16 patients with scrub typhus-related central nervous system infections in South Korea, investigators observed eschar formation in only three patients (18.8%), and the most common presenting symptoms

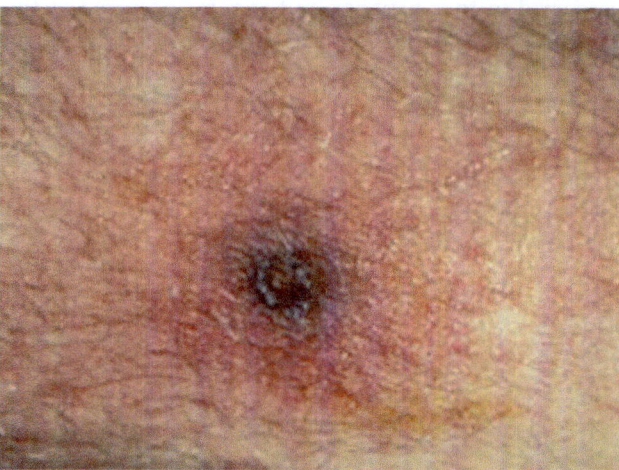

Figure 4.4 Eschar following the bite of a scrub typhus-infected larval ***Leptotrombidium*** species chigger. *(CDC Public domain.)*

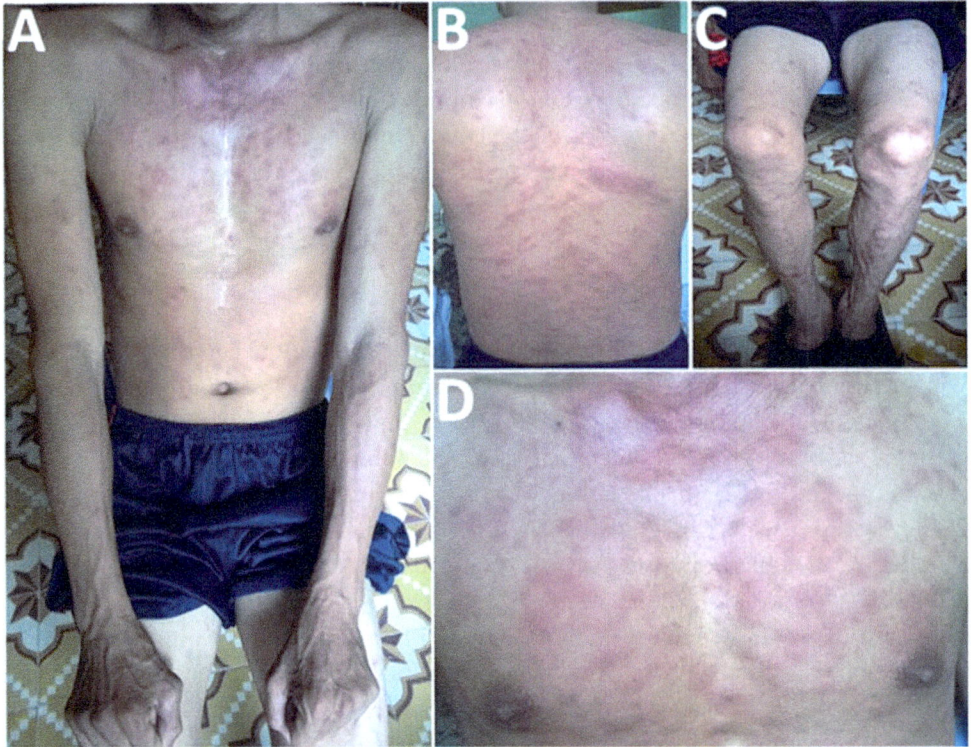

Figure 4.5 Scrub typhus centrifugal rash in a Vietnamese patient with scrub typhus. The rash is papular and centrally located over the abdomen and back. The rash may be overlooked if minimally present. (A) Mid-chest. (B) Mid-back. (C) Mid-leg (knee). (D) Close-up mid-chest. *(CDC. Public domain.)*

were headache (81.3%) and fever (81.3%) (Lee et al., 2017). Among patients with encephalitis, altered consciousness occurred in four patients, and seizures occurred in five patients (Lee et al., 2017). Fatal complications of scrub typhus may include adult respiratory distress syndrome (especially in older patients), hypotensive shock, acute renal failure, encephalomyelitis, myelitis, and disseminated intravascular coagulation (McClain et al., 2009; Rodkvamtook et al., 2013; Lee et al., 2017).

Laboratory diagnosis

Like rickettsialpox, laboratory diagnosis is based on polymerase chain reaction (PCR) on blood, eschar swabs, lymph node aspirates, and biopsies of eschars, rashes, or lymph nodes to detect pathogen DNA. Diagnostic serology including immunofluorescence and immunoperoxidase studies have now replaced the old Weil-Felix tests to detect cross-

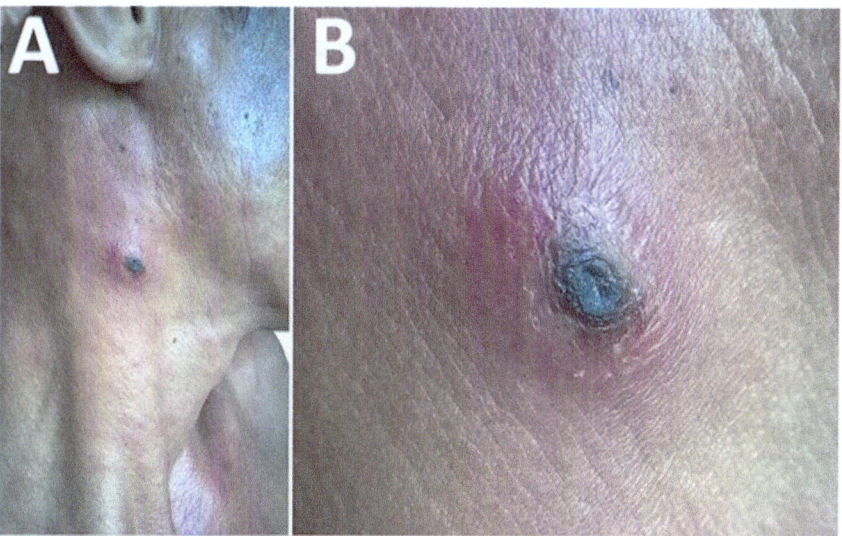

Figure 4.6 *Leptotrombidium* larval mite bite eschar in a Vietnamese patient with dual genotype scrub typhus. (A) Eschar, right neck. (B) Close-up of eschar. *(CDC. Public domain.)*

reacting antibodies to *Proteusmirabilis* OX-K (McClain et al., 2009). Several strains should be included the diagnostic serology because of the genetic variability locally and regionally (Fig. 4.6). In addition, an enzyme-linked immunosorbent assay (ELISA) using recombinant 56 kDa-type specific antigens from multiple strains of *O. tsutsugamushi* was developed in 2019 for the detections of scrub typhus infection (Yang et al., 2019).

Treatment

Oral doxycycline is the preferred antibiotic for scrub typhus in both adults and children with oral chloramphenicol as an effective alternative in case of poor response to doxycycline (Phimda et al., 2007). The CDC and others have advised that short courses of doxycycline for up to 10 days do not cause tooth staining or weaken tooth enamel in children (Todd et al., 2015).

The dosage for doxycycline is 100 mg orally twice a day for 7 days and may be administered in an accelerated fashion over a minimum of 3 days (Phimda et al., 2007). The dosage for chloramphenicol is 50—75 mg/kg/day in four divided doses (Phimda et al., 2007). Other alternative drugs for scrub typhus include rifampin, 600—800 mg/day and azithromycin, 500 mg on the first day and 250 mg/day afterward for 7 days (Phimda et al., 2007). Weekly doses of 200 mg of doxycycline can prevent *O. tsutsugamushi* infections (McClain et al., 2009; Phimda et al., 2007).

Empirical treatment with doxycycline in patients with undifferentiated non-malaria fever with eschar

A wide range of pathogens can cause undifferentiated nonmalaria fevers (Camprubí-Ferrer et al., 2023). Many of these febrile illnesses are caused by pathogens that respond to antibiotic treatment with doxycycline. Febrile illnesses occur in 13% of returning travelers, and up to one-third of the cases remain undiagnosed (Camprubí-Ferrer et al., 2023). The rickettsial diseases, Q fever, bartonellosis, and leptospirosis, are febrile illnesses that occur in returning travelers and are all responsive to doxycycline (Camprubí-Ferrer et al., 2023). Rickettsialpox and scrub typhus are also responsive to doxycycline and present with fever and associated bite eschars.

There is some evidence to support empirical treatment with doxycycline at least in returning travelers with febrile illnesses not caused by malaria or dengue (Camprubí-Ferrer et al., 2023). In a prospective, European multicenter cohort study of 347 returning travelers with undifferentiated nonmalaria fever, 31% (n = 106) were subsequently diagnosed with doxycycline-responding illnesses (Camprubí-Ferrer et al., 2023). The main causes of doxycycline-responding illnesses included rickettsial diseases in 52% (n = 55), Q fever in 15% (n = 15), bartonellosis in 12% (n = 13), and leptospirosis in 10% (n = 10) (Camprubí-Ferrer et al., 2023). The only predictive factor significantly associated with a doxycycline-responding illness was a febrile presentation in association with an eschar (OR = 40, 95% CI = 5-322) (Camprubí-Ferrer et al., 2023).

Although there is no clear consensus on the use of empirical antibiotic treatment in undifferentiated nonmalaria febrile illnesses, consideration should be given to the empirical treatment of undifferentiated nonmalaria fevers associated with eschars with doxycycline in scrub typhus-endemic regions and during outbreaks of rickettsialpox.

Prevention and control of scrub typhus

Preventive strategies include avoidance of high-risk mite island areas of grassland during the late summer and early autumn and the application of synthetic pyrethroid insecticides, such as permethrin, on clothing, shoes, tents, tarps, hammocks, and sleeping bags. In addition to permethrin-impregnated or sprayed clothing, other personal protective measures should include the topical applications of 10%−30% N, N-diethyl-meta-toluamide (DEET, also known as N, N-diethyl-3-methyl-benzamide), or 10%−20% picaridin (also known as icaridin) to skin surfaces in high-risk areas, such as the wrists, ankles, knees, and waists. Combination preparations of insect repellents and sunscreens are not recommended because sunscreens require more frequent applications than insect repellents and may potentiate insect repellant toxicity, especially in children.

There are no vaccines for the primary prevention of scrub typhus or rickettsialpox. Weekly doses of 200 mg of doxycycline can prevent *O. tsutsugamushi* infections (McClain et al., 2009).

Rickettsialpox and scrub typhus as widely distributed and neglected mite-transmitted infectious diseases

Rickettsialpox and scrub typhus are mite-transmitted infectious diseases (IDs) that are widely distributed geographically and neglected clinically. Rickettsialpox is widely distributed for two reasons. First, its animal reservoir, the common house mouse, and its mouse mite vector are ubiquitous in their distributions. Second, subclinical and doxycycline-cured cases of rickettsialpox are often underreported. Scrub typhus is also widely distributed by a global population of potential larval mite vectors. New cases are now reported from the Middle East and South America. These cases are far removed from the Tsutsugamushi Triangle of Asia and northern Australia. Rickettsialpox and scrub typhus are not included among the WHO's list of neglected tropical diseases. Neglect of these mite-transmitted IDs is further evidenced by a lack of research and new drug development as compared with mosquito-borne and tick-borne IDs. In addition, there are no vaccines to prevent rickettsialpox and scrub typhus. Targeted research into mite-transmitted IDs, new drug development to counter increasing doxycycline resistance and replace chloramphenicol, and vaccines, especially for scrub typhus, are needed now.

References

Camprubí-Ferrer, D., Oteo, J.A., Bottieau, E., Genton, B., Balerdi-Sarasola, L., Portillo, A., Cobuccio, L., Van Den Broucke, S., Santibáñez, S., Cadar, D., Rodriguez-Valero, N., Almuedo-Riera, A., Subirà, C., d'Acremont, V., Martinez, M.J., Roldán, M., Navero-Castillejos, J., Van Esbroeck, M., Muñoz, J., 2023. Doxycycline responding illnesses in returning travellers with undifferentiated non-malaria fever: a European multicentre prospective cohort study. Journal of Travel Medicine 30 (1), 1–9. https://doi.org/10.1093/jtm/taac094.

Eisermann, P., Rauch, J., Reuter, S., Eberwein, L., Mehlhoop, U., Allartz, P., Muntau, B., Tappe, D., 2020. Complex cytokine responses in imported scrub typhus cases, Germany, 2010–2018. The American Journal of Tropical Medicine and Hygiene 102 (1), 63–68. https://doi.org/10.4269/ajtmh.19-0498.

Lee, H.S., Sunwoo, J.S., Ahn, S.J., Moon, J., Lim, J.A., Jun, J.S., Lee, W.J., Lee, S.T., Jung, K.H., Park, K.I., Jung, K.Y., Lee, S.K., Chu, K., 2017. Central nervous system infection associated with orientia tsutsugamushi in South Korea. The American Journal of Tropical Medicine and Hygiene 97 (4), 1094–1098. https://doi.org/10.4269/ajtmh.17-0077.

McClain, D., Dana, A.N., Goldenberg, G., 2009. Mite infestations. Dermatologic Therapy 22 (4), 327–346. https://doi.org/10.1111/j.1529-8019.2009.01245.x.

Phimda, K., Hoontrakul, S., Suttinont, C., Chareonwat, S., Losuwanaluk, K., Chueasuwanchai, S., Chierakul, W., Suwancharoen, D., Silpasakorn, S., Saisongkorh, W., Peacock, S.J., Day, N.P.J., Suputtamongkol, Y., 2007. Doxycycline versus azithromycin for treatment of leptospirosis and scrub typhus. Antimicrobial Agents and Chemotherapy 51 (9), 3259–3263. https://doi.org/10.1128/AAC.00508-07.

Rodkvamtook, W., Kuttasingkee, N., Linsuwanon, P., 2013. Emerg. Infect. Dis. 24 (2), 361–365.

Todd, S.R., Dahlgren, F.S., Traeger, M.S., Beltrán-Aguilar, E.D., Marianos, D.W., Hamilton, C., McQuiston, J.H., Regan, J.J., 2015. No visible dental staining in children treated with doxycycline for suspected rocky mountain spotted fever. The Journal of Pediatrics 166 (5), 1246–1251. https://doi.org/10.1016/j.jpeds.2015.02.015.

Weitzel, T., Dittrich, S., López, J., Phuklia, W., Martinez-Valdebenito, C., Velásquez, K., Blacksell, S.D., Paris, D.H., Abarca, K., 2016. Endemic scrub typhus in South America. New England Journal of Medicine 375 (10), 954–961. https://doi.org/10.1056/NEJMoa1603657.

Yang, S.L., Tsai, K.H., Chen, H.F., Luo, J.Y., Shu, P.Y., 2019. Evaluation of enzyme-linked immunosorbent assay using recombinant 56-kDa type-specific antigens derived from multiple orientia tsutsugamushi strains for detection of scrub typhus infection. The American Journal of Tropical Medicine and Hygiene 100 (3), 532–539. https://doi.org/10.4269/ajtmh.18-0391.

Yoo, J.S., Kim, D., Choi, H.Y., Yoo, S., Hwang, J.H., Hwang, J.H., Choi, S.H., Achangwa, C., Ryu, S., Lee, C.S., 2022. Prevalence rate and distribution of eschar in patients with scrub typhus. The American Journal of Tropical Medicine and Hygiene 106 (5), 1358–1362. https://doi.org/10.4269/ajtmh.21-1129.

Zangpo, T., Phuentshok, Y., Dorji, K., Dorjee, C., Dorjee, S., Jolly, P., Morris, R., Marquetoux, N., McKenzie, J., 2023. Environmental, occupational, and demographic risk factors for clinical scrub typhus, Bhutan. Emerging Infectious Diseases 29 (5), 909–918. https://doi.org/10.3201/eid2905.221430.

Further reading

Rodkvamtook, W., Kuttasingkee, N., Linsuwanon, P., et al., 2018. Scrub typhus outbreak in chonburi province, Central Thailand, 2013. Emerging Infectious Diseases 24 (2), 361–365.

CHAPTER 5

Scabies (scabies mites)

Definitions

Scabies, an infestation by the itch or scabies mite, *Sarcoptes scabiei* var. *hominis,* remains a major public health problem throughout the developing world (Fig. 5.1). Scabies in its most severe form, crusted or Norwegian scabies (Fig. 5.2), has now become a significant reemerging ectoparasitosis in the developed world, especially among homeless people, refugees, institutionalized older adults, individuals with intellectual disabilities, including Down syndrome, and immunocompromised individuals (Romani et al., 2017).

The human scabies or itch mite is not visible to the unaided eye, but the linear tunnels made by female mites for egg laying may be visible in areas with thin skin, such as the inside of the wrists.

Epidemiology

Scabies occurs worldwide in both sexes, at all ages, and among all ethnic and socioeconomic groups. The worldwide annual prevalence of scabies has been estimated to be about 100 million cases with most cases confined to tropical countries with the South Pacific region particularly impacted (Romani et al., 2017). In industrialized countries, scabies is more often associated with crowding, refugee status, homelessness, and institutionalization (Romani et al., 2017; Otero et al., 2004). In resource-poor settings in the tropics, scabies is hyperendemic and reaches prevalences as high as 25% in the general population and 50% in children (Romani et al., 2017).

In addition to the South Pacific Island chains, especially the Fiji, Polynesian, and Solomon Islands, other hyperendemic regions for scabies include sub-Saharan Africa, India, and the Native Aboriginal regions of tropical northwestern Australia. In these high-risk regions, impetigo occurs commonly especially among children due to scratching of the lesions and may lead to complications of Group A streptococcal infections including septicemia, glomerulonephritis, and rheumatic heart disease (Romani et al., 2017). The World Health Organization has now designated scabies as a neglected tropical disease and has sponsored mass drug administration programs with topicals such as permethrin or oral treatment with ivermectin to reduce the disease burden of scabies and its associated incidence of impetigo (Romani et al., 2017).

Infestations with crusted (Norwegian) scabies are more prevalent among several specific high-risk groups including men who have sex with men, patients treated in sexually

Ectoparasitic Diseases
ISBN 978-0-443-26724-6
https://doi.org/10.1016/B978-0-443-26724-6.00005-9

Figure 5.1 The scabies or itch mite, *Sarcoptes scabiei* var. *hominis*, female, length 0.30–0.45 mm. *(CDC, public domain.)*

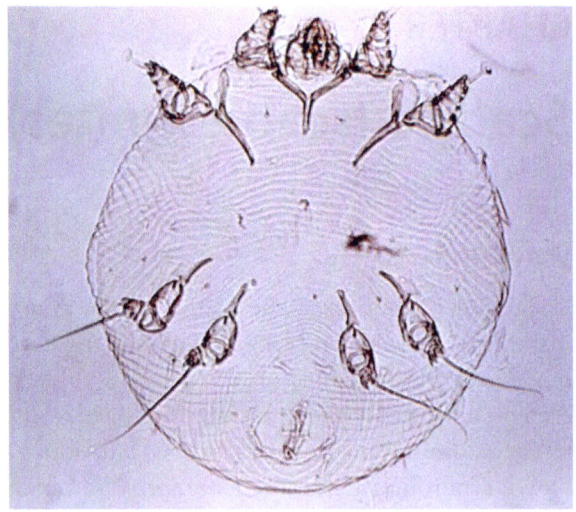

Figure 5.2 Crusted scabies on both hands in an immunocompromised patient. *(Wikipedia.)*

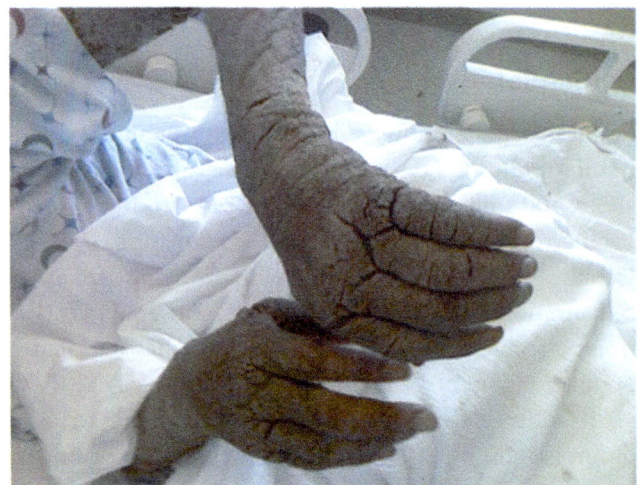

transmitted disease clinics; patients in long-term care, acute care, and skilled nursing facilities; homeless individuals with the acquired immunodeficiency syndrome (AIDS); and patients with human T-cell lymphotropic virus type 1 (HTLV-1) infections (Otero et al., 2004; Bravo et al., 2005; del Giudice et al., 1997). All high-risk patients with crusted scabies should be assessed for human immunodeficiency virus (HIV) and HTLV-1 infections (Bravo et al., 2005; del Giudice et al., 1997). In a prospective study of 23 patients with crusted scabies in Peru, HTLV-1 infection was diagnosed in 16 (69.6%) by enzyme-linked immunosorbent assay and confirmed by Western immunoblot analysis (Bravo et al., 2005). In addition to HTLV-1 infection, other significant comorbid features for crusted scabies in the Peruvian study included corticosteroid therapy (8.6%), malnutrition (8.6%), and Down syndrome (4.3%) (Bravo et al., 2005).

Transmission

In contrast to ectoparasitic fleas and flies, scabies mites cannot jump or fly, but they can crawl at a rate of 2.5 cm/minute on warm, moist skin (Fig. 5.1) (Arlian et al., 1984). They can survive for 24–36 hours at room temperature and average humidity and remain capable of infesting humans (Arlian et al., 1984). Scabies is most easily transmitted by skin-to-skin contact, as with sex partners and children playing, as well as by healthcare providers examining highly infectious patients with crusted scabies (Arlian et al., 1984). High-risk sexual behaviors for contracting scabies include multiple sexual contacts and men who have sex with men (Otero et al., 2004). Scabies mites have not been demonstrated to transmit HIV, HTLV-1, or any other infectious agent (Bravo et al., 2005; del Giudice et al., 1997). Increased mite burdens as in crusted scabies and closer human contacts increase the risks of scabies transmission to a greater extent than indirect contacts with fomites, such as shared bedding, personal grooming items, and clothing (Arlian et al., 1984). Although rare, indirect transmission of scabies occurs and is more common in immunocompromised hosts with AIDS, in family members of an index atypical (crusted) case, and within crowded institutional settings (Arlian et al., 1984).

Several nonhuman species of sarcoptic mites can cause animal scabies or scabietic mange with itching, inflammation, and hair loss. Animal scabies occurs commonly in domestic pets and animals, especially in cats, dogs, rabbits, pigs, horses, and camels. Immunocompromised individuals may also contract animal scabies from domestic animals, most often dogs, with sarcoptic mange. Animal scabies mites are facultative ectoparasites in humans and cannot effectively complete their life cycles in human or "*dead-end*" hosts. Infections are usually self-limited in humans but can be treated successfully, if indicated, with 5% permethrin lotion, 10% crotamiton cream or lotion, or oral ivermectin.

Clinical manifestations

The human scabies mite is an obligate parasite and completes its entire life cycle on its human hosts, as females burrow intradermally to lay eggs and larvae emerge and mature to reinfest the same or new hosts. Female mites burrow preferentially into the thinner areas of the epidermis by dissolving the stratum corneum with proteolytic secretions. Burrows are usually no deeper than the stratum granulosum (Fig. 5.3). Female mites then lay their eggs at the end of their tunneled burrows, which are typically 5–10 mm long (Fig. 5.4). Larvae hatch 2–3 days after eggs are laid. The entire

Figure 5.3 Scabies mites in a skin biopsy. Photomicrograph of *Sarcoptes scabiei* in a skin biopsy at moderate power (40 X) stained with hematoxylin and eosin showing both an adult (green arrow) and an egg (blue arrow). Note also the presence of cuticular spines (black arrow) on the adult. *(CDC. Available at: https://www.cdc.gov/dpdx/scabies/images/2/scabies_tissue_BAM2.jpg.)*

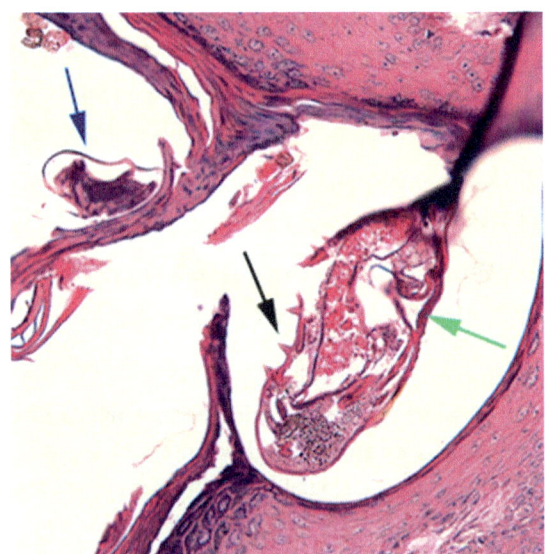

Figure 5.4 Classic scabies on the sides and interdigital web spaces of the fingers caused by burrowing scabies mites and immune reactions to the mites and their feces, ova, and disintegrating body fragments and exoskeletons.

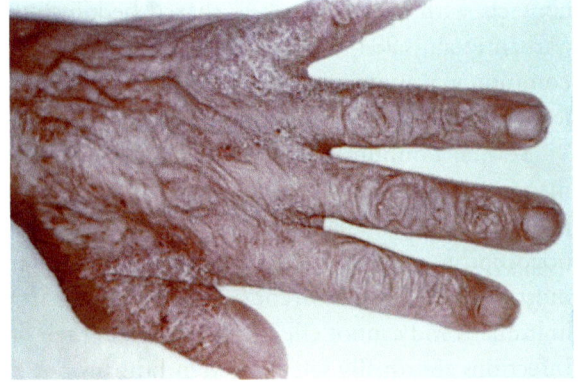

incubation period from eggs to adult mites lasts 14—15 days. The human incubation period from initial infection to symptom development is 3—6 weeks in initial infections and 1—3 days in reinfections as a result of prior sensitization to mite antigens.

Classic or ordinary scabies manifests as generalized, intense nocturnal itching in a characteristic topographic distribution as 10—15 fertile female mites are transferred from infected patients to new hosts. The skin eruptions in reinfections and atypical forms of scabies are more intense and exacerbated by hypersensitivity reactions to prior-encountered mite antigens.

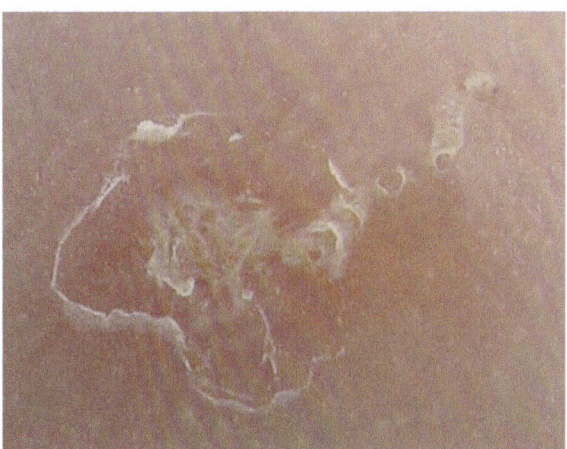

Figure 5.5 The linear burrows of a female scabies mite. *(Wikipedia.)*

In classic scabies, the preferred distribution of skin eruptions includes hairless areas with a thin stratum corneum, such as the sides and interdigital web spaces of fingers and toes, popliteal fossae, flexor surfaces of the wrists, buttocks, and female breasts (Fig. 5.4). Although inflammatory pruritic papules are present at most infested sites, the pathognomonic linear to serpiginous intradermal burrows, 5–10 mm long, dotted with fecaliths (pellets) or scybala, and terminating in raised papules hiding ovipositing females, may be absent (Fig. 5.5). Nonspecific secondary lesions occur commonly as the result of scratching and secondary infection and include self-inflicted excoriation, eczematization, lichenification, and impetigo (Romani et al., 2017).

Bullous scabies is a rare subtype of classic scabies, with only 44 cases reported to date (Zhao et al., 2016). The highly pruritic bullous lesions resemble bullous pemphigoid and most commonly cluster on the trunk and extremities but may involve the genitals, feet, thighs, inguinal folds, and neck (Zhao et al., 2016). Facial and mucosal involvement has not been reported (Zhao et al., 2016). Risk factors for bullous scabies include male sex and advanced age (Zhao et al., 2016). To date, all cases have been successfully treated with available antiscabietic therapies (Zhao et al., 2016).

In addition to classic and bullous scabies, there are three atypical forms of scabies, especially in high-risk institutionalized or immunocompromised individuals with HIV or HTLV-1 infections. The atypical forms of scabies include scalp scabies in infants, crusted (Norwegian) scabies in institutionalized and immunocompromised individuals and in high-risk populations such as Aboriginal populations in remote areas of desert and tropical northwestern Australia, and sexually transmitted nodular scabies. Scabietic nodules develop in 7%–10% of patients with scabies infections, usually in men on the penis and scrotum, and appear as darkened, tender nodules 5–20 mm in diameter, often

Figure 5.6 Nodular scabies presenting as three red, raised, tender lesions on the dorsum of the hand. A female scabies burrow is present on top of the middle nodule. *(Wikipedia.)*

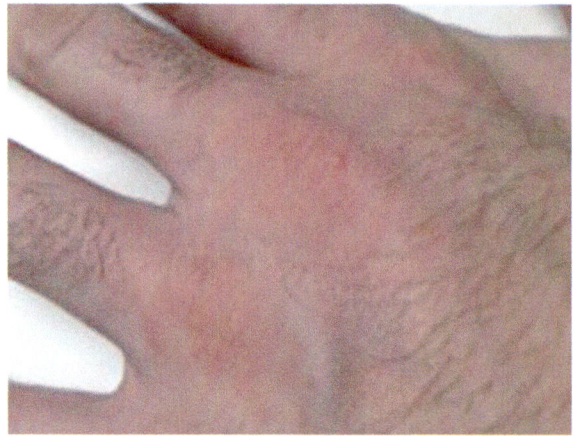

with a raised female mite burrow on top (Fig. 5.6 and 5.7). The atypical forms of scabies are compared with classic or ordinary scabies and stratified by high-risk human host populations, clinical manifestations, and differential diagnoses in Table 5.1.

Immune responses in scabies

The host immune and inflammatory responses characterizing the different clinical manifestations of scabies are complex and remain poorly understood (Bhat et al., 2017).

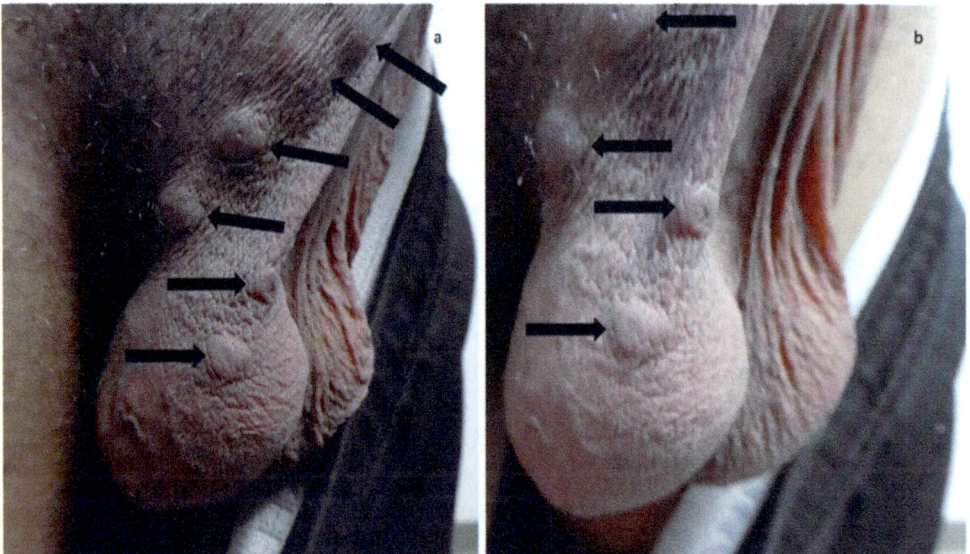

Figure 5.7 Nodular scabies on the male scrotum. Nodules (black arrows) on a male scrotum are characteristic of nodular scabies in the male which is often sexually transmitted. *(CDC.)*

Table 5.1 Different presenting forms of scabies.

Presenting form of scabies	Specific high-risk populations	Clinical manifestations	Limited differential diagnoses
Classic (ordinary) scabies (scabies vulgaris)	Infants and children; sexually active adults; men who have sex with men	Intense generalized pruritus, worse at night; inflammatory pruritic papules localized to finger webs, flexor aspects of wrists, elbows, axillae, buttocks, genitalia, female breasts; lesions and pruritus spare the face, head, and neck; secondary lesions include eczematization, excoriation, impetigo	Dermatitis herpetiformis, drug reactions, eczema, pediculosis corporis, lichen planus, pityriasis rosea
Scalp scabies	Infants and children; institutionalized older adults; AIDS patients; patients with preexisting crusted scabies	Atypical crusted papular lesions of the scalp, face, palms, and soles	Dermatomyositis, ringworm, seborrheic dermatitis
Crusted scabies (Norwegian scabies, scabies norvegica, scabies crustosa)	Institutionalized older adults; institutionalized developmentally disabled (Down syndrome) individuals; homeless people, especially HIV-positive; all immunocompromised patients, particularly those with AIDS or positive for HIV or HTLV-1; transplant recipients; patients on prolonged systemic corticosteroid therapy and chemotherapy	Psoriasiform hyperkeratotic papular lesions of the scalp, face, neck, hands, feet, with extensive nail involvement; eczematization and impetigo common	Contact dermatitis, drug reactions, eczema, erythroderma, ichthyosis, psoriasis

Continued

Table 5.1 Different presenting forms of scabies.—cont'd

Presenting form of scabies	Specific high-risk populations	Clinical manifestations	Limited differential diagnoses
Nodular scabies	Sexually active adults; men who have sex with men; HIV-positive men > HIV-positive women	Violaceous pruritic nodules localized to male genitalia, groin, axillae, representing hypersensitivity reaction to mite antigens	Acropustulosis, atopic dermatitis, Darier disease, lupus erythematosus, lymphomatoid papulosis, papular urticaria, necrotizing vasculitis, secondary syphilis

AIDS, Acquired immunodeficiency syndrome; *HIV,* human immunodeficiency virus; *HTLV-1,* human T-cell lymphotropic virus type 1.
Adapted from Diaz, J.H., 2023. Scabies. Chapter 4. In Diaz, JH. *Mite-Human Encounters: Nuisances, Vectors, Parasites, Allergens, and Commensals,* Elsevier, Philadelphia. Elsevier publication.

Recent investigations in porcine models of scabies have enabled researchers to begin to separate the immune and inflammatory responses responsible for the clinical manifestations of classic or ordinary scabies from the immunological responses responsible for the clinical manifestations of crusted scabies (Table 5.2) (Bhat et al., 2017).

The underlying molecular mechanisms responsible for the increased production of T cells, cytokines, and immunoglobulins in crusted scabies remain unknown, but experimental evidence in animal models and humans suggests that susceptibility to crusted scabies occurs in two forms (Bhat et al., 2017). The most well-known form of crusted scabies is associated with immunosuppressive conditions including HIV, HTLV-1, organ transplant antirejection therapy, psoriasis, and chemotherapy, including chemotherapy for noncancerous conditions, such as methotrexate therapy for psoriasis (Bhat et al., 2017; Khurana et al., 2022). Nevertheless, some patients without any recognized immunodeficiency can also develop crusted scabies suggesting an immunity-related genetic predisposition increasing susceptibility to crusted scabies (Bhat et al., 2017). For example, the Native Aboriginal population of Australia appear to be more susceptible to crusted scabies than the White population of Australia (Gramp et al., 2021).

A comparative model of crusted scabies has been studied in porcine models infested with the same number of scabies mites in which some pigs developed classic or ordinary scabies and others developed crusted scabies (Bhat et al., 2017). The study of immune responses and genetic susceptibilities in scabies in humans and in animal models, especially in pigs that are natural hosts for scabies mites and can develop either classic or

Table 5.2 Immune responses in classic or ordinary scabies versus crusted scabies.

Immune responses	Classic or ordinary scabies	Crusted scabies
Cellular responses	CD4 T cells, eosinophils, macrophages	Mostly CD8 T cells, increased Gamma-delta T cells, more eosinophils, few macrophages
Humoral responses	B-cell subsets within normal ranges	B-cell subsets within normal ranges
Th1/Th2-mediated cytokine responses	Th1-mediated with increased production of Th1 cytokines: IFN gamma, IL-2, TNF-alpha. Increased production of IL-10.	Th2-mediated with increased production of Th2 cytokines: IL-4, IL-5, and IL-13. Increased production of Th 17-associated cytokines: IL-17, IL-23. Decreased production of IL-10.
Immunoglobulin responses	Variable increases in the levels of total IgG, IgA, IgE, and IgM. Increased levels of scabies-specific IgE, IgG, and IgA.	Increased levels of total IgG, IgG1, IgG2, IgG3, IgG4, IgE, and IgA. Increased levels of scabies-specific IgG4, IgE, and Ig A.

Adapted from Bhat, S.A., Mounsey, K.E., Liu, X., et al., 2017. Host immune responses to the itch mite Sarcoptes scabiei, in humans. Parasites and Vectors 10, 385. https://doi.org/10.1186/s13071-017-2320-4.

crusted scabies, may contribute to developing new diagnostic tests, novel chemotherapeutics, and new strategies for disease control in susceptible populations.

Diagnosis

Although newer diagnostic methods are under investigation, the diagnosis of scabies is made predominantly by epidemiologic considerations and clinical observations. A clinical diagnosis may be confirmed by low-power microscopic examination of a burrow skin scraping that excavates the female mite, 0.2—0.5 mm in length, translucent with brown legs, and too small to be seen with the unassisted eye (Fig. 5.3) (Leung and Miller, 2011; Micali et al., 2015). Eggs (0.02—0.03 mm in diameter), smaller eggshell fragments, and fecaliths or pellets may also be identified in microscopic specimens of burrow scrapings (Fig. 5.3) (Leung and Miller, 2011). Potassium hydroxide should not be used to mount the burrow scrapings because it can dissolve mite fecaliths.

As noted, failure to identify pathognomonic burrows and to find mites is common, particularly in initial cases with low mite burdens, and does not rule out scabies. One of the simplest and often overlooked bedside tests to identify scabies mite burrows is the burrow ink test (BIT). In the BIT, fountain pen ink or any colored indicator liquid, such as methylene blue dye, is gently rubbed on skin surfaces with suspected scabies and then wiped off with an alcohol pad to reveal the indicator-highlighted wavy tunnels made by the burrowing female mite in the stratum corneum.

In atypical scabies cases, skin biopsy may help confirm the diagnosis (Leung and Miller, 2011). Although untested in controlled trials in large study populations, newer diagnostic methods for scabies include enhanced microscopic techniques (e.g., epiluminescence microscopy, computed or digital dermoscopy, and videodermoscopy), immunologic detection of specific scabies antibodies by enzyme-linked immunosorbent assay (ELISA), and molecular identification of scabies DNA by polymerase chain reaction (PCR) assay (Leung and Miller, 2011; Micali et al., 2015; Argenziano et al., 1997; Prins et al., 2004).

More recently, two immunoreactive muscle protein allergens in scabies mites, tropomyosin and paramyosin, have been assessed for immunoreactivity by IgE antibodies in human sera. IgE binding to the allergens was confirmed by ELISA in vitro and could represent a more specific serological method for the diagnosis of scabies in clinical practice (Naz et al., 2017).

Handheld dermoscopy (also known as dermatoscopy) is an accurate test that requires a dermatoscope and a trained microscopist (Prins et al., 2004). The simplest dermatoscopes consist of a low-power (10×) magnifier, a nonpolarized light source, and a liquid medium between the light source and a transparent lens to limit skin reflection (Micali et al., 2015; Prins et al., 2004). More sophisticated dermatoscopes, such as digital epiluminescence dermatoscopes, rely on polarized light rather than a liquid medium to reduce skin surface reflection. Epiluminescence dermatoscopes can be wirelessly linked to computers for videodermoscopy and display screens for real-time imaging and video capturing of scabies lesions (Argenziano et al., 1997; Prins et al., 2004). In a small trial, videomicroscopy was noninferior to videodermoscopy, which may be useful for diagnostic testing in settings with scarce resources (Micali et al., 2015; Argenziano et al., 1997; Prins et al., 2004). Serologic and molecular methods for diagnosing scabies are under development and are not universally available (Delaunay et al., 2020; Chng et al., 2021; Bae et al., 2007). At the present time, epidemiologic considerations and clinical observations, often aided by bedside techniques such as the BIT and handheld dermoscopy, remain the most rapid and practical methods for diagnosing scabies (Leung and Miller, 2011; Micali et al., 2015).

Therapy

Topical or oral scabicides should be used to treat infested persons and their close personal contacts simultaneously, regardless of the presence of symptoms. Currently recommended treatment options for scabies are listed in Table 5.3. In a review on the treatment of scabies, Strong and Johnstone (Singal and Thami, 2006) noted that both topical 5%

Table 5.3 Recommended treatment for scabies.

Scabicides	FDA approved?	Pregnancy Category[a]	Dosing schedule	Safety profile	Contraindications
5% permethrin cream (Actin, Nix, Elimite)	Yes	B	Apply from neck down; wash off after 8–14 hours; good residual activity, but second application recommended after 1 wk	Excellent; itching and stinging on application	Prior allergic reactions; infants <2 mo of age; breastfeeding
1% lindane lotion or cream	Yes	B	Apply 30–60 mL from neck down; wash off after 8–12 hours; no residual activity, increasing drug resistance	Potential for central nervous system toxicity from organochloride poisoning, usually manifesting as seizures, with overapplication and ingestions	Preexisting seizure disorder; infants and children <6 mo of age; pregnancy; breastfeeding
10% crotamiton cream or lotion (Eurax)	Yes	C	Apply from neck down on 2 consecutive nights; wash off 24 hours after second application	Excellent; exacerbates pruritus	None
2%–10% sulfur in petrolatum ointments	No	C	Apply for 2–3 days, then wash	Excellent;	Preexisting sulfur allergy
10%–25% benzoyl benzoate lotion	No	None	Two applications for 24 hours with 1-day to 1-wk interval	Irritant; exacerbates pruritus; can induce contact irritant dermatitis and pruritic cutaneous xerosis	Preexisting eczema

Continued

Table 5.3 Recommended treatment for scabies.—cont'd

Scabicides	FDA approved?	Pregnancy Category[a]	Dosing schedule	Safety profile	Contraindications
0.5% malathion lotion (Ovide), 1% malathion shampoo (unavailable in United States)	No	B	95% ovicidal; rapid (5 minutes) killing; good residual activity; increasing drug resistance	Flammable 78% isopropyl alcohol vehicle stings eyes, skin, mucosa; increasing drug resistance; organophosphate poisoning risk with overapplication and ingestions	Infants and children <6 mo of age; pregnancy; breastfeeding
Ivermectin (Stromectol)	Yes	C	200-µg/kg single PO dose, may be repeated in 14–15 days; not ovicidal, second dose on day 14 or 15 highly recommended; recommended for endemic or epidemic scabies in institutions and refugee camps	Excellent; may cause nausea and vomiting; take on empty stomach with water	Safety in pregnancy uncertain; probably safe during breastfeeding; not recommended for children <5 yr of age or weighing <15 kg

[a]US Food and Drug Administration safety in pregnancy categories: A, safety established; B, presumed safe; C, uncertain safety; D, unsafe; X, highly unsafe. PO, Per os (orally).

Adapted from Diaz, J.H., 2023. Scabies. Chapter 4. In Diaz, J.H. *Mite-Human Encounters: Nuisances, Vectors, Parasites, Allergens, and Commensals*, Elsevier, Philadelphia. Elsevier publication.

permethrin and oral ivermectin were most effective for individual infections, more research would be needed to compare the effectiveness of malathion with permethrin for individual infections, and there was insufficient evidence at the present time to recommend specific miticides to control community and institutional outbreaks of scabies.

The most effective topical agents for scabies are 5% permethrin cream and 1% lindane cream or lotion, with permethrin safer and slightly more effective than lindane, an organochlorine pesticide. The overapplication or accidental ingestion of lindane can cause seizures and sudden death, especially in children (Currie and McCarthy, 2010; Sule and Thacher, 2007; Richards, 2021). The other topical agents for scabies include 10%–25% benzoyl benzoate lotions, 10% crotamiton cream or lotion, 2%–10% sulfur in petrolatum ointments, and 0.8% ivermectin lotion (see Table 5.3) (Sule and Thacher, 2007; Richards, 2021; Usha and Gopalakrishnannair, 2000).

The topical agents for scabies may not be well accepted or tolerated by some patients for many reasons, including severe burning and stinging (with 25% benzyl benzoate and 5% permethrin) in cases of secondarily excoriated or eczematous infections and inability of demented or disabled patients to comply with complicated application regimens. In such cases, two doses of oral ivermectin, 200 µg/kg/dose taken with food, once on day 1 with the second given between days 8 and 15, may be a more acceptable and equally effective alternative (Sule and Thacher, 2007).

In a 2007 prospective trial, Sule and Thacher (2007) compared the effectiveness of oral ivermectin, 200 µg/kg/dose, with topical 25% benzoyl benzoate and monosulfiram soap in 210 Nigerian patients 5–65 years of age with scabies. Subjects with persistent lesions received a second course of therapy after 2 weeks. The investigators observed resolution of all lesions in 77 of 98 subjects (79%) treated with ivermectin and in 60 of 102 subjects (59%) treated topically ($P = .003$). The scabies cure rate at 4 weeks was 95% in the ivermectin group and 86% in the topical treatment group ($P = .04$). The investigators concluded that oral ivermectin was as effective as topical treatment with benzyl benzoate and monosulfiram in scabies and led to more rapid improvement. Ivermectin, however, is not ovicidal, and a second course of oral treatment at adult mite maturation time of 14–15 days is now recommended (Sule and Thacher, 2007; Richards, 2021; Usha and Gopalakrishnannair, 2000).

In a prospective trial comparing oral ivermectin with topical 5% permethrin in scabies, Usha and Gopalakrishnan Nair (2000) reported a 70% cure rate with a single dose of ivermectin, compared with a 95% cure rate with topical 5% permethrin ($P < .003$), but a second ivermectin dose, 200 µg/kg, taken 2 weeks later, increased the cure rate to 95%. Nevertheless, the US Centers for Disease Control and Prevention (CDC) recommends topical 5% permethrin cream or lotion as first-line therapy for scabies, especially in initial classic infections.

Scabies mite drug resistance to both topical 5% permethrin preparations and oral iver-mectin has emerged in severe outbreaks of crusted scabies in nursing homes and in the hyperendemic international regions noted (Romani et al., 2015). As a result, the manage-ment of crusted scabies may require combined, intense scabicidal therapies in high-risk community and institutional outbreaks (Romani et al., 2015).

Currie and McCarthy (2010) have recommended both 5% topical permethrin every 2–3 days for 1–2 weeks and oral ivermectin, 200 µg/kg/dose, taken with food and administered as three doses (days 1, 2, and 8), five doses (days 1, 2, 8, 9, and 15), or seven doses, depending on the severity of the infection. For refractory institutional and com-munity outbreaks, the authors recommended combined therapy with topical permethrin and oral ivermectin for all symptomatic cases with classic or crusted scabies and a single oral dose of ivermectin, 200 µg/kg, for all exposed, asymptomatic residents, visitors, and staff (Currie and McCarthy, 2010).

Scabicide drug resistance

The emerging resistance of the scabies mite to commonly used standard treatments, spe-cifically topical permethrin and oral ivermectin, will limit the future therapeutic useful-ness of these agents and encourage the development of new and effective scabicidal agents (Mounsey et al., 2008; Romani et al., 2015). Tea tree oil (TTO) has already demonstrated scabicidal effects against scabies mites in vitro and has been used as an effec-tive topical adjunct for treating crusted scabies not responding to standard therapies.[25]

Managing large outbreaks of scabies

In conclusion, a variety of topical agents are effective in scabies, but are expensive to deploy and cumbersome to apply in those nonadherent to topicals and in large popula-tions, such as in refugee camps and crowded communities and institutions. In these cases, and in all cases of crusted scabies, oral ivermectin remains the recommended treatment of choice (Richards, 2021).

Prevention and control

Prevention and control strategies for scabies include: (1) aggressive treatment of infested patients and all close household, institutional, and sexual contacts, especially in cases of highly infectious crusted scabies; (2) disposal or hot wash-dry sterilization (by machine washing and drying at 60°C [140°F] or higher) of all contaminated clothing and bedding of index cases; (3) provision of improved access for personal hygiene and health care for all displaced, homeless, or institutionalized persons; and (4) aggressive control of out-breaks of zoonotic scabies with the potential for human transmission caused by the sar-coptic mange mites of domestic animals, especially cats, dogs, camels, pigs, and horses.

Scabies-associated impetigo

As noted, epidemic outbreaks of scabies that are often associated with impetigo, especially in children, are difficult to control, and frequently affect isolated, impoverished communities. Indigenous populations uniquely predisposed to community outbreaks of scabies include island communities throughout the South Pacific, especially in the Polynesian and Solomon Islands, and the Aboriginal communities of northwestern Australia.

In a prospective study designed to control endemic scabies in isolated island communities, Romani and coworkers (Romani et al., 2017) randomly assigned three Polynesian Island communities in Fiji to one of three different drug treatment interventions for mass scabies control: (1) topical permethrin to affected persons and their contacts (standard care group, $n = 803$); (2) mass topical permethrin administration (permethrin group, $n = 532$); and (3) mass administration of oral ivermectin (ivermectin group, $n = 716$) (Romani et al., 2017). Although the prevalence of scabies declined significantly in all three groups, the greatest decline was observed in the ivermectin group (relative reduction 94% from prevalence of 32.1%—1.9%) (Romani et al., 2017). The prevalence of impetigo also declined significantly in all three groups, with the greatest decline again in the ivermectin group (relative reduction 67%) (Romani et al., 2017). In addition to improvements in living standards, mass administration of scabicides, especially oral ivermectin, may be effective for the population-based control of endemic scabies and associated impetigo (Romani et al., 2017).

Conclusions

All patients with scabies and their close household, institutional, and sexual contacts should be informed that scabies is a transmissible ectoparasitic infection and that several topical treatments and an effective oral treatment are now readily available and highly effective (Table 5.2). Future molecular investigations of scabies mite biology and genetic drug resistance are needed to permit the development of better diagnostic tools and treatment strategies for human scabies, especially atypical scabies.

References

Argenziano, G., Fabbrocini, G., Delfino, M., 1997. Epiluminescence microscopy: a new approach to in vivo detection of sarcoptes scabiei. Archives of Dermatology 133 (6), 751—753. https://doi.org/10.1001/archderm.133.6.751.

Arlian, L.G., Runyan, R.A., Achar, S., Estes, S.A., 1984. Survival and infestivity of Sarcoptes scabiei var. canis and var. hominis. Journal of the American Academy of Dermatology 11 (2), 210—215. https://doi.org/10.1016/s0190-9622(84)70151-4.

Bae, Kim, J.Y., Jung, Cha, Jeon, et al., 2007. Diagnostic value of the molecular detection of Sarcoptes scabiei from a skin scraping in patients with suspected scabies. PLoS Neglected Tropical Diseases 14 (4). https://doi.org/10.1371/journal.pntd.0008229Strong.

Bhat, S.A., Mounsey, K.E., Liu, X., Walton, S.F., 2017. Host immune responses to the itch mite, Sarcoptes scabiei, in humans. Parasites & Vectors 10 (1). https://doi.org/10.1186/s13071-017-2320-4.

Bravo, F., Gotuzzo, E., Blas, M., Cairampoma, R., Catacora, J., Navarro, P., Ballona, R., Castillo, W.J., Castillo, W., 2005. Norwegian scabies in Peru: the impact of human T cell lymphotropic virus type I infection. The American Journal of Tropical Medicine and Hygiene 72 (6), 855−857. https://doi.org/10.4269/ajtmh.2005.72.855.

Chng, L., Holt, D.C., Field, M., Francis, J.R., Tilakaratne, D., Dekkers, M.H., Robinson, G., Mounsey, K., Pavlos, R., Bowen, A.C., Fischer, K., Papenfuss, A.T., Gasser, R.B., Korhonen, P.K., Currie, B.J., McCarthy, J.S., Pasay, C., 2021. Molecular diagnosis of scabies using a novel probe-based polymerase chain reaction assay targeting high-copy number repetitive sequences in the sarcoptes scabiei genome. PLoS Neglected Tropical Diseases 15 (2). https://doi.org/10.1371/journal.pntd.0009149.

Currie, B.J., McCarthy, J.S., 2010. Permethrin and ivermectin for scabies. New England Journal of Medicine 362 (8), 717−725. https://doi.org/10.1056/NEJMct0910329.

del Giudice, P., Marie, D.S., Gérard, Y., Couppié, P., Pradinaud, R., 1997. Is crusted (Norwegian) scabies a marker of adult T cell leukemia/lymphoma in human T lymphotropic virus type I-seropositive patients? The Journal of Infectious Diseases 176 (4), 1090−1092. https://doi.org/10.1086/516518.

Delaunay, P., Hérissé, A.L., Hasseine, L., Chiaverini, C., Tran, A., Mary, C., Del Giudice, P., Marty, P., Akhoundi, M., Hubiche, T., 2020. Scabies polymerase chain reaction with standardized dry swab sampling: an easy tool for cluster diagnosis of human scabies. British Journal of Dermatology 182 (1), 197−201. https://doi.org/10.1111/bjd.18017.

Gramp, P., Gramp, D., Marks, M., 2021. Scabies in remote aboriginal and torres strait islander populations in Australia: a narrative review. PLoS Neglected Tropical Diseases 15 (9). https://doi.org/10.1371/journal.pntd.0009751.

Khurana, A., Muddebihal, A., Ahuja, S.B., 2022. Severe, recurrent crusted scabies in a psoriatic on methotrexate. The American Journal of Tropical Medicine and Hygiene 1−2. https://doi.org/10.4269/ajtmh.22.0008.

Leung, V., Miller, M., 2011. Detection of scabies: a systematic review of diagnostic methods. The Canadian Journal of Infectious Diseases & Medical Microbiology 22 (4), 143−146. https://doi.org/10.1155/2011/698494.

Micali, G., Lacarrubba, F., Verzì, A.E., Nasca, M.R., 2015. Low-cost equipment for diagnosis and management of endemic scabies outbreaks in underserved populations. Clinical Infectious Diseases 60 (2), 327−329. https://doi.org/10.1093/cid/ciu826.

Mounsey, K.E., Holt, D., McCarthy, J., Currie, B.J., Walton, S.F., 2008. Scabies: molecular perspectives and therapeutic implications in the face of emerging drug resistance. Future Microbiology 3 (1), 57−66. https://doi.org/10.2217/17460913.3.1.57.

Naz, S., Desclozeaux, M., Mounsey, K.E., Chaudhry, F.R., Walton, S.F., 2017. Characterization of Sarcoptes scabiei tropomyosin and paramyosin: immunoreactive allergens in scabies. The American Journal of Tropical Medicine and Hygiene 97 (3), 851−860. https://doi.org/10.4269/ajtmh.16-0976.

Otero, L., Varela, J.A., Espinosa, E., Sànchez, C., Junquera, M.L., Del Valle, A., Vàzquez, F., 2004. Sarcoptes scabiei in a sexually transmitted infections unit: a 15-year study. Sexually Transmitted Diseases 31 (12), 761−765. https://doi.org/10.1097/01.olq.0000145853.35574.18.

Prins, C., Stucki, L., French, L., Saurat, J.H., Braun, R.P., 2004. Dermoscopy for the in vivo detection of Sarcoptes scabiei. Dermatology 208 (3), 241−243. https://doi.org/10.1159/000077310.

Richards, R.N., 2021. Scabies: diagnostic and therapeutic update. Journal of Cutaneous Medicine and Surgery 25 (1), 95−101. https://doi.org/10.1177/1203475420960446.

Romani, L., Whitfeld, M.J., Koroivueta, J., Kama, M., Wand, H., Tikoduadua, L., Tuicakau, M., Koroi, A., Andrews, R., Kaldor, J.M., Steer, A.C., 2015. Mass drug administration for scabies control in a population with endemic disease. New England Journal of Medicine 373 (24), 2305−2313. https://doi.org/10.1056/NEJMoa1500987.

Romani, L., Whitfeld, M.J., Koroivueta, J., Kama, M., Wand, H., Tikoduadua, L., Tuicakau, M., Koroi, A., Ritova, R., Andrews, R., Kaldor, J.M., Steer, A.C., 2017. The epidemiology of scabies and impetigo in relation to demographic and residential characteristics: baseline findings from the skin health intervention Fiji Trial. The American Journal of Tropical Medicine and Hygiene 97 (3), 845−850. https://doi.org/10.4269/ajtmh.16-0753.

Singal, A., Thami, G.P., 2006. Lindane neurotoxicity in childhood. American Journal of Therapeutics 13 (3), 277−280. https://doi.org/10.1097/01.mjt.0000212707.81034.c6.

Sule, H.M., Thacher, T.D., 2007. Comparison of ivermectin and benzyl benzoate lotion for scabies in Nigerian patients. The American Journal of Tropical Medicine and Hygiene 76 (2), 392−395. https://doi.org/10.4269/ajtmh.2007.76.392.

Usha, V., Gopalakrishnannair, T., 2000. A comparative study of oral ivermectin and topical permethrin cream in the treatment of scabies, . Journal of the American Academy of Dermatology 42 (2), 236−240. https://doi.org/10.1016/s0190-9622(00)90131-2.

Zhao, Y.-K., Liu, J.-H., Luo, D.-Q., Sarkar, R., Tang, W., Huang, M.-X., 2016. Bullous scabies. The American Journal of Tropical Medicine and Hygiene 95 (3), 689−693. https://doi.org/10.4269/ajtmh.16-0273.

CHAPTER 6

Rickettsialpox (rat mites)

Reservoirs and vectors

Rickettsialpox is caused by the Gram-negative, intracellular, spotted fever group rickettsial bacterium, *Rickettsia akari*, with a worldwide rodent reservoir in the common house mouse (*Mus musculus*). Rickettsialpox is transmitted to humans by bites from infected house mouse mites, *Liponyssoides sanguineus* (Fig. 6.1).

The causative bacterium of rickettsialpox is *Rickettsia akari*, which is transmitted to humans by bites from infected house mice mites.

Life cycle and feeding behavior

The house mouse mite's life cycle begins with a larval form hatched from an egg that undergoes two nymph stages before maturing into an adult. Nymphs and adult mites feed on house mice every 3—4 days for 1—2 hours before dropping off engorged (McClain et al., 2009). Gravid adult females lay eggs after feeding completing the life cycle. *R. akari* bacteria are passed transovarily from females to eggs and are maintained throughout the larval and nymphal developmental stages by transstadial transmission (McClain et al., 2009).

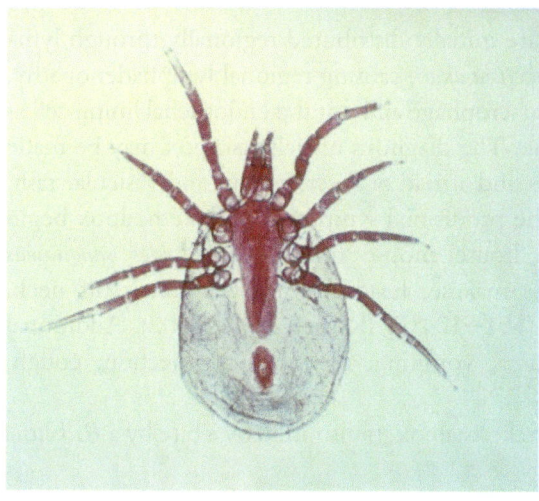

Figure 6.1 The adult house mouse mite, ***Liponyssoides sanguineus,*** the mite vector of rickettsialpox. *(United States Centers for Disease Control and Prevention. Public Health Image Library (PHIL). PHIL ID 5447. Public domain. No copyright permission required. Available at https://phil.cdc.gov/details.aspx?pid=5447. Wikipedia. Public domain.)*

Ectoparasitic Diseases
ISBN 978-0-443-26724-6
https://doi.org/10.1016/B978-0-443-26724-6.00006-0

Epidemiology

The disease ecology of rickettsialpox is characterized by a worldwide epizootic cycle of asymptomatic maintenance of *R. akari* transmitted by house mouse mites in a rodent reservoir of house mice. Although the common house mouse, *Mus musculus*, is considered the preferred rodent reservoir host for mite-transmitted rickettsialpox, other rodent reservoirs have been suspected outside of the United States, but remain unconfirmed, including the Korean vole, Mongolian gerbil, and Egyptian gerbil (Krusell et al., 2002; McClain et al., 2009).

Although nymph and adult mouse mites typically blood-feed on house mice every 3—4 days, they can go for week-long periods without feeding. This feeding—starvation cycling behavior resulted in cluster outbreaks of rickettsialpox in apartment complexes in large US cities, including New York, Boston, Cleveland, Philadelphia, and Pittsburgh, following mice extermination programs that encouraged house mouse mites to seek alternative human hosts for blood feeding (and Fig. 6.1) (Krusell et al., 2002; Ozturk et al., 2003).

Investigators now agree that rickettsialpox is an internationally underreported infection for many reasons including: (1) The worldwide distribution of house mice and their mites; (2) additional suspected rodent reservoirs of *R akari*; (3) a high seroprevalence of *R. akari* infection in domestic animals, especially dogs, in large cities; (4) a high prevalence of undiagnosed, empirically treated cases of rickettsialpox susceptible to doxycycline and a broad range of other antibiotics; and (5) an unknown prevalence of patients with subclinical rickettsialpox who recover without treatment (Krusell et al., 2002; McClain et al., 2009; Ozturk et al., 2003).

Clinical manifestations

Once injected into the host, rickettsiae are initially distributed regionally through lymphatics with many species, including *Rickettsia akari*, causing regional lymphadenopathy. The intracellular target of *R. akari* is the macrophage and not the endothelial lining cell as with other spotted fever group rickettsiae. The diagnosis of rickettsialpox may be made on the history of house mouse exposures and a triad of fever, eschar, and vesicular rash. The incubation period is 7—14 days. The prodromal symptoms of rickettsialpox begin 2—3 days after a painless bite by a house mouse mite, *Liponyssoides sanguineus* (Fig. 6.2). Common symptoms include malaise, headache, photophobia, stiff neck, myalgia, and high fever, 38.3—40.0°C (101—104°F) (Krusell et al., 2002). Additional prodromal symptoms may include nausea, vomiting, conjunctival injection, cough, and pharyngitis (Krusell et al., 2002).

The eschar is the inoculation site for rickettsialpox, transmitted by a bite by a *Rickettsia akari*-infected house mouse mite.

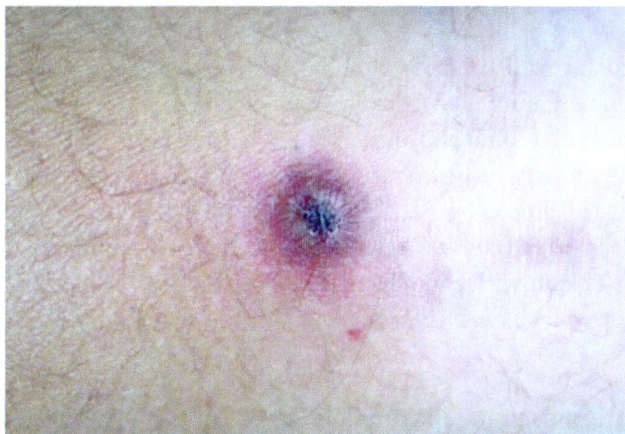

Figure 6.2 The mite bite eschar of rickettsialpox with a black scab surrounded by reddish-purplish erythema. *(Krusell, A., Comer, J.A., Sexton, D.J., 2002. Rickettsialpox in North Carolina: A case report. Emerg Infect Dis 8 (7), 727–729. United States Centers for Disease Control and Prevention. Public domain. No copyright permission required. Available at https://www.ncbi.nlm.nih.gov/pmc/articles/PMC2730333/pdf/01-0501_FinalD.pdf.)*

Eschar phase

The tick bite eschar is the classic hallmark of infection. It follows the house mite bite by 2–3 days and precedes the rash by 1–3 days. The eschar is umbilicated with surrounding reddish-purplish erythema, crusts over in 1–2 days, and heals later without significant scarring within 2–3 weeks (Fig. 6.2) (Krusell et al., 2002).

Rash phase

The rash phase is delayed and begins several days after the onset of the prodromal phase and starts with maculopapules that progress to papulovesicular lesions that eventually darken, scab over, crust, and fall off within 10–12 days without scarring (Figs. 6.2 and 6.3) (Krusell et al., 2002). Patients usually have 20–40 papulovesicular lesions, distributed primarily on the trunk and upper extremities, sparing the palms and soles. This is in contrast to other spotted fever group rickettsioses, such as Rocky Mountain spotted fever (RMSF), which cause lesions on palms and soles.

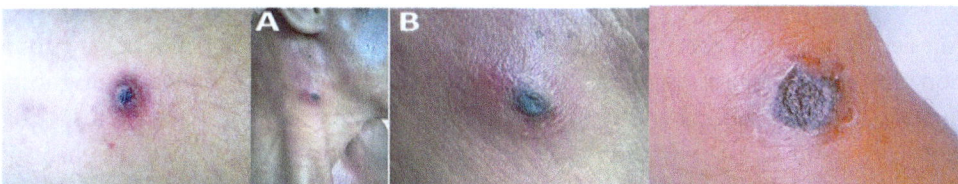

Figure 6.3 The mite bite eschars of rickettsialpox and scrub typhus and the inoculation eschar of anthrax all resemble each other and can be differentiated by historical details of exposures and laboratory tests on eschar swabs. Left: Rickettsialpox house mite bite eschar. *(Wikipedia. Public domain. Center A, B: Scrub typhus. CDC. Right: Cutaneous anthrax inoculation. Available at: https://en.wikipedia.org/wiki/Rickettsialpox#/media/File:Rickettsialpox_lesion.jpg. https://wwwnc.cdc.gov/eid/article/24/8/17-1622-f1.)*

Differential diagnosis

The diagnosis of rickettsialpox may be made on the history of house mouse exposures, on the delayed clinical manifestations as differentiated from chickenpox, and on the presence of the eschar as differentiated from scrub typhus and anthrax (Figs. 6.2 and 6.3). The cutaneous manifestations of rickettsialpox may be distinguished from chickenpox and other infections causing vesicular rashes (smallpox, herpes zoster, and herpes simplex) by the appearance of one of more eschars at mite bite sites before the rash starts. The cutaneous manifestations of rickettsialpox also begin with papules and not vesicles as in chickenpox. Rickettsialpox has a single crop of vesicles, and chickenpox has successive crops of vesicles (Krusell et al., 2002).

Differentiating among inoculation eschars: Rickettsialpox, scrub typhus, tick-borne rickettsiae, and anthrax

The incubation period, prodromal manifestations, and eschar of rickettsialpox resemble those of inoculation anthrax, larval trombiculid-mite transmitted scrub typhus, *R. parkeri* and other endemic tick bite-transmitted spotted fevers in the United States, African tick bite fever in East Africa, and Queensland tick typhus in Australia. Inoculation or cutaneous anthrax is characterized by a dark eschar that is not followed by a vesicular rash (Fig. 6.3). Cutaneous anthrax can be rapidly excluded in the diagnosis of *R. akari* infection by Gram stain, direct immunofluorescent antibody testing, or polymerase chain reaction (PCR) assay on swab samples of vesicular fluid in the base of the eschar.

In mite-borne scrub typhus and other tickborne rickettsial cases, an eschar forms at the arthropod bite site within 3—7 days. Fever, chills, severe headache, regional lymphadenopathy, and truncal maculopapular progressing to vesiculopustular rash follow the eschar's appearance. Scrub typhus and other tick-borne infections with eschars can also be ruled out by their geographic distributions and by serological and molecular testing of samples obtained from eschar swabs, draining vesicles or pustules, and lymph node aspirates.

Laboratory diagnosis

Transient leukopenia, thrombocytopenia, and elevated hepatic transaminases are common abnormal laboratory findings (Krusell et al., 2002). Positive laboratory diagnostic findings can begin at the bite site where eschar swabs and biopsies may reveal *R. akari* antibodies upon direct immunofluorescent antibody testing. Swabs of the eschar and weeping vesicles will also permit detection of *R. akari* DNA by PCR (Figs. 6.2 and 6.3). During the febrile phase, blood cultures may isolate *R. akari*, and serological tests may detect IgM and later IgG antibody titers to rickettsial antigens 7—15 days after onset of the illness. Cross-reactivity leading to positive serology will occur in cases of prior RMSF caused by *Rickettsia rickettsii* (Krusell et al., 2002).

Therapy

Rickettsialpox may resolve on its own with supportive treatment only and without antibiotic therapy in uncomplicated cases. However, antibiotic therapy is recommended in all cases in order to shorten the course of illness and to prevent complications including interstitial pneumonia, chronically elevated hepatic transaminases, and central nervous system involvement.

Although *R. akari* is sensitive to many antibiotics, doxycycline is the preferred antibiotic for treatment with an initial oral loading dose of 200 mg, followed by an oral maintenance dose of 100 mg every 12 hours for 7 days (Krusell et al., 2002; Ozturk et al., 2003; Paddock et al., 2003). Erythromycin, azithromycin, and tetracycline may also be effective in treating rickettsialpox, but are not recommended as first-line treatments. Chloramphenicol is an effective alternative antibiotic, but is also not recommended due to its bone marrow and fetal toxicities.

Prevention and control

Prevention and control strategies include house mouse rodent control and house mite vector extermination programs.

References

Krusell, A., Comer, J.A., Sexton, D.J., 2002. Rickettsialpox in North Carolina: a case report. Emerging Infectious Diseases 8 (7), 727–728. https://doi.org/10.3201/eid0807.010501.

McClain, D., Dana, A.N., Goldenberg, G., 2009. Mite infestations. Dermatologic Therapy 22 (4), 327–346. https://doi.org/10.1111/j.1529-8019.2009.01245.x.

Ozturk, M.K., Gunes, T., Kose, M., Coker, C., Radulovic, S., 2003. Rickettsialpox in Turkey [6]. Emerging Infectious Diseases 9 (11), 1498–1499. https://doi.org/10.3201/eid0911.030224.

Paddock, C.D., Zaki, S.R., Koss, T., Singleton, J., Sumner, J.W., Comer, J.A., Eremeeva, M.E., Dasch, G.A., Cherry, B., Childs, J.E., 2003. Rickettsialpox in New York City: a persistent urban zoonosis. Annals of the New York Academy of Sciences 990, 36–44. https://doi.org/10.1111/j.1749-6632.2003.tb07334.x.

CHAPTER 7

Animal (zoonotic) and insect mites

Bites from several animal and insect mite species can cause bothersome erythematous and pruritic papules with urticarial wheals progressing to papulovesicular eruptions. The most common domestic animals harboring species-specific mites that attack humans as dead-end hosts include pet dogs, cats, and rabbits (McClain et al., 2009). The most common wild animal species harboring mites that bite humans on contact as dead end hosts include bird, snake, and tropical rat mites (McClain et al., 2009). The most common insect mite species that can cause human outbreaks of pruritic dermatitis are primarily from the family Pyemotidae and include the North American hay or grain itch mite, *Pyemotes tritici,* and its close relative, the oak leaf gall mite, *Pyemotes herfsi* (McClain et al., 2009).

Animal (zoonotic) mites

Animal or zoonotic mites do not transmit infectious diseases, but are common causes of annoying infestations with pruritic, erythematous, maculopapular rashes on the extremities of dog and cat owners, bird and snake owners, backpackers, campers, and spelunkers (Table 7.1).

Domestic animal-transmitted cheyletiellosis
Definitions

Cheyletiellosis or "*walking dandruff*" is a common dermatitis of domestic animals that can be transmitted to humans by species-specific mites of dogs (*Cheyletiella yasguri*), cats (*C. blakei*), and rabbits (*C. parasitivorax*) (Elston, 2004; Rivers et al., 1976; Flatt and Wiemers, 1976). Pet animals harboring mite infestations may be asymptomatic, manifest a mild dermatitis with some white dandruff on their backs, or suffer from a heavy pruritic case of dandruff with alopecia (Fig. 7.1) (McClain et al., 2009; Rivers et al., 1976).

Up to 50% of rabbits bred in large colonies for commercial sale during holiday periods may harbor *Cheyletiella* mites (Flatt and Wiemers, 1976).

Life cycle

Cheyletiella mites usually complete their life cycles on one animal host and mature from egg to adult in 3 weeks. Although females and eggs can survive for up to 10 days away from their hosts, males will die within 2 days if separated. As a result, large groups of *Cheyletiella* mites are always found close to their animal hosts, such as on sleeping

Ectoparasitic Diseases
ISBN 978-0-443-26724-6
https://doi.org/10.1016/B978-0-443-26724-6.00007-2

Table 7.1 Mites with exclusive animal (zoonotic) and arthropod host reservoirs.

Latin names	Common names	Host reservoirs	Geographic distributions	Infections or infestations
Cheyletiella species	Domestic animal white dandruff mites	Dogs, cats, and rabbits	Worldwide	White dandruff
Dermanyssus americanum	American bird mite	Birds	Americas	Erythematous papulovesicular dermatitis
Dermanyssus gallinae	Red poultry mite, Chicken mite	Domestic and wild birds	Worldwide	Poultry workers' dermatitis
Eutrombicula alfreddugesi	American chigger mite, Red bug or mite	Birds, rodents, and small mammals	Americas	American chiggers (trombidiosis)
Eutrombicula sarcina	Asian chigger mite	Birds, rodents, and small mammals	Asia, Australia	Asian chiggers (trombidiosis)
Leptotrombidium species	Scrub mites Scrub typhus mites	Birds, rodents, and small mammals	Asia and Eurasia	Scrub typhus infection
Liponyssoides sanguineus	House mouse mite	Common house mice	Worldwide	Rickettsialpox infection
Neotrombicula autumnalis	European harvest mite	Birds, rodents, and small mammals	Europe	European chiggers
Ophionyssus natricis	Snake mite	Reptiles	Worldwide	Erythematous urticarial papulovesicular to pustular dermatitis
Ornithonyssus bacoti	Tropical rat mite	Large rodents	Tropics worldwide	Erythematous urticarial papulovesicular to pustular dermatitis
Ornithonyssus bursa	Tropical fowl mite	Waterfowl, poultry, English sparrow	Worldwide	Erythematous urticarial papulovesicular to pustular dermatitis
Ornithonyssus sylvarium	Northern fowl mite	Domestic fowl, pigeons, sparrows, starlings	Temperate regions worldwide	Erythematous urticarial papulovesicular to pustular dermatitis

Pediculoides ventricosus	European wood beetle mite	Beetles in wood, cane, and wicker furniture, and in straw	Worldwide	Erythematous urticarial papulovesicular dermatitis
Peymotes herfsi	Oak leaf gall mite	Gall-making larvae of oak tree leaves	Worldwide	Erythematous urticarial papulovesicular dermatitis
Peymotes tritici	Grain itch mite	Insects in straw, hay, grain, rice	Worldwide	Grain workers' dermatitis
Psoroptes ovis	Scab mite	Sheep	Worldwide	Erythematous urticarial papulovesicular dermatitis
Sarcoptes scabiei var. *canis*	Canine scabies mite, Dog mite	Domestic and wild dogs	Worldwide	Human mange

Adapted from Diaz, J.H., 2023. Zoonotic (animal) mites and allergies. Chapter 8. In: Diaz, J.H., Elsevier, Philadelphia. Elsevier publication.

Figure 7.1 Severe cheyletiellosis with alopecia in a Labrador retriever. *(From Wikipedia. Public domain.).*

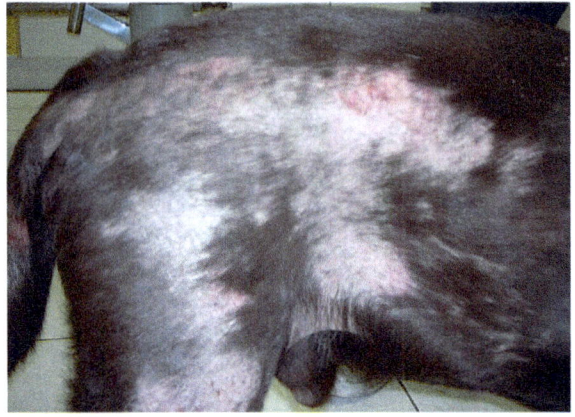

mattresses and pet beds. The six-legged larvae and eight-legged adults do not burrow into the skin like scabies mites and feed on the uppermost keratin layer of the epidermis on debris, tissue juices, and epithelial cells (Elston, 2004; Rivers et al., 1986). *Cheyletiella* mites are very contagious and will bite humans on contact without prolonged feeding and quickly depart to return to their host animals (Fig. 7.2).

Figure 7.2 *Cheyletiella yasguri,* the dog dandruff mite, causes cheyletiellosis or "walking dandruff" in dogs and will bite humans causing a self-limited pruritic, popular dermatitis. *(From Wikipedia. Public domain.).*

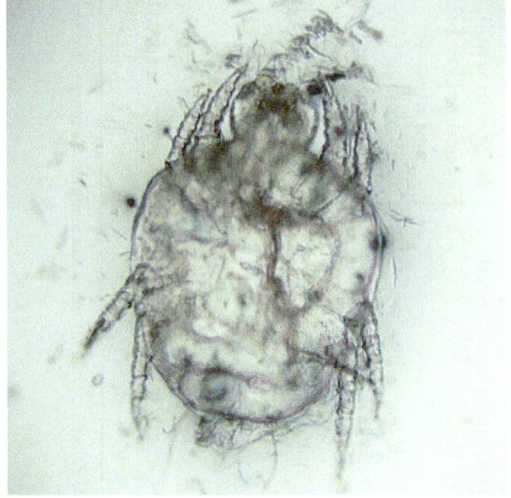

Clinical manifestations of cheyletiellosis

Most cases of cheyletiellosis have been reported in females 40 years of age and younger who present with a grouping of pruritic papules in areas that have been in contact with the infected animal or its contaminated bedding (Elston, 2004; Rivers et al., 1986).

Human infestations with *Cheyletiella* mites will occur in 20% of infected dog, cat, or rabbit owners (Fig. 7.3) (Rivers et al., 1976).

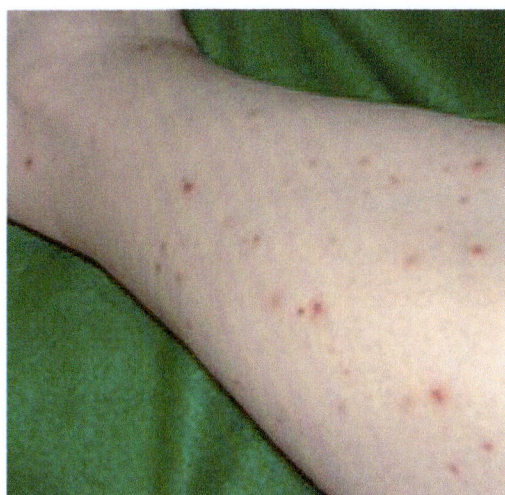

Figure 7.3 Human cheyletiellosis in an infested dog owner who developed a grouping of pruritic papules in areas that were in contact with the infested pet or its contaminated bedding. *(From Wikipedia. Public domain.).*

Complicated infections are less common and characterized by widespread erythematous and pruritic papules associated with urticarial wheals. Systemic manifestations of joint pain and numbness of the fingers have been reported in high-density infestations.

Treatment

If human cheyletiellosis is suspected, a veterinarian should examine the suspect animal looking for eggs or mites and treat the infested animal with ectoparasitic shampoos or sprays containing permethrin and fipronil. Other than symptomatic treatment with topical and oral antihistamines or other antipruritics, such as hydralazine, the pet owners will not require specific treatments as the lesions will disappear within 3 weeks of their pet's successful treatment (Rivers et al., 1986).

Domestic animal scabies in humans (Scabietic mange)

Domestic and stray pets, especially dogs, can become infested with a different kind of zoonotic scabies mite that does not survive or reproduce on humans but causes scabietic mange in animals (Fig. 7.4).

If an animal with scabietic mange has close contact with a person, the animal mite can be transferred to the person's skin, burrow into the superficial epidermis, and cause temporary itching and skin irritation. However, the animal scabies mite cannot reproduce to complete its life cycle on a person and will die on its own in a couple of days causing further inflammation from its feces and disintegrating exoskeleton (Fig. 7.5) (McClain et al., 2009).

Figure 7.4 Severe scabietic mange in a stray street dog in Bali, Indonesia, with potential for human transmission by direct contact. *(From Wikipedia. Public domain.).*

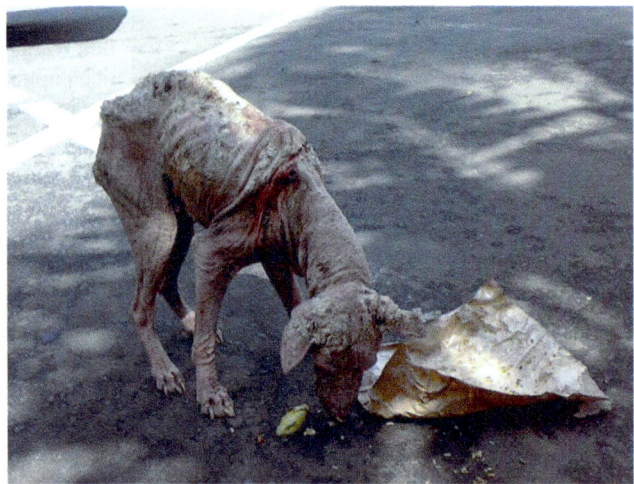

Figure 7.5 Transient human infestation with sarcoptic or scabietic mange following close contact with a mange-infected domestic or stray animal, typically a dog. The animal scabies mite cannot complete its life cycle in human dead-end hosts and will cause temporary, highly pruritic skin eruptions which can be managed symptomatically. *(From Wikipedia. Public domain.).*

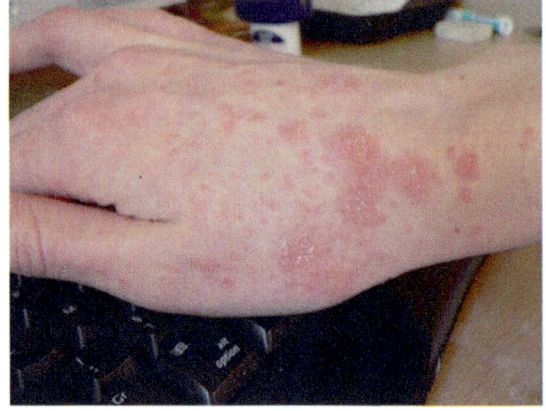

Although the infected person does not need to be treated, the animal should be treated because its scabies mites can continue to burrow into the person's skin and cause symptoms until the animal has been treated successfully, and the zoonotic infestation cleared (McClain et al., 2009).

Zoonotic acariasis: Definitions

Zoonotic acariasis is a human skin disease that is caused by burrowing tissue-juice feeding mites primarily of birds and, to a lesser extent, of bats, rodents, and snakes. The bird or dermanyssid mites (Family Dermanyssidae) infest a broad range of wild birds, including ducks, pigeons, robins, starlings, and swallows, and domestic and pet birds, including chickens, canaries, gerbils, parakeets, and zebra finches (McClain et al., 2009). Avian mite infestations can cause increased mortality in domestic poultry and have a significant negative impact on the poultry industry (Lutsky and Bar-Sela, 1982). Avian mites have caused dermatitis and occupational asthma in poultry workers, dermatitis in pet bird owners, and highly pruritic, erythematous papular rashes in persons closely exposed to nesting birds (Lucky et al., 2001).

Infested wild birds, especially pigeons, nesting on window ledges and window unit air conditioners near bedrooms have caused household outbreaks of avian mite dermatitis (Kong and To, 2006; McClain et al., 2009). The bird mites are nocturnal feeders, do not burrow into the epidermis, bite to tissue juice feed, and depart quickly for their bird hosts and nests (Kong and To, 2006; McClain et al., 2009). Most cases occur during the late spring and early summer when fledgling birds leave their nests and their mites need alternative food sources, such as human dead-end hosts (McClain et al., 2009).

Clinical manifestations of bird mite bites and infestations

The chicken or poultry mite (or red chicken mite), *Dermanyssus gallinae*, is found worldwide on domestic fowl and other birds including pigeons, sparrows, and starlings and is a common cause of dermatitis anywhere chickens are raised or sold (Lutsky and Bar-Sela, 1982). Bites from the red chicken mite are painful and cause a highly pruritic dermatitis, quickly excoriated by scratching, usually on the backs of the hands and forearms in poultry workers (Fig. 7.6) (Lutsky and Bar-Sela, 1982; McClain et al., 2009).

The American bird mite, *Dermanyssus americanus*, rarely bites humans but can cause an acute generalized eczematous dermatitis from bites in the late spring (Kong and To, 2006; McClain et al., 2009). The tropical fowl mite, *Ornithonyssus bursa* (Family Macronyssidae), is a common ectoparasite of pigeons worldwide, inflicts a sharply painful bite, and is a frequent cause of highly pruritic, maculopapular dermatitis of the finger web spaces and axillae in pigeon breeders and fanciers (Fig. 7.7) (McClain et al., 2009).

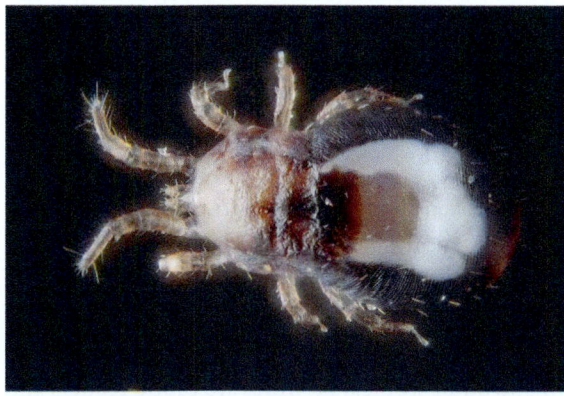

Figure 7.6 The red chicken or poultry mite, *Dermanyssus gallinae*, can inflict painful bites and cause a highly pruritic dermatitis, quickly excoriated by scratching. *(From Wikipedia. Public domain.)*

Figure 7.7 The tropical fowl mite, *Ornithonyssus bursa* (family Macronyssidae), is a common ectoparasite of pigeons worldwide. *(From Wikipedia. Public domain. No copyright permission required.).*

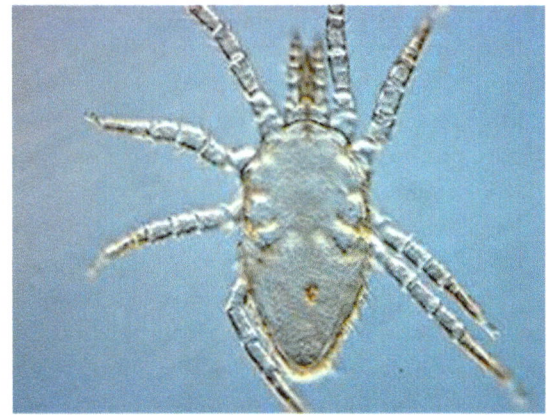

Treatment of avian bites and infestations

Avian mite bites and dermatitis may be treated topically with local anesthetics, such as lidocaine and prilocaine, antipruritics, and antihistamines, such as diphenhydramine, and corticosteroids in persistent cases. Therapy can be supplemented with oral antihistamines, hydralazine, and corticosteroids if indicated. Infestations may require treatment with topical acaricides, such as crotamiton, permethrin, lindane, or malathion.

Prevention and control of avian bites and infestations

The eradication of avian mites requires removal of all infested birds and their nesting materials on window ledges and atop window air conditioning units following topical fumigation with acaricides, and ancillary house cleaning and fumigation with acaricides, such as permethrin, lindane, or malathion.

Rat, bat, and snake mite bites
Definitions

In addition to the tropical fowl mite, *Ornithonyssus bursa* (Family Macronyssidae), other species of macronyssid mites that bite humans include the tropical rat mite, *Ornithonyssus bacoti*, the free-tailed bat mite, *Chiroptonyssus robustipes*, and the snake mite, *Ophionyssus natricis* (Table 7.1) (McClain et al., 2009).

Clinical manifestations

Bites from the tropical rat mite, *Ornithonyssus bacoti,* which is ubiquitous in the temperate areas of Europe and the Americas, can cause a painful bite followed by a papulovesicular dermatitis on the wrists and hands in stockyard and warehouse workers, and in owners of pet rodents, such as hamsters, guinea pigs, and gerbils (Fig. 7.8) (Lucky et al., 2001; McClain et al., 2009).

The first stage nymph (protonymph) and adult tropical rat mites are blood feeders and not tissue juice feeders such as chiggers and other mites (McClain et al., 2009). Engorged

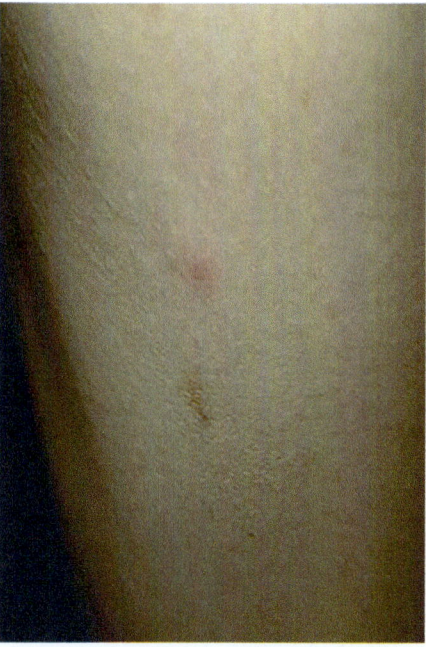

Figure 7.8 Avian mites of birds nesting on window sills and window air conditioning units can gain access to bedrooms through open windows and inflict bite groupings at night typically under bed clothes that are characterized by highly pruritic erythematous macules and papules as shown here on a patient's lateral chest. *(Source: Wikimedia Commons. Public Domain. No copyright permission required. Available at https://commons.wikimedia.org/wiki/File:Mite_bite_on_chest.jpg.)*

with blood, the free-ranging nymph and adult tropical rat mites look more like tiny blood-engorged ticks than mites (Fig. 7.9).

The free-tailed bat mite, *Chiroptonyssus robustipes,* has a limited range of distribution in Central America and the southern United States, bites are rare, and confined to bat handlers, cave explorers, and exterminators (McClain et al., 2009). The snake mite, *Ophionyssus natricis,* infests sylvatic, captive, and exotic snakes in the United States (McClain et al., 2009). Human bite cases have been reported in most states during the spring in snake handlers and owners of exotic snakes, such as imported boas and pythons. A vesiculopapular dermatitis will follow a bite by a snake mite, typically on the upper extremities (Fig. 7.10).

A vesiculopapular dermatitis will follow a bite by a snake mite, typically on the upper extremities.

Treatment of rat, bat, and snake mite bites

The treatment of both rat mite and snake mite dermatitis is entirely symptomatic and may include antihistamines and corticosteroids. Treatment of the human host with acaricides in usually not necessary because the rat mite feeds for a short time and then departs for the

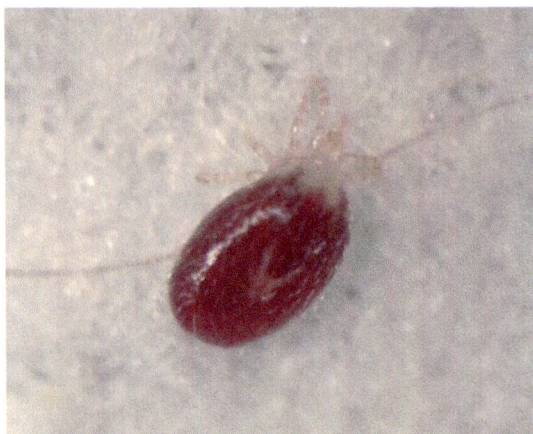

Figure 7.9 An adult tropical rat mite, *Ornithonyssus bacoti*, inflicts a painful bite and is a blood feeder like ticks and not a tissue juice feeder like most mites. Engorged after a recent blood feed, this tropical rat mite looks more like a small tick than a mite. *(From https://messengermountainnews.com/wp-content/uploads/2018/08/rat_mite-300x240.jpg).*

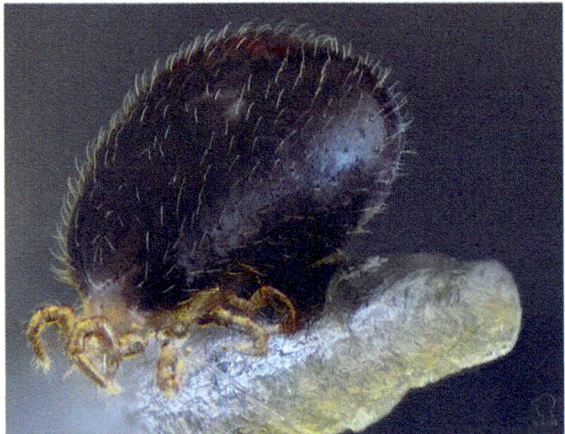

Figure 7.10 The snake mite, *Ophionyssus natricis*, infects sylvatic, captive, and exotic snakes in the United States, human cases have been reported in most states during the spring in snake handlers owners of exotic snakes, such as imported boas and pythons. *(From Wikipedia. Public domain. Author Dack9. Available at https://en.wikipedia.org/wiki/Ophionyssus_natricis#/media/File:%D0%97%D0%BC%D0%B5%D0%B8%D0%BD%D1%8B%D0%B9_%D0%BA%D0%BB%D0%B5%D1%89_%D0%BD%D0%B0_%D0%BA%D0%BE%D0%BD%D1%87%D0%B8%D0%BA%D0%B5_%D0%B8%D0%B3%D0%BB%D1%8B.jpg).*

rat host's nest. Treatment of the human host with acaricides in usually not necessary in snake mite dermatitis as snake mites feed on humans for a short time and then depart.

Prevention and control of rat, bat, and snake mite bites

Rats and bats need to be exterminated and their nesting sites treated with acaricides.

Insect (itch) mites

Several insect mite species, primarily from the family Pyemotidae, can cause bothersome erythematous papulovesicular eruptions following bites. The North American hay or grain itch mite, *Pyemotes tritici,* feeds preferentially on the larvae of insects that infest cane, hay, straw, and some grains, especially rice (Rivers et al., 1976). Hay itch mite dermatitis is characterized by pruritic, maculopapulovesicular eruptions on the limbs and trunk, which resolve rapidly with topical therapy (Betz et al., 1982). A close relative of the hay itch mite, the oak leaf gall mite, *Pyemotes herfsi,* which preferentially feeds on insect larvae in oak trees, caused a large outbreak of plant insect mite dermatitis in a suburban population in Kansas in 2004 (McClain et al., 2009).

Definitions and taxonomy

The pyemotid or insect itch mites (Family Pyemotidae) are ectoparasites of the larvae of beetles, bees, wasps, and moths and other insects that infest trees and stored grains including corn, wheat, barley, rice, beans, peas, cotton seed, straw, and hay (Rivers et al., 1976). The pyemotid mites are oviparous and exhibit an unusual life cycle with the female swelling up to 2 mm in diameter and delivering more than several hundred immature adults with males delivering first. Males then fertilize females who search for a new food source, especially after prolonged grain storage or when environmental conditions deteriorate. The insect itch mites that will attack humans causing community outbreaks of plant insect mite dermatitis include *Pyemotes tritici,* *P. herfsi,* *P. ventricosus,* and *P. zwoelferi* (Rivers et al., 1976; Betz et al., 1982).

  P. tritici, the widely distributed hay or grain itch mite, is the most common pyemotid species to bite humans handling straw or hay for agricultural or decorative purposes, or joy-riders on hay wagons (Fig. 7.11) (Rivers et al., 1976). Workplace outbreaks of pruritic maculopapular dermatitis due to *P. tritici* have been reported among persons handling straw or hay for animal bedding and or using hay or straw to protect furniture for transport and shipping (Rivers et al., 1976).

  Pyemotes herfsi, the oak leaf gall mite, first identified in Europe and now widespread, preys on oak leaf gall-making midge larvae (Fig. 7.12). Galls are abnormal growths that occur on the leaves, twigs, roots, or flowers of many plants. Most galls are caused by irritation and/or stimulation of plant cells due to feeding or egg-laying by insects such as aphids, midges, wasps, and mites.

Figure 7.11 The hay or grain itch mite, *Peymotes tritici*, is the most common pyemotid species mite to bite humans exposed to or handling straw or hay. *(Wikipedia: Public domain.).*

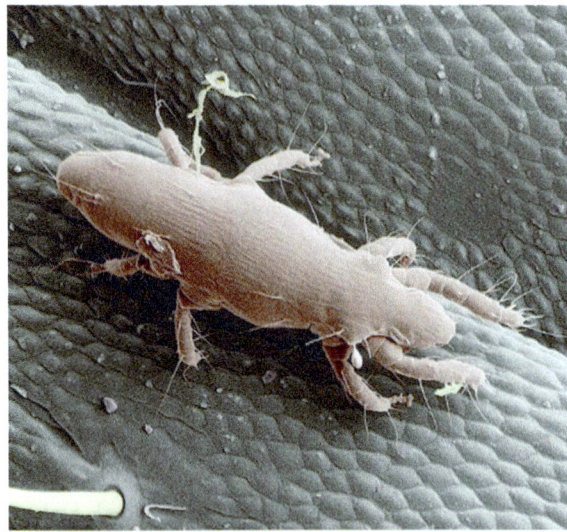

Figure 7.12 The oak leaf gall mites, *Pyemotes herfsi*, such as the one shown here, infested a pin oak tree grove in Kansas in 2004, and their bites caused intensely pruritic maculopapular eruptions in hundreds of suburban residents. *(CDC: Public domain.).*

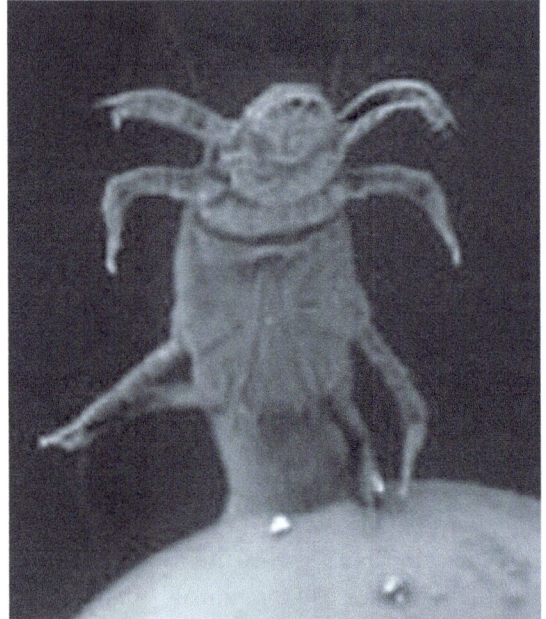

In 2004, oak leaf gall mites infested a grove of pin oaks in a Kansas suburb. Hundreds of residents were attacked by biting mites and developed initial pruritus 10–16 h after suffering mite bites that progressed to an erythematous popular rash with 20% presenting with macules, pustules, and confluent erythema (McClain et al., 2009; Rivers et al., 1976).

The dermatitis was confined to the neck in 50% of the cases as mites dropped from the upper stories of oak trees with the trunks less commonly affected. Systemic symptoms of fever, wheezing, and rhinorrhea were absent in all cases, and the rash resolved within a week in all patients (Fig. 7.13). An intensive investigation by state and federal public health officials confirmed *Pyemotes herfsi*, the oak leaf gall mite, as the cause of the community outbreak of dermatitis and dispelled rumors of chemical releases (McClain et al., 2009; Rivers et al., 1976).

Three separate outbreaks of mite bite dermatitis affecting over 100 persons were caused by another species of insect itch mite, *Pyemotes ventricosus,* and reported from Spain in 2000 (Fig. 7.14) (Rivers et al., 1976).

A similar outbreak, also suggestive of *P. ventricosus* mite bite—induced dermatitis, was reported in southeastern France in 2006 (Rivers et al., 1976). The dermatitis was characterized by solitary to multiple, highly erythematous pruritic macules; some were accompanied by contiguous, linear erythematous macular tracts that resembled comet tails (Fig. 7.15). In a 2007 outbreak investigation of an additional 42 cases of dermatitis with comet tail signs in the same region of France, Del Giudice and coworkers identified *P. ventricosus* mites as causative agents and described the epidemiology and outcomes of *P. ventricosus* infections in homes and humans (Fig. 7.15). The comet tail sign has become a pathognomonic cutaneous biomarker of *P. ventricosus* mite bite—induced dermatitis (Fig. 7.15).

Most residences of index case patients with *P. ventricosus* dermatitis were infested with live furniture beetles, *Anobium punctatum,* which do not bite or infest humans. However, adult *P. ventricosus* mites, common ectoparasites of beetles, were present in stereomicroscopic examination of wood dust beneath beetle-infested furniture. Confocal laser

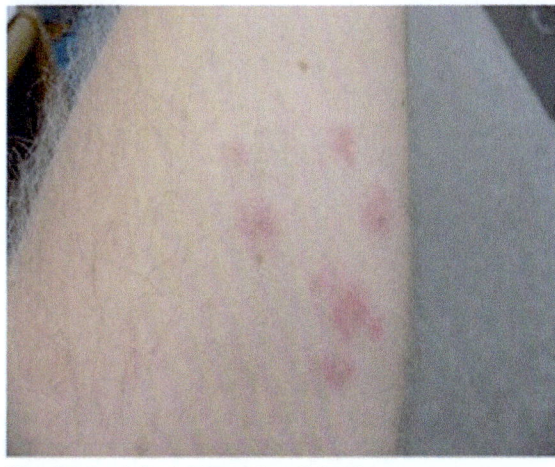

Photo/A Broce, L Zurek, Kansas State University

Figure 7.13 A maculopapular grouping of pruritic bites by oak leaf gall mites, *Peymotes herfsi, occurs* 10—16 h after suffering mite bites and may progress to an erythematous papular rash as shown here presenting with macules, pustules, and confluent erythema (Lutsky and Bar-Sela, 1982). The dermatitis was confined to the neck in 50% of the cases as mites dropped from the upper stories of oak trees with the trunks less commonly affected (Rivers et al., 1976). Systemic symptoms of fever, wheezing, and rhinorrhea were absent in all cases, and the rash resolved within a week in all patients. (*CDC. Public domain.*).

ACARINA > PEDICULOIDIDAE

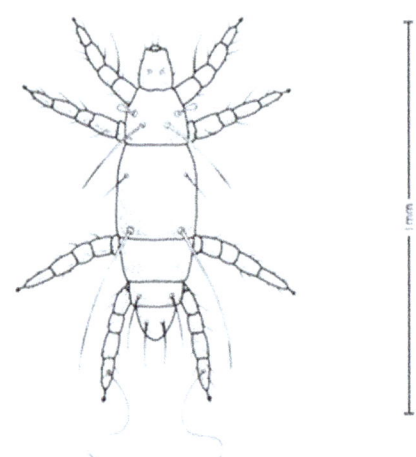

Pyemotes ventricosus
(Newport)
(female, dorsal aspect)

Figure 7.14 *Peymotes ventricosus,* another species of insect itch mites, prefers to feed on wood and grain-boring insects. *(CDC: Public domain.).*

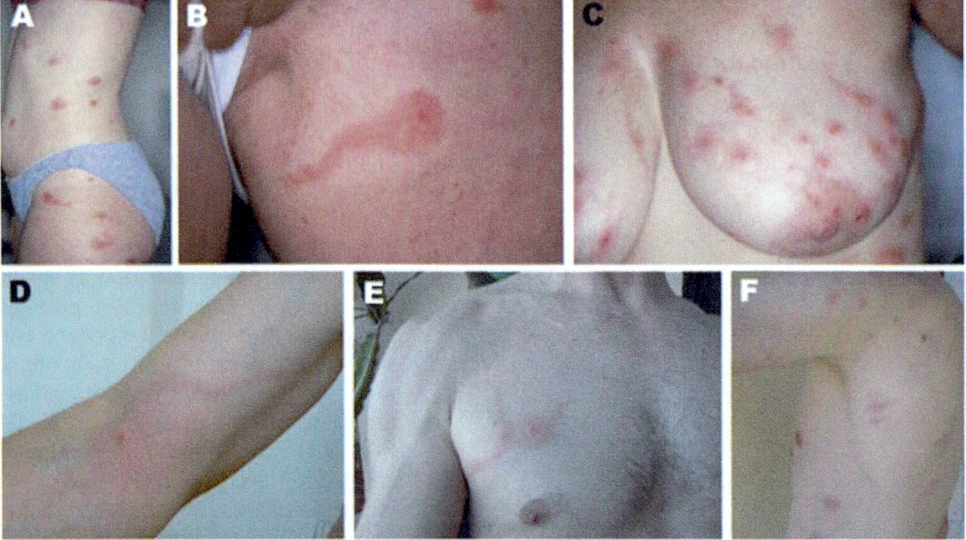

Figure 7.15 Six persons with the skin lesions of *Peymotes ventricosus* dermatitis. The dermatitis was characterized by solitary to multiple, highly erythematous pruritic macules; some were accompanied by contiguous, linear erythematous macular tracts that resembled comet tails. The comet tail sign has become a pathognomonic cutaneous biomarker of *P. ventricosus* mite bite–induced dermatitis. *(CDC Public domain.).*

scanning microscopy of a central microvesicle in a maculopapular lesion on an experimentally infested coinvestigator demonstrated an ovoid foreign body consistent with a *P. ventricosus* mite. Both naturally occurring and experimental infections caused the characteristic maculopapular rash of *P. ventricosus* dermatitis, associated with comet signs (Fig. 7.15). Although oral prednisone (0.5 mg/kg) rapidly relieved pruritus, *P. ventricosus* dermatitis would persist or recur in index case patients until wood beetle-infested furniture was completely removed from households or patients moved permanently vacating their infested residences.

In addition to *P. tritici, P. ventricosus*, and *P. herfsi, Pyemotes zwoelferi* has caused pruritic dermatitis after exposures and was implicated in outbreaks of erythematous papular eruptions in florists and patrons exposed to mite-infested dried flowers (McClain et al., 2009).

Clinical manifestations of pyemotid mite infestations

Numerous bites by pyemotid species mites cause an intensely pruritic dermatitis often called "grain itch," "straw itch," "hay itch," or "furniture repairer's itch," depending on the exposure source. The bites often cluster on the extremities and trunk and are initially painful as the skin is pierced by the mite's sharp chelicerae and two neurotoxic and paralytic venoms, Txp-I and Txp-II, are injected into the bite site (Betz et al., 1982). The venoms are produced by these insect mites in order to disable mobile and flying prey, especially beetles, moths, and moth larvae (Betz et al., 1982). Vesicular urticarial lesions described as varicelliform or chicken pox-like can form at the bite sites and later develop erythematous bases with white wheal centers and a central speck on top representing the offending mite (Betz et al., 1982). Systemic symptoms are unusual but can include malaise, fever, chills, and diarrhea. If the source of the mites is completely removed, the eruption will be self-limited following supportive care and will resolve without scarring in 1—3 weeks.

Treatment

The treatment of pyemotid mite bites is symptomatic with topical antipruritics, such as calamine, antihistamines, such as chlorpheniramine, and corticosteroids for nonresolving lesions. The complete resolution of the lesions will depend on the total elimination of the infesting mites.

Prevention and control of pyemotid mite infestations

In order to eliminate the source of pyemotid mites, the infested areas, such as oak groves, need to be treated with acaricides, such as carbaryl and other carbamates, permethrin, sulfur dust, or methyl bromide gas if permitted by environmental regulations.

References

Betz, T.G., Davis, B.L., Fournier, P.V., Rawlings, J.A., Elliot, L.B., Baggett, D.A., 1982. Occupational dermatitis associated with straw itch mites (Pyemotes ventricosus). JAMA, the Journal of the American Medical Association 247 (20), 2821—2823. https://doi.org/10.1001/jama.1982.03320450055037.

Elston, D.M., 2004. What's eating you? Cheyletiella mites. Cutis 74 (1), 23—24.

Flatt, R.E., Wiemers, J., 1976. A survey of fur mites in domestic rabbits. Laboratory Animal Science 26 (5), 758—761.

Kong, T.K., To, W.K., 2006. Bird-mite infestation. New England Journal of Medicine 354 (16). https://doi.org/10.1056/NEJMicm050608.

Lucky, A.W., Sayers, C.P., Argus, J.D., Lucky, A., 2001. Avian mite bites acquired from a new source - pet gerbils: report of 2 cases and review of the literature. Archives of Dermatology 137 (2), 167—170.

Lutsky, I., Bar-Sela, S., 1982. Northern fowl mite (Ornithonyssus sylviarum) in occupational asthma of poultry workers. The Lancet 320 (8303), 874—875. https://doi.org/10.1016/s0140-6736(82)90834-0.

McClain, D., Dana, A.N., Goldenberg, G., 2009. Mite infestations. Dermatologic Therapy 22 (4), 327—346. https://doi.org/10.1111/j.1529-8019.2009.01245.x.

Rivers, J.K., Martin, J., Pukay, B., Flatt, R.E., Wiemers, J., Mcclain, D., Dana, A.N., Goldenberg, G., Lucky, A.W., Sayers, C., Argus, J.D., Lucky, A., Betz, T.G., Davis, B.L., Fournier, P.V., Rawlings, J.A., Elliot, L.E., Baggett, D., Giudice, P.D., Blanc-Amrane, V., Bahadoran, P., 1976. Preliminary characteristics of toxins from the straw itch mite, Peymotes tritici, which induce paralysis in the larvae of a moth. MMWR Morbidity and Mortality Weekly Report 15 (4), 327—346.

Rivers, J.K., Martin, J., Pukay, B., 1986. Walking dandruff and Cheyletiella dermatitis. Journal of the American Academy of Dermatology 15 (5), 1130—1133. https://doi.org/10.1016/S0190-9622(86)70280-6.

CHAPTER 8

Plant, food, dust, and follicle mites and allergies

Plant, food, and food storage mites

Definitions and taxonomy

Plant, food, and food storage mites feed on plants, plant bulbs, fungi, and the insects on stored foods, including grains, dried fruits and vegetables, cheeses, and cured, processed, and smoked meats and fish. These mites belong to three families, Acaridae, Carboglyphidae, and Glycyphagidae (McClain et al., 2009). They prefer warm, moist environments with a relative humidity of 80% and a temperature between 23 and 30°C (McClain et al., 2009). They are significant causes of contact dermatitis, inhalational allergy, and bronchial asthma in exposed workers in several industries including agriculture, grain and food storage, baking, cheese production and storage, meat and seafood smoking and processing, furniture manufacturing and repair, and horticulture (Table 8.1).

Clinical manifestations of plant, food, and storage mite infestations

The atopic and contact dermatitis caused by plant, food, and stored food mites may occur following bites or by close contact with mite-infected foods, especially cheeses and dried fruits and vegetables. Anaphylaxis may occur if the mites or mite-contaminated foods or their aerosols are contacted, inhaled, or swallowed by atopic individuals (McClain et al., 2009).

The most commonly encountered plant, food, and storage mites and the clinical manifestations of their infestations include the following (McClain et al., 2009). (1) *Acarussiro* species in stored dried fruits and vegetables, which causes contact dermatitis in agricultural workers and grocers. (2) *Tyrophagus longior* in coconut kernals (copra), which causes a papulopustular eruption in coconut handlers, known as "copra itch" (Figs. 8.1 and 8.2). (3) *Tyrophagus putrescentiae* in smoked and cured ham and fish, stored cheeses, and dried fruits and vegetables, which causes allergic dermatitis in food handlers. (4) *Tyrolichus casei* (formerly *Tyrophagus casei*) in stored cheeses, which causes a contact dermatitis in cheese handlers. (5) *Suidasia nesbitti* in wheat pollard, a by-product of flour milling from grains, which causes a contact dermatitis in bakers, known as "wheat pollard itch". (6) *Carpoglyphuslactis*, the date or fig mite, which causes scabies-like eruptions with erythematous papules and scabs in date and fig handlers. (7) *Rhgizoglyphus* species, the bulb mite, which causes contact dermatitis in plant bulb handlers and horticulturalists.

Ectoparasitic Diseases
ISBN 978-0-443-26724-6
https://doi.org/10.1016/B978-0-443-26724-6.00008-4

Table 8.1 Mites with exclusive plant, food, storage, and house dust host reservoirs.

Latinnames	Common names	Host reservoirs	Geographic distributions	Infestations
Acarus farris	Grain mite	Cereal, flour, grain, rice, hay	Worldwide	Bakers' itch contact dermatitis in bakers and hay workers
Acarus siro (formerly Tyrophagus siro)	Grocers' itch mite	Stored plant products, grains, cheeses	Worldwide	Grocers' itch; Bakers' itch; Vanillism; Contact and inhalational allergies in agricultural workers, bakers, and cheese producers
Bryobiapraetiosa	Clover mite	Clover, ivy, grasses, fruit trees	Worldwide	Will invade homes with close by vegetation, such as ivy-covered exterior walls and fencing. Do not bite humans.
Carpoglyphus lactis	Cheese mite Fruit mite	Dried cheesesDried fruits	Worldwide	Cheese and fruit workers' dermatitis
Dermatophagoides farina	American house dust mite	House dust	Worldwide	Contact dermatitis and inhalational allergy-asthma
Dermatophagoides pteronyssinus	European house dust mite	House dust	Worldwide	Contact dermatitis and inhalational allergy-asthma
Glyciphagus destructus	Hay mite	Cut hay	Worldwide	Hay wagon riders' allergy
Glyciphagus domesticus	Date mite Furniture mite	Dried dates, figs, and insects in wood and furniture	Worldwide	Contact dermatitis in dried fruit workers, scabies-like erythematous papules with scabs possible in dried fruit workers

Species	Common name	Source	Distribution	Disease
Lepidoglyphus destructus	Cosmopolitan food mite	Stored dried foods	Worldwide	Storage mite dermatitis
Suidasia nesbitti	Wheat pollard mite	Flour milled from wheat and other grains	Worldwide	Wheat pollard itch contact dermatitis
Tyrolichus casei (formerly Tyrophagus casei)	Cheese mite	Dried cheeses	Worldwide	Cheese workers' dermatitis Storage mite dermatitis
Tyrophagus longior	Mold mite Coconut mite	Coconut kernel (copra)	Worldwide	Papulopustular "copra itch" in coconut processors
Tyrophagus putrescentiae	Cheese mite Cheese mold mite	Cured ham, cheeses, smoked herring, dried fruits, grains, mushrooms, plant bulbs	Worldwide	Allergic dermatitis and occupational inhalational allergies in food and grain workers
Rhizoglyphus species	Bulb mite Flower bulb mite	Flower and plant bulbs	Worldwide	Storage mite dermatitis, Bulb dermatitis

Adapted from Diaz, J.H. 2023. Plant, food, food storage, and dust mites and allergies. Chapter 10. Mite–Human Encounters: Nuisances, Vectors, Parasites, Allergens, and Commensals, Elsevier, Philadelphia.

A

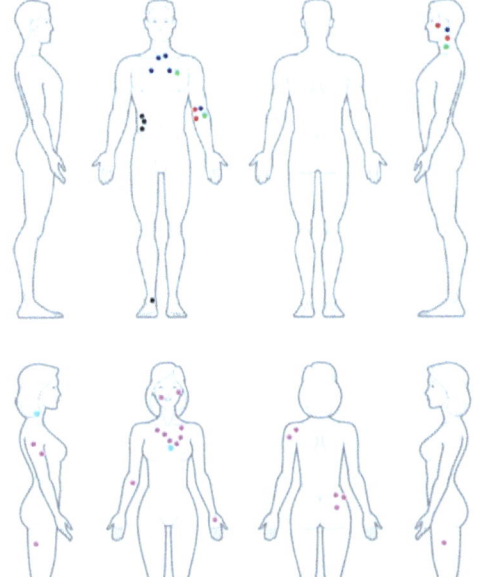

Locations and frequencies of erythematous papules of 4 male cases

Location	Frequencies of erythematous papules			
	Case 2	Case 3	Case 5	Case 6
Body	0	2	3	1
Neck	1	2	0	1
Face	1	1	0	0
Arms	2	1	0	1
Angles	0	0	1	0

Locations and frequencies of erythematous papules of 2 female cases

Location	Frequencies of erythematous papules	
	Case 1	Case 4
Body	9	1
Neck	0	1
Face	2	0
Arms	4	0
Hands	1	0
Legs	10	0

B

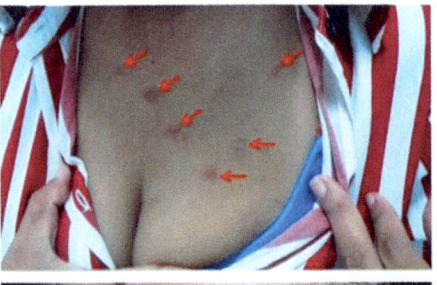

Erythematous papules on the chest (red arrows) of case no 1

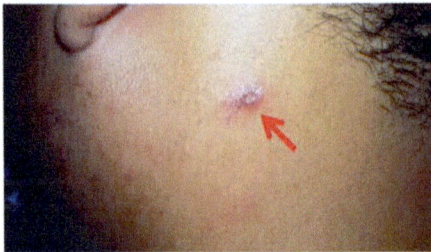

Erythematous papule with central punctum at neck (red arrow) of case no 3

Figure 8.1 *Tyrophagus longior*, the coconut mite, is found in coconut kernels (copra) and causes a papulopustular eruption in coconut handlers, known as "copra itch." The figures depict a descriptive epidemiological and clinical investigation of a copra itch outbreak in a Thai family of seven (four males, three females) living among stored coconuts and attacked by copra mites, *Tyrophagus longior*. *(From Elsevier article. Available at: https://ars.els-cdn.com/content/image/1-s2.0-S2214250918300350-gr1.jpg).*

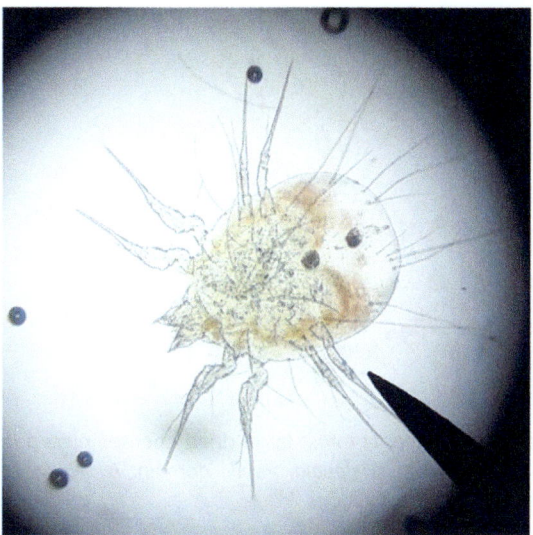

Figure 8.2 A copra mite, *Tyrophagus longior*, identified among coconuts in a Thai household and responsible for an outbreak of copra itch in seven family members living in the household. *(From Elsevier article. Available at: https://ars.els-cdn.com/content/image/1-s2.0-S2214250918300350-gr2_lrg.jpg).*

(8) *Glyciphagus domesticus*, the furniture mite, causes an atopic vesicular dermatitis in woodworkers restoring wood beetle-infested furniture.

Treatment of plant, food, and storage mite infestations

Plant, food, and food storage mite allergic and contact dermatitis may be treated symptomatically with oral antipruritics, such as diphenhydramine and hydralazine, and antiinflammatory agents, such as corticosteroids. The dermatitis is self-limited following both domestic and occupational exposures as long as the source of the mite infestation is completely eliminated. Inhalational exposures causing wheezing and bronchial asthma will require treatment with oral and possibly intravenous bronchodilators and corticosteroids. Anaphylactic reactions will require emergency management with parenteral vasopressors, such as self-administered intramuscular epinephrine.

Prevention and control of plant, food, and storage mite infestations

The prevention and control of plant, food, and storage mite infestations will require spraying of contaminated areas with residual pesticides including permethrin, other pyrethroids, and more toxic carbamate, organophosphate (malathion), and organochlorine (lindane) pesticides (Collins, 2006). Alternative arcaricidal strategies should be considered in order to reduce all toxic pesticide exposures and pesticide resistance including growth regulators, inorganic dusts, such as diatomaceous earth, and plant-derived acaricides (Collins, 2006). Cheese mites can be controlled preferentially by encasing cheeses in thin layers of paraffin in a process known as cheese waxing (Fig. 8.3) (Wilkin, 1973).

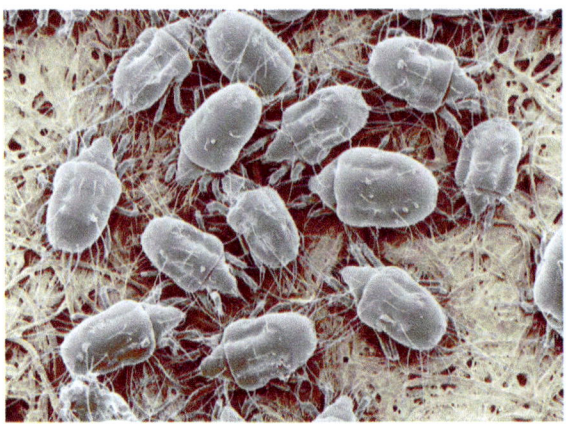

Figure 8.3 Cheese mites, *Tyrophagus putrescentiae*, commonly infest large dried cheeses placed in cold storage without cheese waxing with paraffin. *(From Wikipedia. Public domain. Available at: https://en.wikipedia.org/wiki/Cheese_mite#/media/File:Cheese_mite.jpg).*

Dust mites and dust mite allergies

Definitions and taxonomy

Dust mites are distributed worldwide, can trigger allergic contact dermatitis, atopic dermatitis, and inhalational allergies, and belong primarily to four families of mites, the Acaridae, Chlortoglyphidae, Glyciphagidae, and Pyroglyphidae (McClain et al., 2009). More than 10 species of dust mites from these four families have been identified in house dust, the most common of which are the American (*Dermatophagoides farina*) and the European (*Dermatophagoides pteronyssinus*) house dust mites, both are distributed worldwide despite their designations as American and European (McClain et al., 2009). The European house dust mite, *D. pteronyssinus* is shown in Fig. 8.4.

Another species of dust mite, the pillow or feather mite, *Dermatophagoides scheremetewskyi*, is not as commonly encountered as the American and European dust mites, but is also distributed worldwide (McClain et al., 2009). Multiple bites by the pillow mite cause feather pillow dermatitis, which presents clinically as erythematous papules on the face, neck, and hands of atopic individuals sleeping on mite-infested feather pillows.

Feeding behavior and life cycle

Dust mites are the smallest adult mites ($\leq$0.3–0.5 mm) and rarely seen microscopically, but easily aerosolized when beds are made and pillows fluffed. Typically, there are 30–40 mites per gram of house dust, but this number can increase significantly during bedmaking, drapery adjusting, and pillow fluffing (Jacquet, 2013). Dust mites prefer to feed on sloughed human epithelial cells, semen, and other human debris, but they will also feed on mold, fungal spores, pollen, feathers, and animal dander. They can live for up to

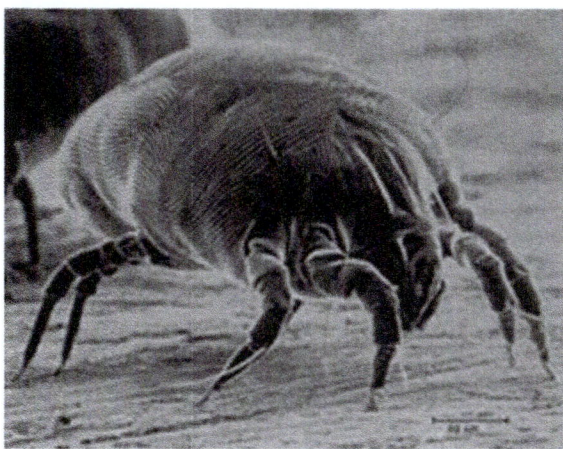

Figure 8.4 The European house dust mite, *Dermatophagoides pteronyssinus*. (From Wikimedia. Public domain. Available at: https://commons.wikimedia.org/wiki/File:House_Dust_Mite.jpg#/media/File: House_Dust_Mite.jpg).

2 months, especially in a high humidity environment with a relative humidity or 75% or greater and temperatures at or above 25°C (Jacquet, 2013).

Female dust mites lay one to three eggs a day, which hatch within 7—14 days to release six-legged larvae that pass through two nymph stages before becoming eight-legged adults. The egg-to-egg life cycle takes 3—4 weeks.

The immune response to dust mite allergens

House dust mites do not bite, sting, or transmit infectious diseases, but their presence in households can induce a variety of allergenic responses including allergic rhinitis, asthma, and childhood eczema. The exact mechanisms responsible for the various immune responses to dust mites remain incompletely understood because of the range of allergens contributed to house dust by dust mites (Jacquet, 2013). The major allergens contributed to house dust by dust mites include feces, ova, body parts and fragments, and exoskeletons (Jacquet, 2013; Lacey et al., 2016; Foley et al., 2021).

Recent studies have suggested that sensitizations to house dust mite allergens trigger exacerbated allergen-induced inflammation of the skin and airway mucosa in atopic subjects resulting in atopic dermatitis, allergic rhinitis, and bronchial asthma (Jacquet, 2013). Initially, the Th2- allergic response to house dust mite allergens was considered mediated only by allergen B- and T-cell epitopes to promote allergen-specific IgE production as well as to release cytokines IL-4, IL-5, and IL-13 in order to recruit inflammatory cells (Jacquet, 2013).

New evidence today suggests that house dust mites are carriers not only for allergenic proteins contained in their ova, exoskeletons, feces, and body segments and parts but are also carriers of microbial adjuvant antigens, specifically bacterial endosymbionts (Jacquet, 2013) (Fig. 8.5).

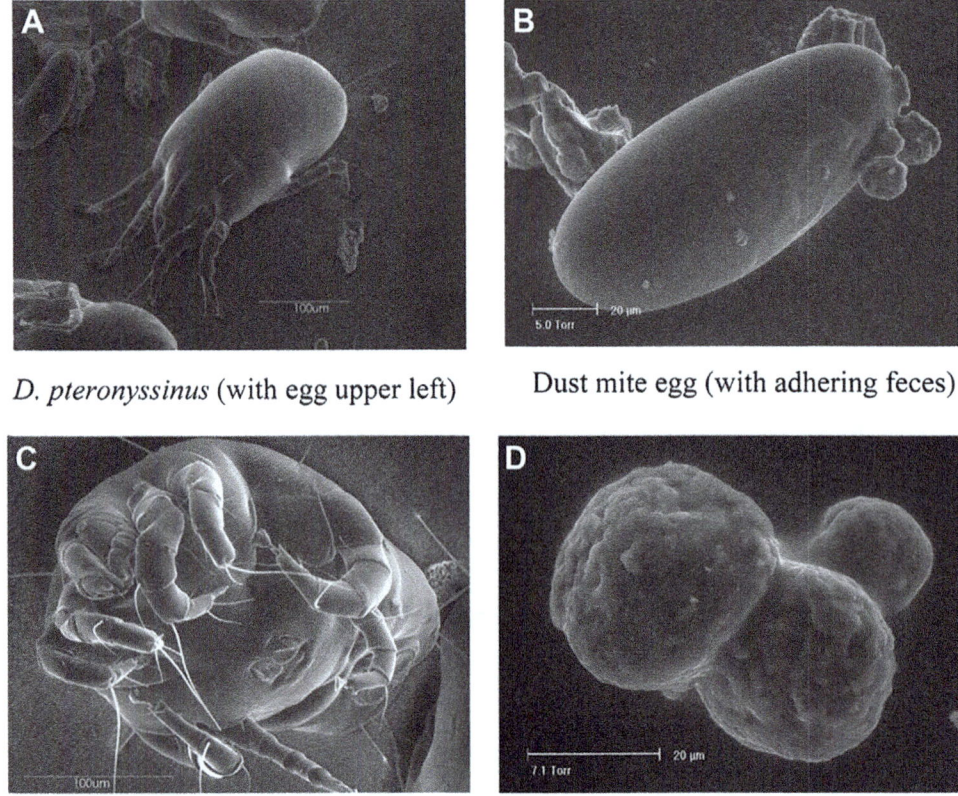

D. pteronyssinus (with egg upper left)   Dust mite egg (with adhering feces)

D. pteronyssinus (ventral view)   Dust mite feces

Figure 8.5 House dust mites present many allergens to the immune system including the allergenic proteins contained in their ova, exoskeletons, feces, and disintegrating body segments and parts. *(Source: From CDC. Public domain. Available at: https://stacks.cdc.gov/view/cdc/43223).*

The allergenic proteins released by house dust mites and their endosymbionts act in concert to stimulate complex, innate signaling pathways leading to allergy (Jacquet, 2013). House dust mite allergy is then initiated by the following three mechanisms, initial IgE secretion by B cells, followed by eosinophil recruitment, and later bronchial airway mucosal remodeling (Jacquet, 2013).

DNA-dependent protein kinase (DNA-PK), an enzyme that repairs breaks in DNA, also plays a major role in house dust mite allergy. DNA-PK is activated in dendritic cells by the major house dust antigens and dust mite endosymbionts and generates reactive oxygen species (ROS), which regulate antigen presentation through Th2-mediated inflammatory responses (Fig. 8.6) (Chung and Levine, 2015). DNA-PK inhibitors have now been demonstrated to block the development of house dust mite-induced bronchial asthma and treat ongoing airway hyperreactivity (Chung and Levine, 2015).

Proposed Role of DNA-PK Activation in House Dust Mite-induced Asthma

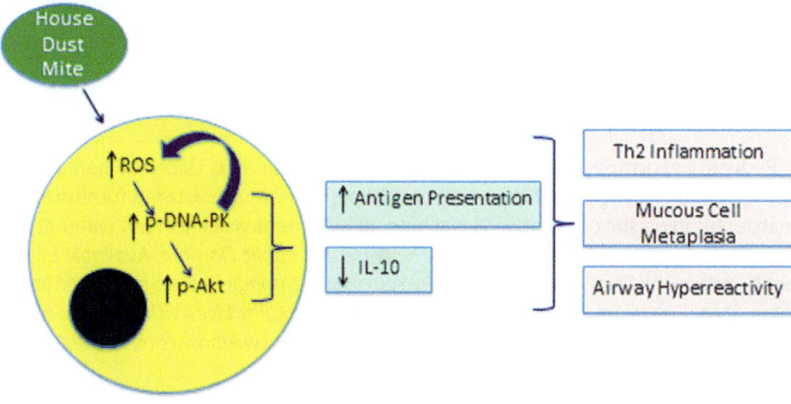

Figure 8.6 DNA-dependent protein kinase (DNA-PK), an enzyme that repairs breaks in DNA, also plays a major role in house dust mite allergy. DNA-PK is activated in dendritic cells by the major house dust antigens and dust mite endosymbionts and generates reactive oxygen species (ROS), which regulate antigen presentation via Th2-mediated inflammatory responses (Figure 10.6). DNA-PK inhibitors have now been demonstrated to block the development of house dust mite-induced bronchial asthma and treat ongoing airway hyperreactivity. (Chung and Levine, 2015) *(Source: From NIH. Public domain. Available at: https://irp.nih.gov/blog/post/2016/05/collaboration-identifies-role-of-dna-pk-in-asthma).*

The treatment, prevention, and control of dust mite allergies

House dust mite allergy is best managed with a combination of immunotherapy with mite antigen extracts and intense efforts to minimize the number of dust mites in the household. Although contact and inhalational allergies to dust mites can be initially managed symptomatically with combinations of topical and oral antihistamines for dermatitis and oral and parenteral bronchodilators and steroids for wheezing and asthmatic reactions, the best management strategies for environmental dust mite infestations are avoidance and reduction of dust mites and their allergens in households (McClain et al., 2009; "Indoor air pollutants and toxic materials. Health Housing Reference Manual," no date).

Avoidance strategies include discarding old mattresses, throw rugs, carpets, draperies, and upholstered sofas and lounge chairs that retain moisture and food and other organic and human debris welcoming dust mite infestations and collecting dust mite allergens, especially in bedrooms (McClain et al., 2009; "Indoor air pollutants and toxic materials. Health Housing Reference Manual," no date). Dust mites are most numerous in mattresses, old wool carpets, and blackout draperies, and, therefore, are more often found in bedrooms than in other rooms.

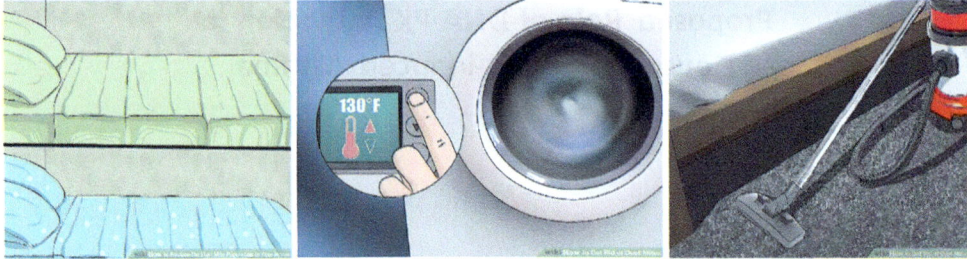

Figure 8.7 Reducing exposure to dust mite allergens in a bedroom as depicted here requires several steps including (1) eliminating throw rugs, carpets, draperies, and upholstered furniture, encasing pillows and mattresses in plastic coverings; (2) washing all bed linens weekly in hot water at 130° F (54.4° C), and (3) weekly vacuuming. *(Source: From Wiki How Health. Public Domain. Available at: https://www.wikihow.health/Reduce-the-Dust-Mite-Population-in-Your-Home#/Image:Reduce-the-Dust-Mite-Population-in-Your-Home-Step-1-Version-2.jpg; https://www.wikihow.health/Live-With-Allergies-to-Dust-Mites#/Image:Live-With-Allergies-to-Dust-Mites-Step-8.jpg; https://www.wikihow.com/Get-Rid-of-Dust-Mites#/Image:Get-Rid-of-Dust-Mites-Step-3-Version-4.jpg).*

Household temperatures should be reduced below 25°C. and humidity levels should be reduced to 40%–50% relative humidity levels with continuous air conditioning if necessary. Air conditioning intakes should be snugly fitted with HEPA filters that are changed monthly ("Indoor air pollutants and toxic materials. Health Housing Reference Manual," no date). Mite allergens and mite populations in homes can also be reduced by weekly vacuuming, encasing pillows and mattresses in plastic coverings, and washing all bed linens weekly in hot water at 130°F (54.4°C.) (Fig. 8.7).

Follicle mites

Scabies and follicle mites are the only exclusively human ectoparasitic mites without host animal reservoirs. They cannot transmit infectious diseases. Less serious but more common than scabies is infestation with the human *Demodex* follicle mites. *Demodex folliculorum* inhabits hair follicles, and *Demodex brevis* inhabits sebaceous glands. These diminutive (0.1–0.4 mm) mites are regarded as commensals because they feed on sebum and exfoliated skin while lodged in hair follicles and sebaceous gland pores (Lacey et al., 2016; Foley et al., 2021). Follicle mites can, however, revert to pathogen status when host immunocompetency is compromised or suppressed.

Follicle mites as commensals

Demodex, follicle, or face mites are ubiquitous human commensal organisms that cluster in hair follicles and sebaceous glands on the forehead, nose, eyelids, eyebrows, cheeks, and nasolabial folds and have even been found living in earwax. However, in heavy infestations or during immunocompromised conditions, follicle mites may be found in

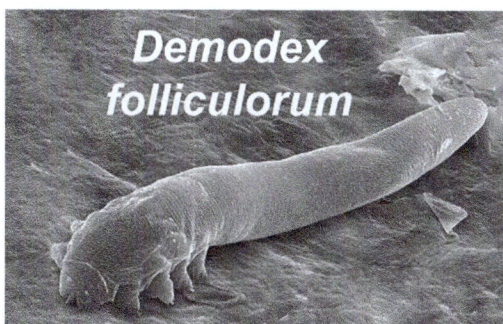

Figure 8.8 Demodex folliculorum follicle mite removed from its insertion in a hair follicle, scanning electron micrograph. Length, 0.2–0.4 mm. *(Source: From Wikipedia Commons. Public domain. Available at: https://upload.wikimedia.org/wikipedia/commons/a/a7/Demodex_folliculorum_SEM_crop.jpg).*

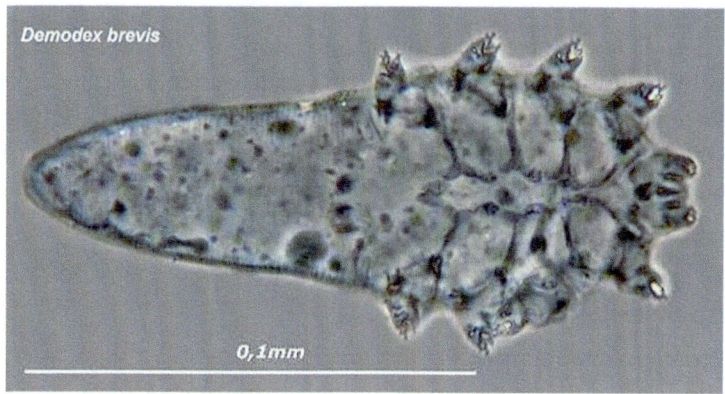

Figure 8.9 Demodex brevis follicle mite removed from its insertion in a sebaceous gland. Length 0.1–0.2 mm. *(Source: From Wikipedia. Public domain. Available at: https://en.wikipedia.org/wiki/Demodex_brevis#/media/File:Demodex_Brevis.jpg).*

ectopic areas including the ear canals, perioral mucosa, anterior chest wall, and other regions (McClain et al., 2009).

Demodex folliculorum lives in hair follicles, has a length of 0.2–0.4 mm, and has an elongated body covered with transverse striations and four pairs of short legs Fig. 8.8 (McClain et al., 2009).

Demodex brevis is considered a short close relative of the elongated *Demodex folliculorum* and inhabits sebaceous glands. *D. brevis* is stubby with a length of only 0.1–0.2 mm and, like *D. folliculorum*, has four pairs of short legs, and its short body is covered with transverse striations Fig. 8.9.

Demodex follicle mites are considered commensals because they clear hair follicle shafts and sebaceous gland pores of excessive sebum and exfoliated skin (Foley et al., 2021). Follicle mites can, however, revert to pathogen status when host immunocompetency is suppressed by many conditions including cancer chemotherapy, corticosteroid therapy, and human immunodeficiency virus (HIV) infection (Foley et al., 2021).

Life cycle of follicle mites

The life cycle of follicle mites begins as females lay eggs within hair follicles or sebaceous glands that hatch into larvae with six legs, which molt to become nymphs and later adults with four paired legs. All of the developmental stages of *Demodex* mites occur over an egg-to-egg cycle of 14—18 days within the confines of hair follicles or sebaceous glands. The exact mode of initial transmission of *Demodex* mites is unknown, but skin surface biopsies have implicated initial transmission from mother to newborn at birth and later by close human contact (Lacey et al., 2016).

Demodex mite prevalence is high on skin surface biopsies and rises with age with a 40%—50% prevalence in adults over age 50 (Lacey et al., 2016). Along eyelashes, *Demodex* presence has been reported in 18% of individuals aged 21—35, rising with age to 33% in individuals over 65 years of age (Lacey et al., 2016).

In some cases, *Demodex* presence with inflammation or demodecidosis may be precipitated in females overusing heavy, cream-based facial cosmetics and in adolescents with increased sebaceous gland activity and acne (McClain et al., 2009). Immunosuppressing conditions known to increase *Demodex* mite activity with inflammation include chronic stress, advancing age, organ transplantation, steroid therapy, cancer, cancer chemotherapy, and HIV infection (McClain et al., 2009; Lacey et al., 2016).

Immune responses to follicle mites

The human immune system tolerates low numbers of *Demodex* mites very well, but as mite population density increases, mites modulate the innate immune response, and can cause local inflammation or demodecidosis (DeDulanto and Camacho-Martinez, 1979). The immune modulating responses created by increasing numbers of follicle mites include downregulating T-cell responses, increasing cytokine responses by interleukins and tumor necrosis factor, and inducing an increase in toll-like receptors on keratinocytes and sebocytes (DeDulanto and Camacho-Martinez, 1979). Although an increasing *Demodex* presence does occur with age and immunosuppression, *Demodex* density usually causes few adverse symptoms, unless infections are associated with acne, blepharitis, impetigo, rosacea, or seborrheic dermatitis (DeDulanto and Camacho-Martinez, 1979; Gao et al., 2005).

Although the human commensal relationship with *Demodex* mites is most common, the exact sequence of immune mechanisms responsible for inciting allergic or pathogenic reactions to *Demodex* mites remains unknown (Lacey et al., 2016; Foley et al., 2021). However, in order to assess potential pathogenicity from an increasing *Demodex* mite presence and activity, mite presence and number can be accurately assessed by microscopic follicle mite counts. Pathogenicity requires the presence of five or more mites per single low-power (10×) microscopic field prepared with potassium hydroxide, or more than five mites per cm (Collins, 2006) in a standardized skin biopsy (McClain et al., 2009).

Clinical manifestations of follicle mite infestations

During conditions of mite overpopulation or immunosuppression, commensal *Demodex* colonization can become pathological and result in the following four significant skin diseases: (1) Pityriasis folliculorum, (2) rosacea-like demodicidosis, (3) demodicosis gravis, and (4) *Demodex* blepharitis (McClain et al., 2009; DeDulanto and Camacho-Martinez, 1979; Gao et al., 2005). Pityriasis folliculorum is a skin condition characterized by faint facial erythema with a burning sensation and fine scaly follicular plugging caused by the overuse of heavy moisturizing facial creams by middle-aged women (McClain et al., 2009).

Rosacea-like demodicidosis is a skin condition that mimics rosacea and is characterized by superficial follicular scale and erythematous vesiculopustules that line the lateral and central face (McClain et al., 2009; DeDulanto and Camacho-Martinez, 1979). Unlike rosacea, there are no telangiectasias, and patients deny flushing, persistent erythema, and photosensitivity (Fig. 8.10) (McClain et al., 2009; DeDulanto and Camacho-Martinez, 1979).

Demodicidosis gravis is a skin condition that presents with erythematous papulonodules and dermal granulomas containing mite remnants in giant phagocytic cells that demonstrate caseation necrosis on histology (DeDulanto and Camacho-Martinez, 1979).

Demodex blepharitis presents with an infestation of *Demodex folliculorum* of the eyelashes, artificial eyelash extensions if present, and eyelids in association with dandruff,

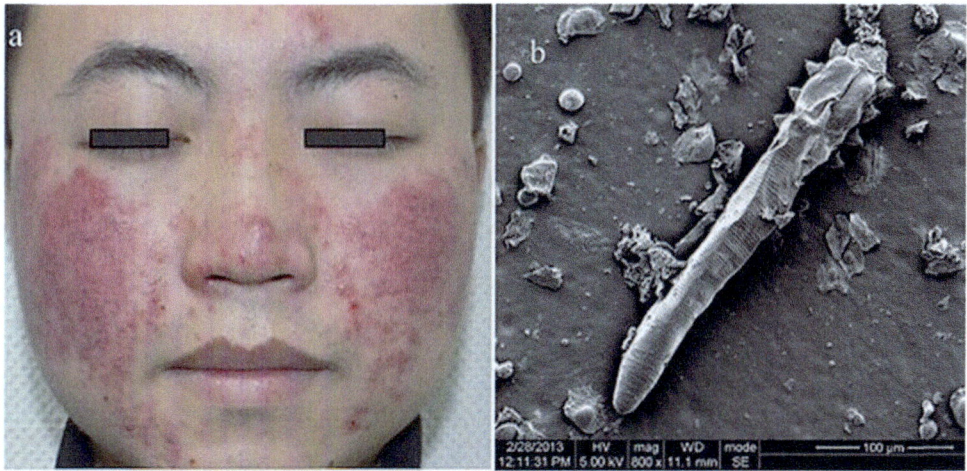

Figure 8.10 A patient with rosacea-like demodicidosis with erythematous vesiculopustules that line the lateral and central face and no telangiectasias. (A.) Central and lateral facial rash sparing the forehead and chin. (B.) *Demodex folliculorum* isolated on a skin scraping of the rash. *(Source: From Wikipedia. Public domain. Available at: https://en.wikipedia.org/wiki/Demodicosis#/media/File:Demodicosis. jpg).*

trichiasis, meibomian gland dysfunction with tearing deficiency, and conjunctival inflammation (Gao et al., 2005).

In patients with HIV, especially when the CD4 count is below 200 per mm (Wilkin, 1973), intensely pruritic *Demodex* eruptions can spread to the face, presternal area, nipples, and interscapular region (Clyti et al., 2006). Other immunocompromising conditions, especially acute myelocytic leukemia, can trigger similar overactive *Demodex* responses (Clyti et al., 2006).

Treatment of follicle mite infestations

Various effective, topical treatments have been used for uncomplicated, but symptomatic demodecidosis including permethrin, ivermectin, metronidazole, lindane, salicylic acid, sulfur, sulfacetamide, and crotamiton (McClain et al., 2009; Gao et al., 2007). Topical sulfur followed by 5% permethrin are recommended as initial topical treatments. Effective oral medications have included ivermectin, ivermectin combined with topical permethrin, and oral metronidazole and ivermectin (McClain et al., 2009; Clyti et al., 2006; Gao et al., 2007). Metronidazole combined with ivermectin is recommended for oral treatment of demodecidosis in patients with HIV infections (McClain et al., 2009; Clyti et al., 2006; Gao et al., 2007). Topical tea tree oil 50% weekly and daily tea tree shampoo are recommended for the treatment of demodecidosis of the eyelids, eyebrows, or eyelashes (Gao et al., 2005).

References

Chung, J., Levine, S., 2015. Dendritic cells induce th2-mediated airway inflammatory responses to house dust mite via DNA-dependent protein kinase. Nature Communications. https://doi.org/10.1038/ncomms.7224.

Clyti, E., Nacher, M., Sainte-Marie, D., Pradinaud, R., Couppie, P., 2006. Ivermectin treatment of three cases of demodecidosis during human immunodeficiency virus infection. International Journal of Dermatology 45 (9), 1066—1068. https://doi.org/10.1111/j.1365-4632.2006.02924.x.

Collins, D.A., 2006. A review of alternatives to organophosphorus compounds for the control of storage mites. Journal of Stored Products Research 42 (4), 395—426. https://doi.org/10.1016/j.jspr.2005.08.001.

DeDulanto, F., Camacho-Martinez, F., 1979. Demodicidosis gravis. Annals Dermatologie Venereologica 106, 699—704.

Foley, R., Kelly, P., Gatault, S., Powell, F., 2021. Demodex: a skin resident in man and his best friend. Journal of the European Academy of Dermatology and Venereology 35 (1), 62—72. https://doi.org/10.1111/jdv.16461.

Gao, Y.Y., Di Pascuale, M.A., Elizondo, A., Tseng, S.C.G., 2007. Clinical treatment of ocular demodecosis by lid scrub with tea tree oil. Cornea 26 (2), 136—143. https://doi.org/10.1097/01.ico.0000244870.62384.79.

Gao, Y.Y., Di Pascuale, M.A., Li, W., Liu, D.T.S., Baradaran-Rafii, A., Elizondo, A., Kawakita, T., Raju, V.K., Tseng, S.C.G., 2005. High prevalence of Demodex in eyelashes with cylindrical dandruff. Investigative Ophthalmology & Visual Science 46 (9), 3089—3094. https://doi.org/10.1167/iovs.05-0275.

Indoor air pollutants and toxic materials. Health Housing Reference Manual. US Centers for Disease Control and Prevention.

Jacquet, A., 2013. Innate immune responses in house dust mite allergy. ISRN Allergy 2013, 1–18. https://doi.org/10.1155/2013/735031.

Lacey, N., Russell-Hallinan, A., Powell, F.C., 2016. Study of demodex mites: Challenges and solutions. Journal of the European Academy of Dermatology and Venereology 30 (5), 764–775. https://doi.org/10.1111/jdv.13517.

McClain, D., Dana, A.N., Goldenberg, G., 2009. Mite infestations. Dermatologic Therapy 22 (4), 327–346. https://doi.org/10.1111/j.1529-8019.2009.01245.x.

Wilkin, D.R., 1973. Resistance to lindane in Acarus siro from an English cheese store. Journal of Stored Products Research 9 (2), 101–104. https://doi.org/10.1016/0022-474x(73)90016-7.

CHAPTER 9

Myiasis, murine typhus, tungiasis, and plague (flies and fleas)

Myiasis

Myiasis is an ectoparasitic infestation of viable or necrotic tissues caused by the dipterous larvae of higher flies and may be broadly classified as obligatory or facultative myiasis. In obligatory myiasis, maggots must live and feed on human or animal hosts as part of their life cycle. In facultative myiasis, normally free-living maggots that preferentially feed on carrion and decaying organic matter attack and feed on the necrotic sores and wounds of living human and animal hosts. Maggot therapy with blowfly and bottlefly larvae is still used today to débride necrotic wounds.

Myiasis may be further stratified clinically as furuncular (subcutaneous) myiasis, wound (superficial cutaneous) myiasis, cavitary (atrial or invasive) myiasis, intestinal myiasis, urinary myiasis, and vaginal myiasis. Furuncular myiasis is the most common clinical manifestation of myiasis and occurs when one or more larvae penetrate the skin, causing pustular lesions that resemble boils or furuncles. Larval maggots can also infest external orifices, sores, or open traumatic or surgical wounds, causing cavitary and wound myiasis. Cavitary myiasis is usually caused by screwworm larvae that can penetrate festering wounds or invade the orbits, nostrils, or external ear canals (Figs. 9.1 and 9.2). Intestinal myiasis is caused by the accidental ingestion of maggot-contaminated food and is characterized by self-limited nausea, vomiting, and diarrhea. Genitourinary myiasis, like intestinal myiasis, is uncommon and may

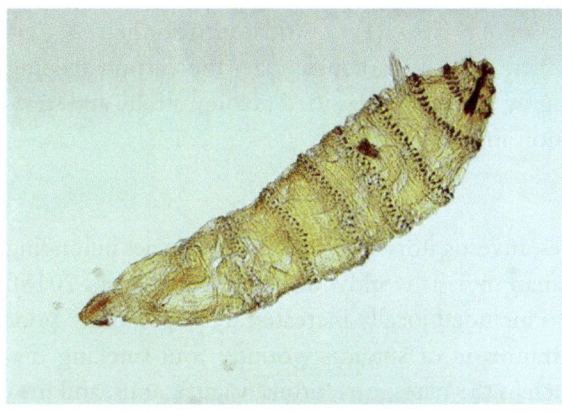

Figure 9.1 First-stage (instar) larva of a ***Cuterebra*** spp. botfly native to North America. capable of causing myiasis. Note the rows of anterior hooklets that can anchor the feeding larva to the dermis. *(From Centers for Disease Control and Prevention. Public health image library: ID #1427; page last reviewed December 20, 2017. https://phil.cdc.gov/details_linked.aspx?pid=1427. No copyright permission required.))*

Ectoparasitic Diseases
ISBN 978-0-443-26724-6,
https://doi.org/10.1016/B978-0-443-26724-6.00009-6

Figure 9.2 Forearm exit site wound (A) of a third-stage (instar) new World screw-worm fly larva or maggot, **Cochliomyia hominivorax** (B). *(From Seppänen M, Virolainen-Julkunen A, Kakko I et al. Myiasis during adventure sports race. Emerg Infect Dis. 2004; 10:137–139. No copyright permission required.)*

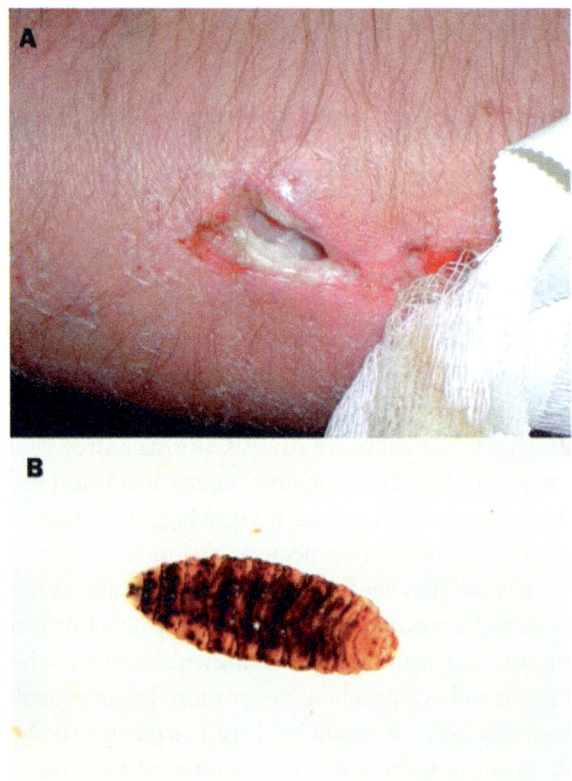

present as dysuria, hematuria, and pyuria, after larval invasion of the urethra (urinary myiasis) or vagina (vaginal myiasis).

Although there are many families of dipterous flies (order Diptera), flies from three families cause most human and animal cases of myiasis: (1) Oestridae, the botflies; (2) Calliphoridae, the screwworms and blowflies; and (3) Sarcophagidae, the carrion-feeding flies. The most common myiasis-causing fly species are classified taxonomically and stratified by clinical type of myiasis infestation in Table 9.1.

Epidemiology

In a retrospective review of human cases, investigators identified 37 fly species belonging to 10 families as capable of causing human myiasis worldwide (Singh and Singh, 2015). The predisposing risk factors for myiasis included locally increased fly populations; poor hygienic conditions; neglected open traumatic or surgical wounds; foul-smelling discharges from natural body openings, such as the nares, ears, orbits, vagina, anus, and urethra; and the presence of nearby domestic animals (Singh and Singh, 2015).

Table 9.1 Myiasis-causing flies.

Family (common family name)	Taxonomic classification	Common name	Geographic distribution	Type of myiasis infestation
Oestridae (botflies)	*Dermatobia hominis*	New World botfly	Caribbean, Central and South America	Furuncular
	Cuterebra spp.	Rodent and rabbit botflies	North America, northern Central America	Furuncular
	Hypoderma sinense	Indian botfly	India, China	Furuncular
Calliphoridae (screwworm flies, blowflies)	*Cordylobia anthropophaga*	Tumbu fly	Africa	Furuncular
	Cordylobia rodhaini	Lund fly	Africa	Furuncular
	Auchmeromyia senegalensis	Congo floor mat fly	Africa	Superficial cutaneous (no tissue invasion)
	Cochliomyia hominivorax	New World screwworm	Southern North America, Central and South America	Wound, cavitary
	Chrysomyia bezziana			Wound, cavitary
	Lucilia spp.	Old World screwworm	Africa, Asia	Wound, cavitary
	Calliphora spp.	Greenbottle blowflies	Worldwide	Wound (used for maggot therapy)
		Bluebottle blowflies	Worldwide	Wound (used for maggot therapy)
Sarcophagidae (carrion flies)	*Sarcophaga carnaria*		Africa	Wound, cavitary, gastrointestinal
	Wohlfahrtia magnifica		Africa	Wound, cavitary, gastrointestinal

Adapted from Diaz JH: Section K. Chapter 295. Myiasis and Tungiasis. In Mandell GL, Bennett JE, Dolin R, Eds. *Principles and Practice of Infectious Diseases*, Seventh Edition, Elsevier, Philadelphia, 2009: 3637–3641. Elsevier publication.

In an epidemiologic study of myiasis cases in Brazil, investigators found myiasis to be more prevalent in impoverished populations (62%) among males (61%), in adults older than 51 years of age (42%), and in children younger than 10 years of age (34%) (Marquez et al., 2007). The predominant causative agent of furuncular myiasis in Brazil was *Dermatobia hominis,* the New World human botfly, and the predominant causative agent of cavitary myiasis was *Cochliomyia macellaria,* an indigenous species of New World screwworm (Marquez et al., 2007).

In a case series from Peru, investigators identified nine cases of myiasis during the reporting period 2012−15-with four cases caused by *Dermatobia hominis* and five cases caused by *Cochliomyia hominivorax*. Peruvian investigators were the first to report significant demographic, epidemiological, and clinical differences in myiasis due to the two most common species of flies causing myiasis in northern Peru (Failoc-Rojas et al., 2018).

Dermatobia hominis caused furuncular myiasis in young, healthy patients and children (mean age, 33.0 ± 31 years) living in tropical regions of Peru. On the other hand, *Cochliomyia hominivorax* caused cavitary myiasis in older patients (mean age, 73.4 ± 6.1 years) with one or more comorbidities living in nontropical regions of Peru (Failoc-Rojas et al., 2018). Comorbidities for cavitary myiasis included diabetes mellitus, cancer, tuberculosis, nasal polyps, and draining wounds, such as ulcerating breast cancers and tracheostomy stomas (Failoc-Rojas et al., 2018). All patients with either type of myiasis were treated with ivermectin, antibiotics and, in some cases, antiinflammatory drugs (Failoc-Rojas et al., 2018).

In addition to poverty and neglected hygiene, atrophic rhinitis and facial leprosy may also predispose patients to cavitary myiasis (Serafim et al., 2020). Atrophic rhinitis can attract gravid flies that deposit their eggs intranasally on foul-smelling, crusty and bloody secretions (Serafim et al., 2020). An enlarged nasal cavity and a reduced sneeze reflex provides safe harbor for the feeding maggots with less risk of expulsion (Serafim et al., 2020).

Facial leprosy can cause painless ulceration of the nasal cavity with erosion into the paranasal air sinuses (Serafim et al., 2020). Resulting inflammation produces purulent secretions in immunosuppressed patients with reduced intranasal sensation, impaired sneezing reflex, and an inability to clean the nose properly due to loss of manual dexterity (Serafim et al., 2020). Brazilian investigators reported a severe case of nasal myiasis in an 89-year-old male with lepromatous leprosy that resulted in nasal septal perforation, atrophy of the inferior and middle nasal turbinates, and erosion of the bony walls of the nose, hard palate, and ethmoidal air cells (Serafim et al., 2020). Clinicians performed an endoscopic sinusectomy in order to clear the eroded nasal cavity of more than 300 maggots (Serafim et al., 2020). In addition to *D. hominis* and

Cochliomyia spp., *Cordylobia* and *Cuterebra* spp. of botflies can also cause furuncular myiasis in North America, Africa, and Asia (Fig. 9.1) (Plotinsky et al., 2007; Shorter et al., 1997; Yasukawa and Dass, 2020).

This is a *Cuterebra* species botfly larva that burrowed into the skin after botfly eggs were deposited on the skin (Fig. 9.1). The botfly larva has just emerged from its development in a dermal pocket.

Clinical manifestations

The most common forms of human myiasis worldwide are furuncular myiasis and cavitary (invasive) myiasis. Furuncular myiasis is most often caused by subcutaneous larval invasion by the tumbu fly, *Cordylobia anthropophaga,* in Africa, and the New World human botfly, *Dermatobia hominis,* in the subtropical and tropical areas of the Americas (Table 9.1) (Yasukawa and Dass, 2020; Lachish et al., 2015). Cavitary myiasis is usually caused by zoonotic screwworm larval deposition in open wounds or exposed, external orifices, such as the nares, ears, and orbits, and may be characterized by deep tissue larval invasion, with secondary infection and extensive tissue necrosis. *Cochliomyia hominivorax,* the New World screwworm, is a common cause of cavitary myiasis in the Americas, and *Chrysomyia bezziana,* the Old World screwworm, is a common cause of cavitary myiasis in Africa, Asia, and Indonesia (Yasukawa and Dass, 2020; Lachish et al., 2015).

Although the clinical manifestations, treatments, and prevention strategies are similar in furuncular myiasis, the mechanisms of larval fly invasion in humans are often different. The gravid female tumbu fly deposits its eggs on moist sandy soil or on wet clothing (e.g., cloth diapers) hung outside to dry. When the human victim dons egg-infested clothing, larvae emerge and rapidly burrow into the skin with sharp mandibles for further development. On the other hand, the female botfly captures blood-feeding insects, usually mosquitoes, in midflight and attaches her eggs to the undersurface of the insect. The intermediate biting vector then delivers the botfly eggs airborne to its next blood meal victims, where the eggs hatch immediately and release their larvae to feed on warm-blooded hosts. Human botfly larvae then rapidly burrow into the skin with sharp mandibles to begin their developmental stages, which can last 6—12 weeks.

In addition to travel history in endemic regions, the mechanisms of larval fly invasion assist in differentiating the cause of furuncular myiasis. In tumbu fly (*Cordylobia anthropophaga)* myiasis, lesions are usually located on body regions covered by clothing, such as the buttocks and trunk. In New World human botfly *(D. hominis)* myiasis, lesions are usually located on exposed areas, such as the scalp, neck, face, and extremities.

After completing three instar stages, the final larval forms of the tumbu fly and human botfly wriggle out of their draining, boil-like, 1–2-cm furuncular swellings; drop to the ground; and pupate in warm, moist soil into adult flies within 9–14 days. Victims may recall a flying insect bite that preceded human botfly-induced furuncular myiasis. While developing in their furuncles, larvae are active, protrude intermittently through draining wounds, and maintain surface contact for respiration with their posterior, paired breathing spiracles. Anterior hooklets anchor the maggots in place subcutaneously, making manual removal, even difficult with forceps (Fig. 9.1).

In 2021, Chinese investigators reported an unusual case of furuncular myiasis associated with an eosinophilic pleural effusion in an afebrile patient presenting with right chest pain, recurrent cough, and hemoptysis (Fan et al., 2021). Chest computed tomography demonstrated a left hydropneumothorax and an atelectatic right lung (Fan et al., 2021). Pertinent laboratory data included peripheral eosinophilia of 37.2% and elevated immunoglobulin A and E levels (Fan et al., 2021).

An ultrasound-guided left-sided thoracentesis yielded a cloudy, yellow exudate filled with eosinophils on microscopy (Fan et al., 2021). Failure to respond to antibiotic treatment led the investigators to suspect an undiagnosed parasitic infection and to institute empiric oral albendazole therapy (Fan et al., 2021). Within a week, tender furuncles containing mobile larvae were detected in the upper arms and shoulders (Fan et al., 2021). The larvae were removed by gentle pressure, suspended in 95% alcohol, and later identified as first stage dipterous fly larvae (Fan et al., 2021). The investigators attributed the eosinophilic pleural effusion to extensive migration of the fly larvae beneath the pleural surfaces that incited a compensatory, systemic eosinophilic response (Fan et al., 2021). They recommended that clinicians consider furuncular myiasis as a cause of eosinophilic pleural effusions in tropical regions with close proximity to domestic animals (Fan et al., 2021).

Therapy

Management strategies for furuncular myiasis include coaxing embedded larvae from furuncles by smothering their respiratory spiracles, often visible in lesions, with sterile transparent wound dressings or occlusive coatings of petrolatum, clear fingernail polish, tobacco tar, pork fat, raw beefsteak, or bacon strips (Loong et al., 1992; Boggild et al., 2002). The injection of lidocaine into draining lesions has also been recommended as a successful extraction technique (Loong et al., 1992; Boggild et al., 2002). Nevertheless, unsuccessful occlusive therapy may fatally asphyxiate larvae and necessitate their surgical or vacuum extraction. Cavitary myiasis must be managed aggressively with surgical débridement and antibiotic therapy for secondary infections to limit tissue damage and disfigurement (Fig. 9.2) (Serafim et al., 2020).

Along with larval removal, all myiasis wounds should be cleansed and conservatively débrided, tetanus prophylaxis administered, and bacterial secondary infections treated with antibiotics. Although *Clostridium tetani* infection of penetrating wounds does occur, tetanus has not been reported in cases of myiasis, but has been reported after ectoparasitic infestations with *Tunga penetrans,* the chigoe (jigger) flea, in Africa and South America(O-bengui, 1989).

Prevention and control

Prevention and control strategies for myiasis should include: (1) control of domestic and livestock animal larval infestations; (2) sanitary disposal of animal carcasses and offal to deny flies their preferred breeding grounds; (3) proper management of any open human wounds or cutaneous infections; (4) cementing floors to deny floor maggot flies their preferred egg-laying surfaces on sandy soils; (5) sleeping on raised beds or cots in screened huts or tents; (6) wearing long-sleeved shirts and pants, which can be pyrethrin or pyrethroid-impregnated; (7) spraying exposed skin with diethyl toluamide (*N,N*-diethyl-meta-toluamide [DEET]) or picaridin-containing insect repellents; and (8) ironing both sides of all clothes and diapers left outside to dry in tumbu fly habitats.

Flea infestations

Fleas of the insect order Siphonaptera are a small group of morphologically similar wingless ectoparasites of warm-blooded animals, including humans. They are not only biting nuisances but also competent vectors of infectious diseases, most notably murine typhus and plague transmitted by rodent and other mammalian fleas (Table 9.2). Although fleas are often classified by their host specificity or the presence of head combs, all fleas can rapidly adapt from animal to human hosts, especially if preferred hosts are exterminated in mass die-offs by disease or by pesticides. Fleas undergo complete metamorphosis from egg to adult stages, with larvae, pupae, and adults exhibiting different morphologies and preferred habitats. Signaled by vibrations and locally rising carbon dioxide levels, adult fleas emerge from egg cases within 1—2 weeks, leap onto the closest mammalian hosts, and begin blood-feeding and reproducing.

Table 9.2 The most common flea-transmitted infectious diseases.

Infectious disease	Causative agent	Flea vector (common name)	Animal reservoir	Major clinical manifestations	Therapy
Bubonic plague	*Yersinia pestis*	*Xenopsylla cheopis* (rat flea); *Oropsylla montana* (squirrel flea); less commonly cat and dog fleas	Rodents (rats, prairie dogs, squirrels); domestic animals (cats > dogs)	Headache, fever, chills, regional lymphadenopathy—draining buboes, pneumonitis (secondary plague pneumonia), septicemia, meningitis; case-fatality rate, 14%	Antibiotic therapy recommended within 24 hours with any of the following effective antibiotics: Tetracyclines, gentamicin, streptomycin, chloramphenicol
Murine typhus	*Rickettsia typhi*	*Xenopsylla cheopis* (rat flea); *Nosopsyllus fasciatus* (northern rat flea); *Oropsylla montana* (squirrel flea)	Rodents (rats and mice)	Fever, headache, maculopapular rash, thrombocytopenia, rarely pneumonitis and encephalitis	Doxycycline, 100 mg bid × 7 –10 days
Flea-borne spotted fever	*Rickettsia felis*	*Ctenocephalides felis* (cat flea)	Rodents (rats, mice, opossums)	Nonspecific fever, headache, maculopapular rash	Tetracyclines (doxycycline)
Cat-scratch fever (disease)	*Bartonella henselae*	*Ctenocephalides felis* (cat flea)	Feral cats (kittens)	Low-grade fever, malaise, regional and rarely multifocal lymphadenopathy, endocarditis; complications more common in HIV infection and include bacillary angiomatosis, peliosis hepatis, neuroretinitis, and encephalopathy	Doxycycline and macrolides (azithromycin) effective; add rifampin for complications

Tungiasis—portal of entry for *Clostridium tetani*	Ectoparasite	*Tunga penetrans* (chigoe or jigger flea)	Humans; domestic animals (dogs > cats and pigs)	Painful white papules with central black pits discharging eggs and feces with lateral pressure, especially on dorsal aspects of toes under toenails and on heels	Surgical extraction of gravid female fleas; ivermectin ineffective in humans and only partially effective in dogs for jigger flea management
		Tunga trimamillata (only in Ecuador and Peru)		Same	Same

Adapted from Diaz JH: Section K. Chapter 295. Myiasis and Tungiasis. In Mandell GL, Bennett JE, Dolin R, Eds. *Principles and Practice of Infectious Diseases*, Seventh Edition, Elsevier, Philadelphia, 2009: 3637–3641. Elsevier publication.

Murine typhus

Murine typhus is an acute, febrile, and generally mild flea-borne infectious disease caused by *Rickettsia typhi*. The most common flea vectors of murine typhus are oriental rat fleas, *Xenopsylla cheopsis*, and cat fleas, *Ctenocephalides felis*, both of which can also transmit *Yersinia pestis*, the causative bacterium of plague (Fig. 9.3).

Plague and murine typhus are transmitted by rat fleas. This is a lateral view of an adult oriental rat flea, *Xenopsylla cheopsis*, the most common vector of murine typhus and plague (Fig. 9.3).

Fleas become infected by blood-feeding on infected animals, such as rodents, opossums, and feral cats. The disease is transmitted to humans most commonly after an infected flea bite, but can also be transmitted by inhalation of aerosols containing infected flea feces or trans-conjunctivally by rubbing infected flea feces into the eyes. Since infected fleas shed rickettsiae in feces, the flea bites the victim, then defecates near the bite wound, and the victim rubs the infected feces, also called flea dirt, into the wound. Murine typhus does not spread person to person like pneumonic plague. Female fleas will pass the rickettsial infection congenitally to their progeny.

Although murine typhus can occur worldwide, most cases are reported from Central and South America, Africa, the Middle East, and Southeast Asia. In the United States, southern California, south Texas, and Hawaii report most cases. The incubation period ranges from 5 to 14 days after the flea bite (mean incubation period = 10 days), and infections range from mild in most cases that resolve without antibiotic treatment to severe and potentially fatal cases in less than 1% of all cases (Doppler et al., 2020).

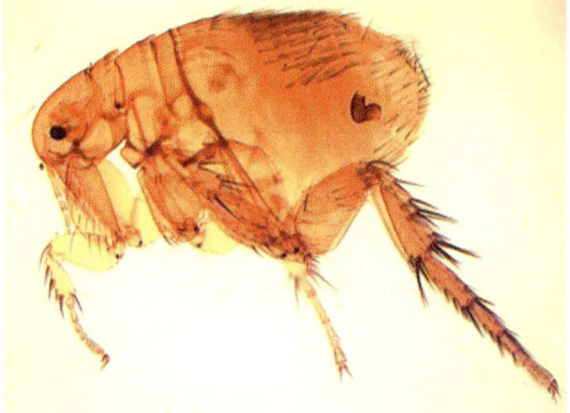

Figure 9.3 Adult oriental rat flea, ***Xenopsylla cheopsis***, the most common vector of murine typhus and plague. *(From Centers for Disease Control and Prevention. https://www.cdc.gov/typhus/murine/index. html. No copyright permission required.)*

Clinical manifestations in mild cases include nonspecific symptoms of fever, malaise, anorexia, headache, cough, abdominal pain, nausea, and vomiting associated with maculopapular rashes in about half of the cases. Moderate-to-severe cases begin with the same early symptoms that progress to later symptoms of febrile chills, myalgia, arthralgia, diarrhea, and pneumonia. Jaundice, coagulopathy, sepsis, and multiorgan failure have been reported in severe cases. The differential diagnosis of murine typhus includes leptospirosis, dengue, brucellosis, ehrlichiosis, and other tick-transmitted infections.

Laboratory diagnostic strategies for confirmation of murine typhus include biopsy of rash, if present, for fluorescent antibody staining for organisms; serological testing for rickettsial antibodies; and polymerase chain reaction (PCR) assays for identification of rickettsial DNA from whole blood, serum, swab, or rash biopsy specimens. Laboratory speciation for *R. typhi* infection will require real-time reverse transcription PCR for specific gene targets, usually only available at reference laboratories.

All cases of murine typhus should be treated with doxycycline. Mild and moderately severe cases may be treated with an oral loading dose of 200 mg of doxycycline followed by 100 mg orally twice a day until the patient has been afebrile for 48 h and has received at least 7 days of treatment. For pediatric and moderate-to-severe cases, intravenous doxycycline may be administered at 2.2 mg/kg/day until fever resolves followed by 2.2 mg/kg/day for a maximum of 7–10 days of treatment. The CDC and others have advised that short courses of doxycycline for up to 10 days do not cause tooth staining or weaken tooth enamel in children (Todd et al., 2015).

In the absence of a vaccine for murine typhus, prevention and control strategies for murine typhus include avoiding contact with infected fleas by applying topical insect repellents, using flea control products for domestic pets, especially cats and dogs; and discouraging potentially infected rodents from residential, work, and recreational spaces by removing nearby brush and debris and sealing all possible openings that encourage rodent entry.

Tungiasis

A currently reemerging, combless, ectoparasitic flea, *Tunga penetrans,* the chigoe or jigger flea, is endemic in the Caribbean and tropical South America, where it originated, and in sub-Saharan Africa, where it was introduced. Tungiasis, a painful, cutaneous infestation with the gravid female jigger flea, is now hyperendemic in underprivileged communities in Africa, South America, and the Caribbean (Ariza et al., 2007; Chadee, 1998; Belaz et al., 2015; Ugbomoiko et al., 2007; Girma et al., 2018). Tungiasis has successfully reemerged in Mexico and Central America; and has been increasingly reported in travelers returning from subtropical and tropical areas worldwide (Ariza et al., 2007; Chadee, 1998; Belaz et al., 2015; Ugbo-moiko et al., 2007; Girma et al., 2018).

Epidemiology

In travelers returning to accessible healthcare infrastructures in developed nations, tungiasis is an exotic infestation, with a minimal parasite burden and a simple surgical cure. However, in the impoverished and underserved rural communities of developing tropical nations, tungiasis is a recurrent infestation with a high parasite burden, causing significant morbidity, including autoamputation of toes and feet.

Myiasis and tungiasis are not rare dermatoses in returning travelers, with most cases acquired in Latin America and Africa. In an outbreak of tungiasis in 13 travelers returning from Madagascar, walking barefoot (100% of cases) and wearing open sandals (62% of cases) were the highest risk factors for tungiasis with a mean clinical incubation period of 15 days or longer than observed in prior case series with incubation periods of 7—12 days (Belaz et al., 2015).

In a community-based cross-sectional study of 366 children, 5—14 years old, in southern Ethiopia, investigators described 215 cases of tungiasis (58.7%) with most lesions on the feet with a similar distribution of cases and lesions in males and females (Girma et al., 2018). The most significant risk factors for tungiasis in children included children of illiterate mothers, children whose mothers had received primary education only, children from cat-owning households, children who only occasionally used footwear, and children who never used footwear (Girma et al., 2018).

Clinical manifestations

Tungiasis is caused by the dermal penetration of the gravid female jigger (chigoe) flea to feed on blood and tissue juices, usually on the feet (or heels), under or near the toenails, or in the interdigital web spaces between the toes (Fig. 9.4). Although the smallest of flea species (1 mm long or shorter), the gravid female jigger flea swells within days with hundreds of developing eggs to 2000 times its size, expelling eggs over a period of 3 weeks or less, and then dying and leaving its shriveled carcass in a contaminated wound tract. Initially, the embedded jigger flea produces a subcutaneous papule or vesicle 6—8 mm in diameter with a central black dot pinpointing its exteriorized segments, including its anus, genital opening, and breathing spiracles (Fig. 9.3 and Fig. 9.4). The papule darkens with intralesional hemorrhage and, if squeezed, extrudes eggs, feces, and internal organs through exteriorized posterior abdominal segments.

Tungiasis is characterized by painful, periungual lesions typically on the toes caused by tissue-feeding gravid female jigger fleas, *Tunga penetrans*.

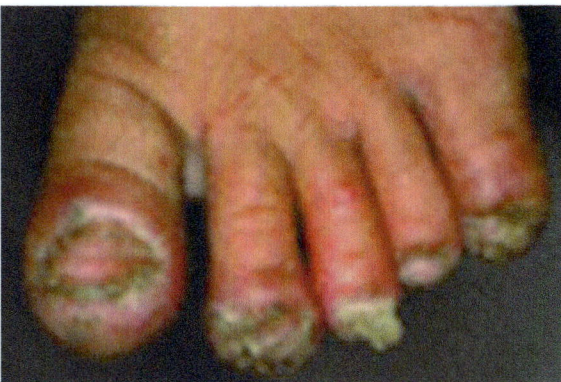

Figure 9.4 Three periungual lesions of tungiasis on the index finger of a 6-year-old girl. These painful lesions were caused by tissue-feeding gravid female jigger fleas, *Tunga penetrans*. *(From Feldmeier H, Eisele M, Sabóia-Moura RC et al. Severe tungiasis in underprivileged communities: case series from Brazil. Emerg Infect Dis. 2003; 9:949–955. No copyright permission required.)*

The differential diagnosis of tungiasis includes bacterial skin infections (impetigo), bacterial and fungal paronychia, cercarial dermatitis, fire ant bites, folliculitis, and scabies. The complications of tungiasis include septicemia, abscesses, fissures, toenail (fingernail) loss, necrotic ulcers, osteomyelitis, and eventual autoamputation of toes and, less often, fingers (Fig. 9.5). Tungiasis is a potential source of entry for tetanus and has been associated with tetanus in nonvaccinated individuals in Africa (Obengui, 1989).

Therapy

Management strategies for tungiasis include extracting all embedded fleas immediately with sterile needles or curettes, administering tetanus prophylaxis, and treating secondary wound infections with appropriate topical or oral antibiotics. Other than surgical extraction, there are no therapeutic options for tungiasis. In a double-blinded, randomized, placebo-controlled trial, investigators demonstrated that a single dose of oral ivermectin, 300 µg/kg repeated at 24 h, had no clinical efficacy compared with placebo as measured by parasite signs of viability or death (Heukelbach et al., 2004).

Given ivermectin's ineffectiveness, there remains a critical need for an effective antiparasitic drug treatment option for tungiasis, especially in superinfestations. Without a standard drug treatment regimen for tungiasis, affected patients can harm themselves by extracting larvae with unsterile instruments and exposing themselves to secondary bacterial infections and bloodborne pathogens. In a search for simple and effective treatments for tungiasis, some investigators have recently recommended topical tea tree oil based on its parsiticidal properties against other ectoparasites, such as head lice and mites (Abrha et al., 2021). Other current investigators found sufficient evidence to continue to recommend to use of occlusive agents and pastes to coax out embedded gravid fleas,

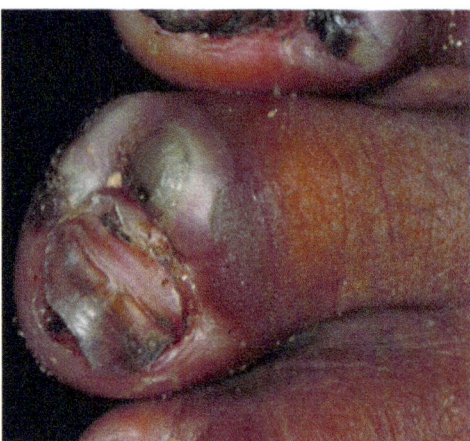

Figure 9.5 Periungual lesion of tungiasis on the fourth toe of a 50-year-old woman. This painfully debilitating lesion on the great toe of a 50-year-old woman was caused by a tissue-feeding gravid female jigger flea, *Tunga penetrans*. The entire great toe nail bed has been elevated by the lesion. *(From Feldmeier H, Eisele M, Sabóia-Moura RC et al. Severe tungiasis in underprivileged communities: case series from Brazil. Emerg Infect Dis. 2003; 9:949–955. No copyright permission required.)*

especially manufactured dimeticone-based products of low viscosity (Tardin Martins et al., 2021).

Prevention and control

In addition to wearing shoes, which can be sprayed with pyrethroid or DEET-containing solutions, and not sitting naked on bare ground, additional preventive strategies for tungiasis include: (1) insecticide treatment of flea-infested domestic and stray animals and pets with 10% pyrethrin or pyrethroid sprays or 1%–4% malathion powder; (2) bathing the feet of domestic and stray dogs and pigs with insecticide solutions, such as 2% trichlorfon; and (3) spraying or dusting households, especially those with dirt or sand floors, with 1%–4% malathion.

Other environmental control strategies for jigger flea infestations include improved stray animal control, especially for cats and dogs; providing cement foundation or slab flooring for dirt-floored homes or building raised homes with solid floors; discouraging stray dogs and cats and other domestic animals, especially pigs, as indoor pets; and spraying rodent and stray animal runways and paths, household unpaved walkways, and dirt floors with solutions containing kerosene, fuel oil, 1% lindane, 1%–4% malathion, or 2% trichlorfon.

Plague

Plague is caused by *Yersina pestis*, a Gram-negative bacillus capable of causing epidemics and pandemics of bubonic, pneumonic, and septicemic plague with high mortality, if not treated with antibiotics. Rodents are the preferred host animal reservoirs for plague bacteria. Infected rodent fleas, especially the oriental rat flea, *Xenopsylla cheopis*, are the arthropod vectors of plague and can transmit plague to other mammals and humans by their blood-feeding bites (Fig. 9.3).

History

There have been three historical plague pandemics beginning with the Justinian Plague in the Sixth Century that killed millions throughout the Roman Empire during the reign of the Emperor Justinian (Raoult et al., 2013). The second pandemic was the Black Death of 14th-century Europe and England with its name derived from septicemic plague-induced hypoperfusion, acrocyanosis, and gangrene of the extremities and nose (Raoult et al., 2013). The third and last pandemic began in China in the late 19th century and killed millions in China and India (Raoult et al., 2013). Plague continues to occur today in arid, rural, regional pockets worldwide including the southwestern United States (US) and, more commonly, in Africa (Madagascar and Uganda) and Asia (India and China) (Raoult et al., 2013). In addition to its animal reservoirs in endemic regions, aerosolized plague is a potential bioterrorism threat.

Ecology

Plague exists in nature in enzootic cycles in endemic regions involving infected rodents and their fleas (Fig. 9.6). Many species of rodents and other wild animals can serve as long-term zoonotic reservoirs of plague including the black rat (*Rattus rattus*), the Norwegian or brown sewer rat (*Rattus norvegicus*), prairie dogs, rock and ground squirrels, chipmunks, mice, voles, and rabbits. Wild and domestic carnivores, especially cats, can become infected with plague by close contact with or eating other small, infected rodents, such as mice and chipmunks. A mass die-off from plague among large numbers of infected rodents, such as in prairie dog colonies, can cause infected fleas to abandon their preferred hosts and to seek alternative blood meals in other mammals and humans (Fig. 9.6). A regional epizootic cycle of plague with animal and human cases tends to occur in the United States during climatic periods with cooler summers that follow wet winters (Kugeler et al., 2015).

This diagram depicts the natural ecology of plague in the United States. Plague exists in nature in enzootic cycles in endemic regions involving infected rodents and their fleas (Left panel) (Fig. 9.6). A mass die-off from plague among large numbers of infected rodents, such as in prairie dog colonies, can cause infected fleas to abandon their preferred hosts and to seek alternative blood meals in other mammals and humans (Right panel).

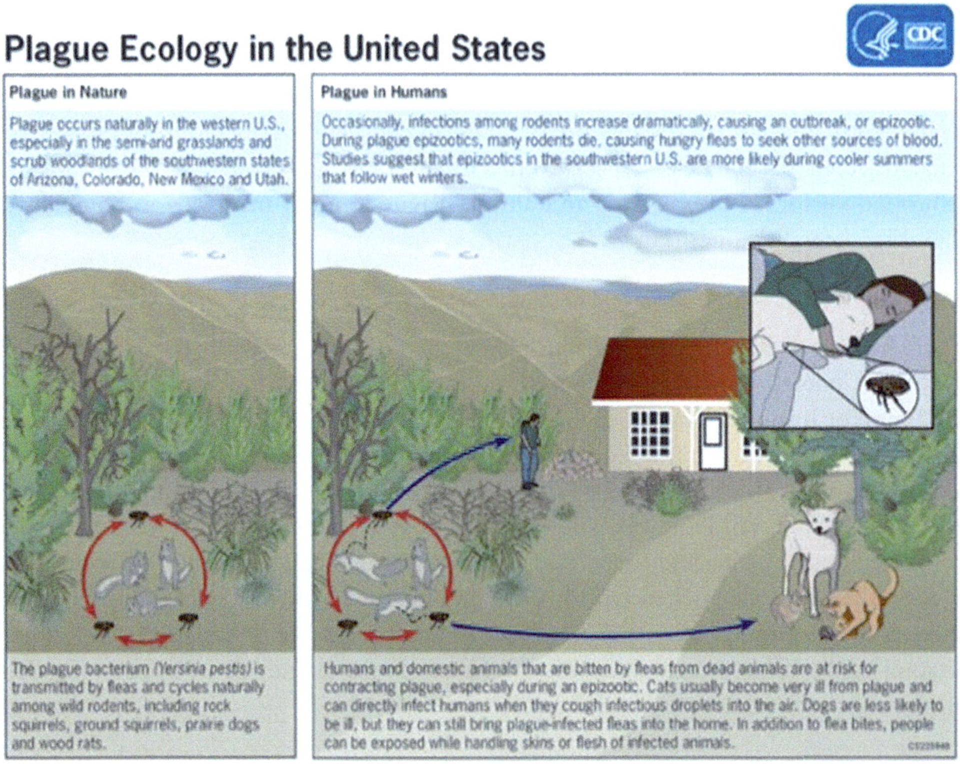

Plague Ecology in the United States

Plague in Nature

Plague occurs naturally in the western U.S., especially in the semi-arid grasslands and scrub woodlands of the southwestern states of Arizona, Colorado, New Mexico and Utah.

Plague in Humans

Occasionally, infections among rodents increase dramatically, causing an outbreak, or epizootic. During plague epizootics, many rodents die, causing hungry fleas to seek other sources of blood. Studies suggest that epizootics in the southwestern U.S. are more likely during cooler summers that follow wet winters.

The plague bacterium (Yersinia pestis) is transmitted by fleas and cycles naturally among wild rodents, including rock squirrels, ground squirrels, prairie dogs and wood rats.

Humans and domestic animals that are bitten by fleas from dead animals are at risk for contracting plague, especially during an epizootic. Cats usually become very ill from plague and can directly infect humans when they cough infectious droplets into the air. Dogs are less likely to be ill, but they can still bring plague-infected fleas into the home. In addition to flea bites, people can be exposed while handling skins or flesh of infected animals.

Figure 9.6 Plague ecology in the United States. Plague exists in nature in enzootic cycles in endemic regions involving infected rodents and their fleas (*Left panel*). A mass die-off from plague among large numbers of infected rodents, such as in prairie dog colonies, can cause infected fleas to abandon their preferred hosts and to seek alternative blood meals in other mammals and humans (*Right panel*). *(From Centers for Disease Control and Prevention. https://www.cdc.gov/plague/transmission/index. html. No copyright permission required.)*

Epidemiology

Plague exhibits a geographic prevalence for warm, arid climates and a seasonal prevalence for the driest seasons, February through August in the United States and September through March in Madagascar. Plague also exhibits a gender preference for males with greater outdoor exposures in endemic regions than females. In the United States, the geographic distribution range of plague is confined to two arid regions: (1) the intersection of the borders of northern New Mexico, northern Arizona, and southern Colorado; and (2) the far West from western Nevada to the Pacific West Coast from southern Oregon to southern California (Fig. 9.7).(Kugeler et al., 2015)

Although flea bites are the most common transmission mechanisms for plague, other mechanisms of transmission include contact, especially with open wounds, with

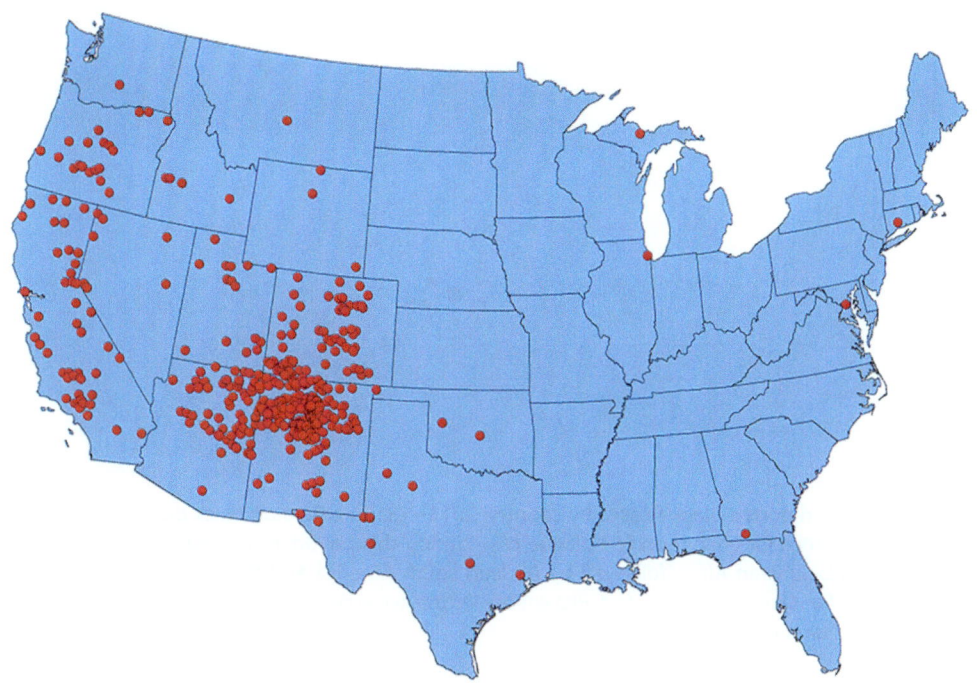

1 dot placed in state of residence for each reported plague case

Figure 9.7 Reported cases of human plague—United States, 1970–2020. One *red dot* is placed in the state of residence for each reported plague case during this period. Most cases of plague are reported from the Pacific Coast and the four corners region of the Southwest where the states of Colorado, Utah, new Mexico, and Arizona share border corners. *(From Centers for Disease Control and Prevention. https://www.cdc.gov/plague/maps/index.html. No copyright permission required.)*

contaminated fluid or tissue from plague-infected wild or domestic animals, consumption of infected animals, and inhalation of infectious respiratory droplets from human or animals, especially cats, with plague pneumonia. Bites and scratches from infected cats can also transmit plague.

Plague can occur in people of all ages, but 50% of United States cases, 80% of which are bubonic plague, occur in young persons, 15–45 years of age, who engage in outdoor activities in endemic areas (Kugeler et al., 2015). An average of seven cases of plague are reported in the United States each year with a range of 1–17 cases per year (Fig. 9.8) (Kugeler et al., 2015).

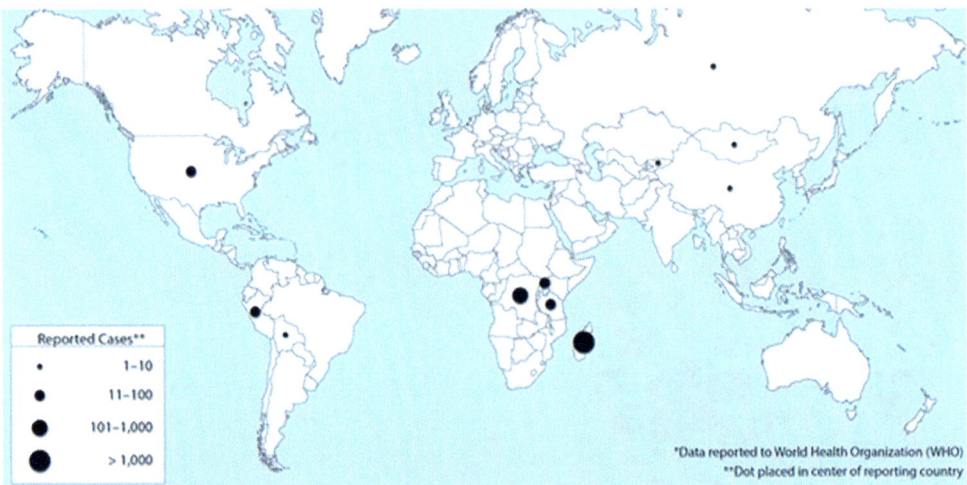

Figure 9.8 WHO-reported plague cases by country, 2013—18. An enlarging black dot is placed in the country of residence for each reported plague case during this period. Most cases of plague are reported from sub-Saharan Africa followed by Andean south America and the western United States. *(From Centers for Disease Control and Prevention. https://www.cdc.gov/plague/maps/index.html. No copyright permission required.)*

In the preantibiotic era, the mortality rate for plague in the United States averaged 66%. In most cases, the mortality was lower for bubonic plague and higher for pneumonic and septicemic plague. With appropriate antibiotic therapy, the overall mortality rate for plague has decreased to 11% in the United States and 8%—10% worldwide according to the World Health Organization (WHO) (Kugeler et al., 2015).

Pathophysiology

When a flea vector blood feeds on a plague-infected rodent, its upper gastrointestinal tract becomes clogged with bacilli causing the flea to bite and feed more often and to regurgitate more *Y. pestis* organisms into new hosts with every bite. Once within the host, *Y. pestis* will avoid human humoral immunity by seeking sanctuary within regional lymph node clusters closest to inoculating flea bites, most commonly among inguinal, axillary, or cervical lymph node groups. Once within lymph nodes, plague bacilli are engulfed by macrophages, propagate until released into the circulation, and incite the three inflammatory, febrile manifestations of plague: bubonic, septicemic, and pneumonic plague.

Clinical manifestations

Although heralding pustular lesions of plague occur at inoculating flea bites in about 25% of cases, they are usually overlooked. Bubonic plague is the most commonly observed clinical manifestation of plague in 80% of patients. Bubonic plague is characterized by painful lymphadenopathy near infected flea bites, and can convert hematogenously to septicemic or pneumonia plague. The incubation period for bubonic plague following an infected flea bite is 2—8 days, but much shorter at 1—3 days for septicemic plague and for pneumonic plague after exposure to *Y. pestis* contaminated respiratory droplets.

Buboes occur in the regional lymph node groupings that drain areas with flea bites, more commonly in the inguinal and axillary regions, than in the cervical node chain (Fig. 9.9). Buboes may be singular or present as clusters of painful, usually nonfluctuant lymph nodes that may suppurate (Fig. 9.9). The regional pain is often so intense that patients avoid movement of the affected extremity or side of the neck. As plague bacteria enter the circulation, buboes will be accompanied by a sudden onset of fever, chills, headache, and weakness. The differential diagnosis of bubonic plague includes all infectious, inflammatory, autoimmune, oncologic, and medication-induced causes of lymphadenopathy or lymphadenitis.

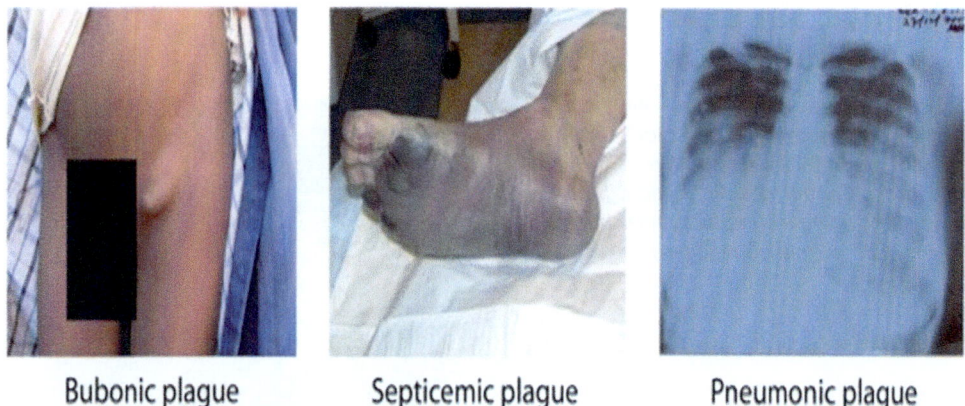

Bubonic plague   Septicemic plague   Pneumonic plague

Figure 9.9 The clinical manifestation of plague include bubonic plague (*Left panel*), septicemic plague with acrocyanosis and gangrene (*middle panel*), and pneumonic plague (*Right panel*, chest X-ray). Bubonic plague, is the most common presenting clinical form of plague. Bubonic plague infects the left inguinal lymph node group in the *left panel*. The plague-transmitting flea bite is most likely on the left leg in this case. (*From Centers for Disease Control and Prevention. https://www.cdc.gov/symptoms/maps/index.html. No copyright permission required.*)

Although bubonic plague may progress to septicemic or pneumonic plague, septicemic plague typically occurs without associated buboes as plague bacteria initially overwhelm humoral immune responses causing tachycardia, hypotension, abdominal pain, hepatosplenomegaly, and coagulopathy progressing to septic shock with high case fatality rates despite antibiotic treatment. Coagulopathy may cause bleeding into skin and tissues with ecchymoses. Septic shock results in vasodilation and peripheral hypoperfusion that may cause acrocyanosis with gangrene of the hands and feet, distal digits, and nasal tip (Black Death) (Fig. 9.10). The differential diagnosis of septicemic plague is very broad and includes all other infectious or inflammatory causes of fever, hypotension, and septic shock.

Primary pneumonic plague may develop from untreated bubonic or septicemic plague, or result secondarily from inhaling infectious droplets from an infected person or animal. Pneumonic plague is characterized by rapidly developing pneumonia with chest pain, dyspnea, and watery, progressing to bloody, sputum with hemoptysis. Pneumonic sepsis can progress to respiratory failure and shock with high case fatality rates despite antibiotic treatment. The differential diagnosis of pneumonic plague is also broad and includes other causes of fever and hemoptysis, such as tuberculosis, bacterial pneumonia, viral bronchitis, pulmonary embolism, and lung cancer.

Pneumonic plague is the most serious manifestation of plague and is the only form of plague that can be transmitted person to person by the inhalation of infectious droplets. Common laboratory abnormalities in plague include significant leukocytosis over 20,000

Figure 9.10 Septicemic plague with distal acrocyanosis from hypoperfusion turning the foot black (black death). *(From Centers for Disease Control and Prevention. https://www.cdc.gov/plague/symptoms/index.html. No copyright permission required.)*

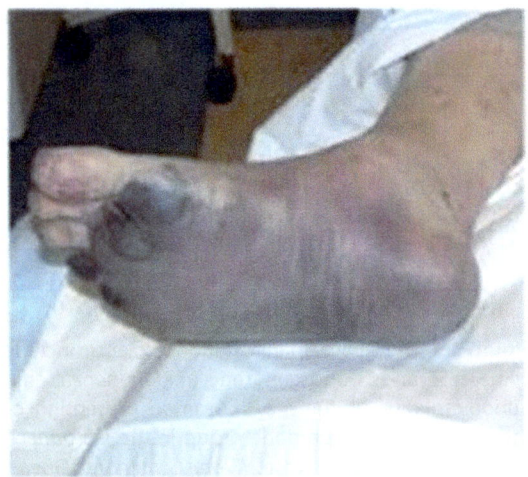

Septicemic plague

per mm (Failoc-Rojas et al., 2018), occasional Dohle bodies within neutrophils, and thrombocytopenia.

Potential complications of delayed treatment include plague meningitis, most commonly, and pharyngitis.

Diagnosis

A presumptive diagnosis of plague should be considered in all cases meeting the following definition: (1) fever following contact with rodents in endemic areas, (2) unexplained painful lymphadenopathy with fever and hypotension, and (3) Gram-negative rods on diagnostic specimens or cultures with a safety-pin shape and bipolar staining with Wright, Giemsa, of Wayson stains (Fig. 9.11). Laboratory personnel should be immediately informed of suspicion of plague in order to receive and analyze diagnostic specimens in a Biosafety Level-3 (BSL-3)-equipped laboratory.

Diagnostic specimens submitted for microscopic examination and culture may include lymph node aspirates from affected buboes, blood cultures, sputum cultures, tracheal and bronchial lavages, bone marrow biopsies, and lymph node and organ biopsies (liver, lung, spleen). In addition to microscopic examination and culture on most media, other laboratory tests often only available in reference labs include acute and convalescent serologic testing for antibodies, rapid direct immunofluorescent antibody testing using the F1 antigen, enzyme linked immunosorbent assay (ELISA), and polymerase chain reaction (PCR) testing to detect plague DNA.

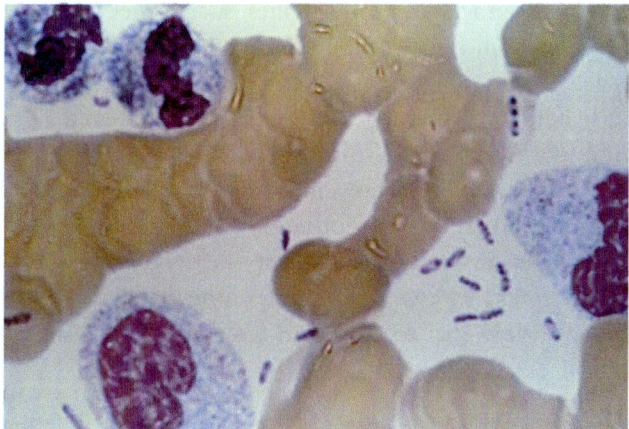

Figure 9.11 Wright-stained peripheral blood sample from a plague victim demonstrating the presence of Yersinia pestis with darkly stained bipolar ends ("safety pins") scattered among red and white blood cells. *(From Centers for Disease Control and Prevention. Public Health Image Library (PHIL). https:// phil.cdc.gov/Details.aspx?pid=2050. No copyright permission required.)*

Therapy

The antibiotic treatment of plague should begin on clinical suspicion and not withheld for laboratory confirmation due to the rapid progression of each disease subtype. Oral or parenteral aminoglycosides are considered first-line treatments with gentamicin now replacing streptomycin. Alternative antibiotics include initially the fluoroquinolones followed by doxycycline, other tetracyclines, and trimethoprim-sulfamethoxazole. Chloramphenicol is the preferred antibiotic for the treatment of plague meningitis. The duration of therapy is 10–14 days. Readers are referred to CDC recommendations for specific doses and routes of administration for the antibiotic treatment of plague with different medications in adults and children (Nelson et al., 2021).

Preexposure chemoprophylaxis is not recommended for first responders and healthcare personnel as long as standard and droplet precautions are followed. Postexposure is recommended for unprotected close contacts with doxycycline, a fluoroquinolone, or trimethoprim-sulfamethoxazole.

Prevention and control

Although new plague vaccines are in development, a plague vaccine is no longer available in the United States. Other prevention and control strategies for plague include the following.

1. Reduce potential rodent habitats around homes, workplaces, and recreational areas by removing brush, rock piles, and firewood.
2. Reduce possible outdoor rodent food supplies, such as pet and wild animal food.
3. Rodent-proof your home and outbuildings by sealing any outside crevices or openings.
4. Wear gloves if handling or skinning a potentially infected animal, such as a rabbit.
5. Wear gloves if disposing of a dead animal.
6. If exposed to fleas, use insect repellents on skin, such as DEET or picaridin, and spray insecticides, such as permethrin, on clothing.
7. Keep fleas off your pets by applying veterinary flea control products.
8. If your pet becomes sick, seek veterinary care immediately.
9. Do not allow dogs or cats that roam free in endemic areas to sleep in your bed.

References

Abrha, S., Tesfaye, W., Thomas, J., 2021. Therapeutic potential of tea tree oil for tungiasis. The American Journal of Tropical Medicine and Hygiene 105 (5), 1157–1162. https://doi.org/10.4269/ajtmh.21-0427.

Ariza, L., Seidenschwang, M., Buckendahl, J., Gomide, M., Feldmeier, H., Heukelbach, J., 2007. Tungiasis: a neglected disease causing severe morbidity in a shantytown in Fortaleza, State of Ceará. Revista da

Sociedade Brasileira de Medicina Tropical 40 (1), 63—67. https://doi.org/10.1590/s0037-8 6822007000100013, 00378682.

Belaz, S., Gay, E., Robert-Gangneux, F., Beaucournu, J.C., Guiguen, C., 2015. Tungiasis outbreak in travelers from Madagascar. Journal of Travel Medicine 22 (4), 263—266. https://doi.org/10.1111/jtm.12217, 17088305.

Boggild, A.K., Keystone, J.S., Kain, K.C., 2002. Furuncular myiasis: a simple and rapid method for extraction of intact Dermatobia hominis larvae. Clinical Infectious Diseases 35 (3), 336—338. https://doi.org/10.1086/341493.

Chadee, D.D., 1998. Tungiasis among five communities south-western Trinidad, in West Indies. Annals of Tropical Medicine and Parasitology 92 (1), 107—113. https://doi.org/10.1080/00034989860238.

Doppler, J.F., Newton, P.N., Lopez, J.E., 2020. A systematic review of the untreated mortality of murine typhus. PLoS Neglected Tropical Diseases 14 (9). https://doi.org/10.1371/journal.pntd.0008641.

Failoc-Rojas, V.E., Molina-Ayasta, C., Salazar-Zuloeta, J., Samame, A., Silva-Diaz, H., 2018. Case Report: myiasis due to cochliomyia hominivorax and dermatobia hominis: clinical and pathological differences between two species in Northern Peru. The American Journal of Tropical Medicine and Hygiene 98 (1), 150—153. https://doi.org/10.4269/ajtmh.16-0437, 00029637.

Fan, T., Zhang, Y., Lv, Y., Chang, J., Bauer, B.A., Yang, J., Wang, C.-W., 2021. Cutaneous myiasis with eosinophilic pleural effusion: a case report. World Journal of Clinical Cases 9 (18), 4803—4809. https://doi.org/10.12998/wjcc.v9.i18.4803.

Girma, M., Astatkie, A., Asnake, S., 2018. Prevalence and risk factors of tungiasis among children of Wensho district, southern Ethiopia. BMC Infectious Diseases 18 (1). https://doi.org/10.1186/s12879-018-3373-5, 14712334.

Heukelbach, J., Franck, S., Feldmeier, H., 2004. Therapy of tungiasis: a double-blinded randomized controlled trial with oral ivermectin. Memórias do Instituto Oswaldo Cruz 99 (8), 873—876. https://doi.org/10.1590/s0074-02762004000800015.

Kugeler, K.J., Staples, J.E., Hinckley, A.F., Gage, K.L., Mead, P.S., 2015. Epidemiology of human plague in the United States, 1900—2012. Emerging Infectious Diseases 21 (1), 16—22. https://doi.org/10.3201/eid2101.140564, 10806059.

Lachish, T., Marhoom, E., Mumcuoglu, K.Y., Tandlich, M., Schwartz, E., 2015. Myiasis in travelers. Journal of Travel Medicine 22 (4), 232—236. https://doi.org/10.1111/jtm.12203, 17088305.

Loong, P.T.L., Lui, H., Buck, H.W., 1992. Cutaneous myiasis: a simple and effective technique for extraction of dermatobia hominis larvae. International Journal of Dermatology 31 (9), 657—659. https://doi.org/10.1111/j.1365-4362.1992.tb03990.x, 13654632.

Marquez, A.T., Mattos, M.D.S., Nascimento, S.B., 2007. Myiasis associated with some socioeconomic factors in five urban areas of the State of Rio de Janeiro. Revista da Sociedade Brasileira de Medicina Tropical 40 (2), 175—180. https://doi.org/10.1590/s0037-86822007000200006, 00378682.

Nelson, C.A., Meaney-Delman, D., Fleck-Derderian, S., Cooley, K.M., Yu, P.A., Mead, P.S., 2021. Antimicrobial treatment and prophylaxis of plague: recommendations for naturally acquired infections and bioterrorism response. MMWR. Recommendations and Reports 70 (3), 1—27. https://doi.org/10.15585/mmwr.rr7003a1.

Obengui, 1989. Tungiasis and tetanus at the university hospital center in Brazzaville. Dakar Medical 34 (1—4), 44—48, 00491101.

Plotinsky, R.N., Talbot, E.A., Davis, H., 2007. Short report: Cuterebra cutaneous myiasis, New Hampshire, 2004. The American Journal of Tropical Medicine and Hygiene 76 (3), 596—597. https://doi.org/10.4269/ajtmh.2007.76.596, 00029637.

Raoult, D., Mouffok, N., Bitam, I., Piarroux, R., Drancourt, M., 2013. Plague: history and contemporary analysis. Journal of Infection 66 (1), 18—26. https://doi.org/10.1016/j.jinf.2012.09.010, 01634453.

Serafim, R.A., Do Espírito Santo, R.B., De Mello, R.A.F., Collin, S.M., Deps, P.D., 2020. Case report: nasal myiasis in an elderly patient with atrophic rhinitis and facial sequelae of leprosy. The American Journal of Tropical Medicine and Hygiene 102 (2), 448—450. https://doi.org/10.4269/ajtmh.19-0708, 00029637.

Shorter, N., Werninghaus, K., Mooney, D., Graham, A., 1997. Furuncular cuterebrid myiasis. Journal of Pediatric Surgery 32 (10), 1511—1513. https://doi.org/10.1016/s0022-3468(97)90579-0, 00223468.

Singh, A., Singh, Z., 2015. Incidence of myiasis among humans—a review. Parasitology Research 114 (9), 3183—3199. https://doi.org/10.1007/s00436-015-4620-y.

Tardin Martins, A.C., de Brito, A.R., Kurizky, P.S., Gonçalves, R.G., Santana, Y.R.T., de Carvalho, F.C.A., Gomes, C.M., Vinetz, J.M., 2021. The efficacy of topical, oral and surgical interventions for the treatment of tungiasis: a systematic review of the literature. PLoS Neglected Tropical Diseases 15 (8). https://doi.org/10.1371/journal.pntd.0009722.

Todd, S.R., Dahlgren, F.S., Traeger, M.S., Beltrán-Aguilar, E.D., Marianos, D.W., Hamilton, C., McQuiston, J.H., Regan, J.J., 2015. No visible dental staining in children treated with doxycycline for suspected rocky mountain spotted fever. The Journal of Pediatrics 166 (5), 1246—1251. https://doi.org/10.1016/j.jpeds.2015.02.015, 10976833.

Ugbomoiko, U.S., Ofoezie, I.E., Heukelbach, J., 2007. Tungiasis: high prevalence, parasite load, and morbidity in a rural community in Lagos State, Nigeria. International Journal of Dermatology 46 (5), 475—481. https://doi.org/10.1111/j.1365-4632.2007.03245.x, 13654632.

Yasukawa, K., Dass, K., 2020. Myiasis due to Cordylobia anthropophaga. The American Journal of Tropical Medicine and Hygiene 102 (2). https://doi.org/10.4269/ajtmh.19-0579, 251-251.

CHAPTER 10

Tick-transmitted bacterial diseases

Introduction

Ticks are the most competent and versatile of all arthropod vectors of zoonotic infectious diseases for several reasons. First, ticks are not afflicted by the microorganisms that they can transmit or the paralytic salivary toxins that they can inject during blood feeding. Second, and unlike mosquitoes, ticks can transmit the broadest range of infectious microbes among all arthropods, including bacteria, viruses, and protozoans. In addition, tick-transmitted coinfections are increasing and complicate differential diagnosis and antimicrobial treatment. Third, ticks can vertically transmit infectious microorganisms congenitally to their offspring of both genders (transovarian transmission) and then transmit asymptomatic carrier infections among all of their generational growth stages (transstadial transmission). Tickborne infectious diseases can also be transmitted to humans by blood transfusions and organ and tissue transplants. In summary, ticks of all ages and both genders may remain infectious for generations without having to reacquire infections from their zoonotic reservoirs, and climatic and behavioral changes place humans and ticks outdoors together for longer periods for disease transmission.

Vector behavior

Ticks exhibit many competitive advantages afforded them by evolving changes in climate and human behavior. The most important advantages include (1) a wider geographic distribution with longer active breeding and blood-feeding seasons as a result of increases in global mean temperatures and humidity; (2) a greater abundance of wild animal reservoir hosts no longer effectively controlled, especially deer and rodents; (3) increased habitat afforded by residential construction in recently cleared woodlands adjacent to pastures, parks, recreational facilities, and residential neighborhoods and school yards frequented by wildlife, domestic animals, and humans; and (4) more vacation and leisure-time activities enjoyed by humans and their domestic pets during prolonged tick activity seasons, especially April through November.

Biology and taxonomy

Ticks are classified into three families: the Ixodidae, or hard ticks; the Argasidae, or soft ticks; and the Nuttalliellidae, a lesser known family with characteristics of both hard and soft ticks. Ixodid ticks have a hard dorsal plate or shield (scutum), which is absent in the

Ectoparasitic Diseases
ISBN 978-0-443-26724-6
https://doi.org/10.1016/B978-0-443-26724-6.00010-2

soft-bodied, argasid ticks. Ixodid ticks also exhibit more sexual dimorphism than argasid ticks, with both genders looking alike. However, all blood-fed ticks, especially females, are capable of enormous expansion, and engorged ixodid females resemble engorged argasid females. Although ticks from all families can serve as infectious disease vectors, the ixodid or hard ticks are responsible for most tickborne diseases in the United States and worldwide.

Ixodid ticks live in open exposed environments, such as woodlands, grasslands, meadows, and scrub brush areas. Argasid ticks prefer to live in more sheltered environments, including rodent burrows, caves, crevices, woodpiles, and uninhabited rural and mountain cabins. Ticks are attracted to warm-blooded hosts by vibration and exhaled carbon dioxide. Ixodid ticks actually "quest" for hosts by climbing onto vegetation with their forelegs outstretched and waving, waiting to embrace passing hosts (Fig. 10.1).

There are four stages in the tick life cycle: egg, six-legged larva, nymph, and adult. With the exception of hollow hypostomes for blood-feeding and clawless palps, adult ticks resemble large mites with eight legs and disk-shaped bodies. Ixodid ticks have mouth parts that are attached anteriorly and visible dorsally. Argasid ticks are leathery and wrinkled in external appearance and have subterminally attached mouthparts that are not visible dorsally. All ticks feed by cutting a small hole in the host's epidermis with their sharp chelicerae and then inserting their hypostomes into the cut painlessly with blood flow maintained in a feeding pool by salivary local anesthetics and anticoagulants. Argasid ticks blood-feed rapidly for minutes to hours and then drop off, while ixodid ticks blood-feed for days (average 6–12 days) before dropping off for mating and egg-laying. Although ticks spend relatively short periods of their long lives mating,

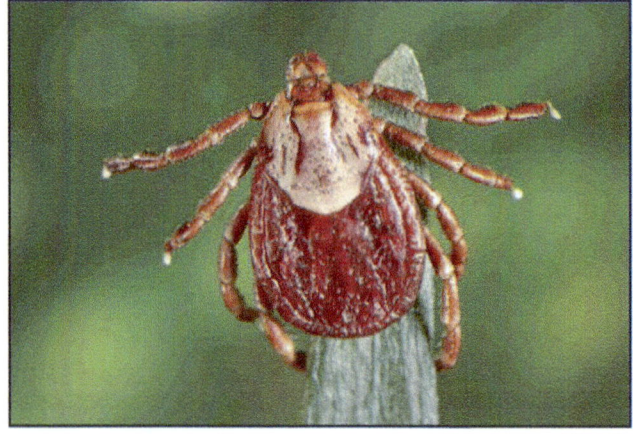

Figure 10.1 Female ***Dermacentor andersoni***, the Rocky mountain wood tick, questing for a host. The Rocky mountain wood tick is the preferred tick vector for *Rickettsia rickettsii*, the causative riskettsial agent of Rocky mountain spotted fever (RMSF) in the USA and the Canadian southwest. Today, most cases of RMSF occur east of the Rocky mountains. *(From Biggs, H.M., Behravesh, C.B., Bradley, K.K., et al. 2016. Diagnosis and management of tickborne rickettsial diseases: Rocky Mountain spotted fever and other spotted fever group rickettsioses, ehrlichioses, and anaplasmosis—United States. MMWR Recomm. Rep. 65, 1–44. CDC. Public Domain. No permission required.)*

egg-laying, and blood-feeding on their hosts, tick feeding behaviors can influence pathogen transmission with longer blood-feeding promoting more effective transmission of pathogens.

Epidemiology

Tickborne infectious diseases have challenged researchers and physicians ever since Theobald Smith (1859—1934) and Frederick Kilbourne (1858—1934) identified the tick as the vector for transmission of *Babesia bigemina,* the apicomplexan hemoprotozoan causing Texas cattle fever (Vannier et al., 1997). The researchers named the pathogen for Victor Babes (1854—1926), who first described babesiosis in cattle with a syndrome of hemolytic anemia, hemoglobinuria, and jaundice (Vannier et al., 1997). The research experiments conducted by Smith and Kilbourne over the period 1889—93 firmly established for the first time the transmission of a pathogen by a tick vector (Vannier et al., 1997).

Later, Howard T. Ricketts, M.D., (1871—1910), first identified the wood tick, *Dermacentor andersoni,* as the vector of Rocky Mountain spotted fever (RMSF) in 1906, and confirmed the insect vector theory of infectious disease transmission (Fig. 10.1).

The emergence and recognition of Lyme disease, or, more specifically, Lyme borreliosis (LB), in the United States in the 1970s, sparked renewed interest in tickborne diseases throughout the United States and Europe. The causative agent of LB was later identified as the spirochete, *Borrelia burgdorferi,* in 1982 (Fig. 10.2). By the early 1990s, LB had become the most common arthropod-borne infectious disease in the United States and Europe Fig. 10.2.

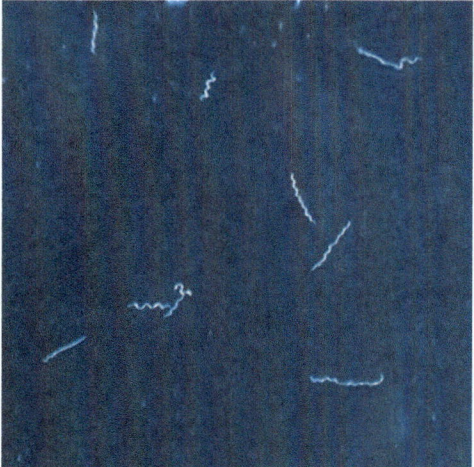

Figure 10.2 *Borrelia burgdorferi,* the causative bacterium of Lyme disease. Note the characteristic coiled spring appearance of a spirochete (peripheral blood smear, immunofluorescence stain under darkfield microscopy, ×1000). *(From Public Health Image Library. Atlanta, G.A. Centers for Disease Control and Prevention. Courtesy Dr. Robert D. Gilmore. CDC Public Domain. No Permission needed.)*

Figure 10.3 *Amblyomma americanum,* the lone star tick, perched on a blade of grass and questing for a host. Shown is the dorsal view of a female lone star tick, *Amblyomma americanum,* the vector of southern tick-associated rash illness (STARI) caused by the spirochete *Borrelia lonestari.* Note the "lone star" mark resembling the Texas lone star in the center of the dorsal shield or scutum. *(From Public Health Image Library. Image 8683. Atlanta, GA: Centers for Disease Control and Prevention. CDC. Public Domain. No Permission needed.)*

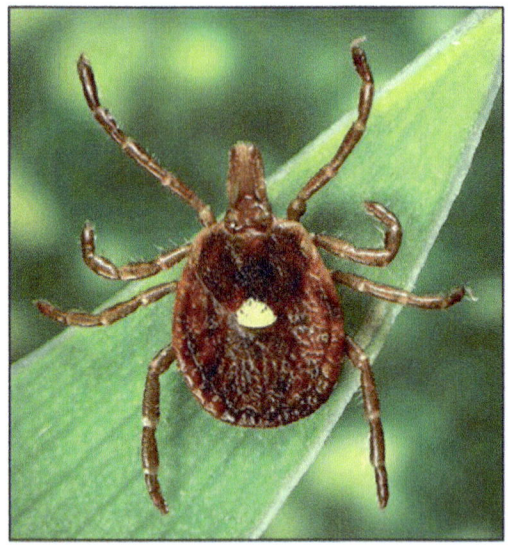

In 1997, investigators described another tickborne illness also characterized by an LB-like erythema migrans rash in North Carolina, a nonendemic area for LB (Vannier et al., 1997). The Lone Star tick, *Amblyomma americanum,* was identified as the vector of the new disease, which was named the southern tick-associated rash illness (STARI) (Fig. 10.3) (Vannier et al., 1997, 2015). The causative pathogen of STARI was identified in 2004 as a new *Borrelia* species and named *B. lonestari* (Kirkland et al., 1997).

By the 1980s and 1990s, the causative agents of the ehrlichioses were recognized as newly emerging, *Rickettsia*-like species, and later, they were completely reorganized into two separate genera, *Anaplasma* and *Ehrlichia.* By 2004, five new spotted fever (SF)-causing rickettsiae were described, four new subspecies of the LB-causing *B. burgdorferi* complex were identified, a new relapsing fever-carrying *Borrelia* species was isolated, and anaplasmosis was exported to Europe from the United States. In a seemingly unending era of discoveries of tick-transmitted diseases, another new and unanticipated vector for RMSF, the brown dog tick, *Rhipicephalus sanguineus* (Fig. 10.4). was identified in the desert Southwest in 2005 and rapidly expanded its range of distribution into Texas and northern Mexico (Masters et al., 2008).

In 2011, the first human cases of relapsing fever caused by tick-transmitted *Borrelia miyamotoi* were reported from Russia. In 2013, 1%—3% of surveyed residents of New England states where LB is hyperendemic were seropositive for prior *B. miyamotoi* infections (Blanton et al., 2008; Varela et al., 2004; Demma et al., 2005). Since 2011, more than 50 patients with acute febrile illnesses resembling LB, but without erythema migrans, have been reported from this region as having *B. miyamotoi* infections (Blanton et al., 2008; Varela et al., 2004; Demma et al., 2005).

In most cases, patients presented with an influenza-like constellation of symptoms including fever, malaise, fatigue, headache, myalgias, and arthralgias. This initial clinical presentation more closely resembled other hard tick—transmitted diseases, such as

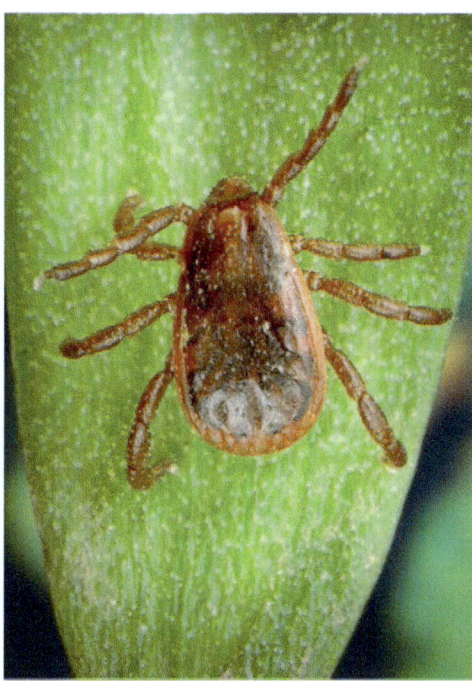

Figure 10.4 *Rhipicephalus sanguineus,* the brown dog tick, perched on a blade of grass and questing for a host. This is a dorsal view of a male tick, a new and unanticipated vector for Rocky mountain spotted fever in addition to the two historical vectors *Dermacentor andersoni,* the Rocky mountain wood tick, and *Dermacentor variabilis,* the American dog tick. *(From Public Health Image Library. Image 7646. Atlanta, GA: Centers for Disease Control and Prevention. CDC. Public Domain. No Permission needed.)*

anaplasmosis and LB without a significant rash. *B. miyamotoi* infections are transmitted by the same ticks that carry Lyme borreliosis: *Ixodes scapularis,* the eastern blacklegged tick (Fig. 10.5), and *Ixodes pacificus,* the western blacklegged tick (Fig. 10.6) (Blanton et al., 2008; Varela et al., 2004; Demma et al., 2005).

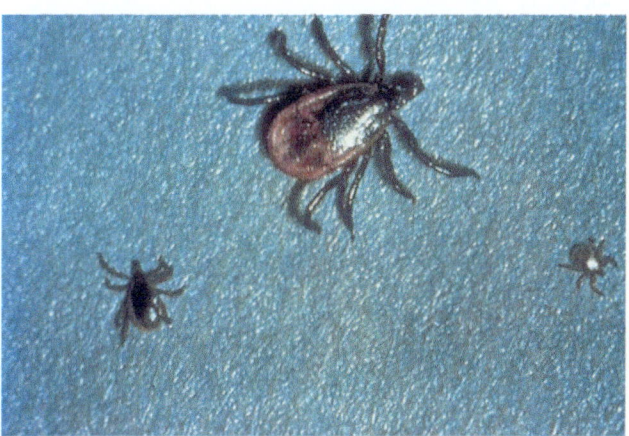

Figure 10.5 *Ixodes scapularis,* the eastern black-legged tick, adult female (top), with two nymphs (below). These are arthropod vectors of babesiosis Lyme disease or Lyme borreliosis (LB), and B. miyamoti, especially the diminutive nymphs, whose bites most often go unnoticed. *(From Public Health Image Library. Image 1205. Atlanta, GA: Centers for Disease Control and Prevention. CDC. Public Domain. No Permission needed.)*

Figure 10.6 A female *Ixodes pacificus*, the western black-legged tick, perched on a blade of grass and questing for a host. *I. pacificus* is the preferred tick vector for the transmission of *Borrelia* spirochetal infections, including *B. burgdorferi*, the causative agent of Lyme borreliosis, and *B. miyamotoi*, the causative agent of a Lyme disease—like borreliosis without the characteristic bull's eye-shaped erythema migrans rash of LB, along the US Pacific coast and west of the Rocky mountains. *(From Biggs, H.M., Behravesh, C.B., Bradley, K.K., et al. 2016. Diagnosis and management of tick-borne rickettsial diseases: Rocky Mountain spotted fever and other spotted fever group rickettsioses, ehrlichioses, and anaplasmosis—United States. MMWR Recomm. Rep. 65, 1—44. CDC. Public Domain. No Permission needed.)*

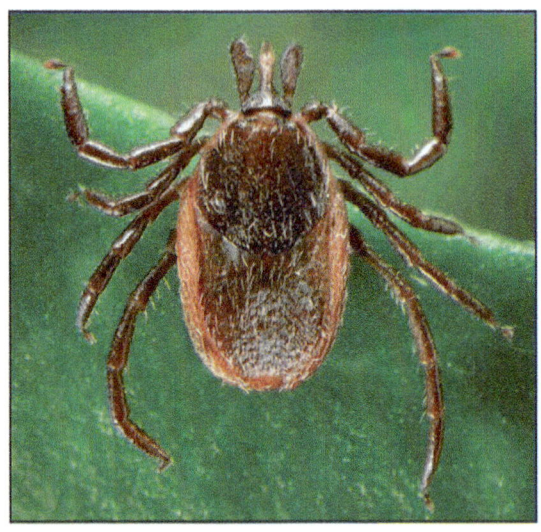

In July 2008, four patients with a tick bite—appearing eschars, lymphadenitis, and regional lymphadenopathy were reported in northern California. An afebrile, "spotless" rickettsial disease was suspected (Krause et al., 2013). Convalescent sera from all four patients exhibited cross-reacting antibodies to *Rickettsia rickettsii,* the RMSF pathogen and to *Rickettsia* 364D (proposed name, *R.philipii*), a newly described SF group rickettsia (Krause et al., 2013). Rickettsia 364D was later detected in a new tick vector, the Pacific Coast tick, *Dermacentor occidentalis* (Fig. 10.7) (Krause et al., 2013).

Figure 10.7 *Dermacentor occidentalis,* the Pacific coast tick, adult female. The Pacific coast tick, has now been identified as the tick vector of *Rickettsia* 364D (*Rickettsia philipii* [proposed]) rickettsiosis in California, which has been described as a "spotless" fever with a tick-bite eschar. *(From Shapiro, M.R., Fritz, C.L., Tait, K., et al. 2010. Rickettsia 364D: a newly recognized cause of eschar-associated illness in California. Clin. Infect. Dis. 50, 541—548; and Centers for Disease Control and Prevention, Atlanta, GA. Photographs courtesy James Gathany. CDC. Public Domain. No Permission needed.)*

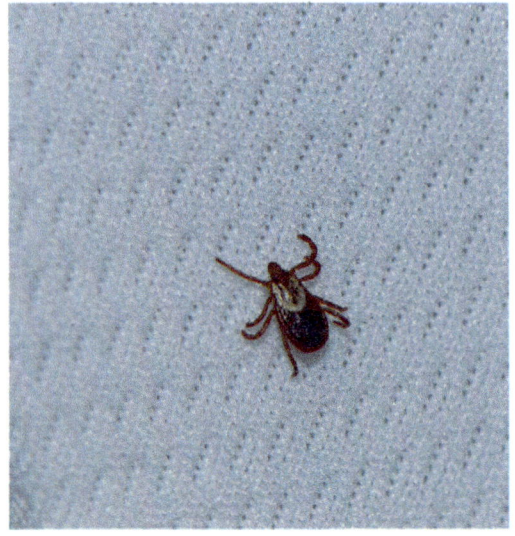

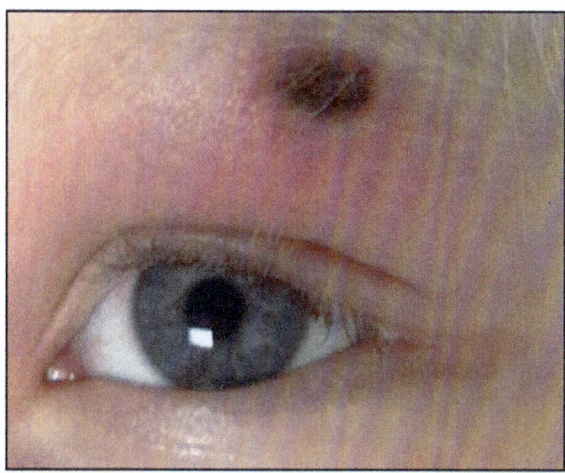

Figure 10.8 Rickettsia 364D eschar. A pediatric patient in California with a tick-bite eschar on the left brow from the newly discovered rickettsial species ***Rickettsia 364D*** transmitted by the bite of an infected Pacific coast tick (***Dermacentor occidentalis***). *(From Biggs, H.M., Behravesh, C.B., Bradley, K.K., et al. 2016. Diagnosis and management of tickborne rickettsial diseases: Rocky Mountain spotted fever and other spotted fever group rickettsioses, ehrlichioses, and anaplasmosis—United States. MMWR Recomm. Rep. 65, 1–44. Photo courtesy Samantha, H., Johnson, M.D., Oakland Children's Hospital and Research Center, Oakland, CA. CDC. Public Domain. No Permission needed.)*

In July 2008, four patients with a tick bite—appearing eschars, lymphadenitis, and regional lymphadenopathy were reported in northern California. An afebrile, "spotless" rickettsial disease was suspected (Krause et al., 2013). Convalescent sera from all four patients exhibited cross-reacting antibodies to *Rickettsia rickettsii,* the RMSF pathogen and to *Rickettsia* 364D (proposed name, *R.philipii*), a newly described SF group rickettsia (Krause et al., 2013). Rickettsia 364D was later detected in a new tick vector, the Pacific Coast tick, *Dermacentor occidentalis* (Fig. 10.7) (Krause et al., 2013) (Fig. 10.8).

Blood product—transmitted infections have now been described for the tickborne rickettsial diseases, Q fever, babesiosis, anaplasmosis, and ehrlichiosis. These diseases have also been transmitted by organ transplants, and Q fever has been transmitted by infectious aerosols from slaughterhouses.

Several tickborne infectious diseases have now been reclassified by the United States Centers for Disease Control and Prevention (CDC) as potential biological terrorism agents, including *Francisella tularensis* (tularemia), a category A agent (highly likely microorganism to be weaponized); *Coxiella burnetii* (Q fever), a category B agent (less likely to be weaponized); and the tickborne encephalitis and hemorrhagic fever viruses, category C agents (least likely to be weaponized) (Otsuki et al., 2020).

Borrelioses

The borrelioses are a large group of tickborne spirochetal diseases caused by several species of *Borrelia,* with unique geographic distributions, tick vectors, and host animal reservoirs. The borrelioses are stratified into three separate epidemiologic and clinical presentations: Lyme borreliosis (LB), southern tick-associated rash illness (STARI), and the tickborne relapsing fevers (TBRFs) (Table 10.1).

Table 10.1 Clinicopathophysiologic comparison of Lyme borreliosis, southern tick-associated rash illness (STARI), and tickborne relapsing fever.

Infectious disease characteristics	Lyme borreliosis	Southern tick-associated rash illness	Tickborne relapsing fever
Microbial agents	*Borrelia burgdorferi* (United States, Europe), *B. afzelii* (Europe, Asia), *B. garinii* (Europe, Asia)	*Borrelia lonestari* has now been isolated from a skin biopsy of a patient with STARI and cultured in vitro from infected *Amblyomma americanum* ticks	*Ornithodoros* species of soft ticks
Preferred tick vectors	*Ixodes* spp. hard ticks	*A. americanum*	*Ornithodoros* spp. soft ticks
Preferred animal reservoirs	Rodents (nymphs); deer, birds (adults)	Lizards	Rodents (nymphs); humans (*B. duttonii* only); deer, birds (adults)
Endemicity	Highly endemic in United States and Europe	Southeastern United States	Highly endemic among vector-populated regions worldwide
Fever ≤39°C (102.2°F)	Very uncommon	Absent; low-grade fever may occur rarely	Present in relapsing episodes 1–3 days each; may reach 43°C (109.4°F)
Relapsing fevers	Not present	Not present	Present
Erythema migrans, or other rash	Present as annular or target-like maculopapular rash (mean diameter, 7 cm); more common on extremities	Present and mimics that of Lyme disease but with a smaller mean diameter of 4.5 cm; more common on trunk	Absent
Arthritis	May be present in untreated (up to 60%) late, or "chronic" infections, manifesting as oligoarthritis	Arthralgias, myalgias, and neck stiffness may occur less commonly than with Lyme disease; no chronic arthritic complications	Neck stiffness, arthralgias, myalgias common, not arthritis

Neurologic manifestations	May be present in up to 15% of cases; include headache, neuritis of cranial nerve (CN) VII (Bell palsy)	Dizziness, headache, memory loss, concentration difficulty may occur; no chronic neurologic complications	Common: Meningitis, meningoencephalitis; neuritis of CN VII (Bell palsy); neuritis of CN VIII (deafness, myelitis, radiculopathy)
Other presenting clinical manifestations	Myocarditis, conduction defects in up to 8% of late-onset and "chronic" cases	Regional lymphadenopathy may occur; chronic complications have not been described	Splenomegaly in most, hepatomegaly in 10% of cases; myocarditis manifesting as prolonged QTc interval
Best screening serodiagnostics	Giemsa- or Wright-stained peripheral smear, phase-contrast, or darkfield microscopy for spirochetes; ELISA, IFA	Epidemiologic and clinical presentation; no screening serodiagnostics available at present; Lyme disease ruled out by ELISA, IFA, western immunoblot	Giemsa- or Wright-stained peripheral smear, phase-contrast, or darkfield microscopy for spirochetes; ELISA, IFA
Best confirmatory diagnostics	In vitro cultivation, western immunoblot, PCR assay	PCR assay on skin biopsy; in vitro cultivation	In vitro cultivation (not recommended; Biosafety level 3 laboratory required), rodent inoculation, PCR assay
Recommended antibiotic therapy	Doxycycline, 100 mg PO bid, or amoxicillin, 500 mg PO tid, for 14–21 d; parenteral therapy for CNS involvement	Doxycycline, 100 mg PO bid, or amoxicillin, 500 mg PO tid, for 14–21 d	Tetracycline, 500 mg or 12.5 mg/kg PO qid, or doxycycline, 100 mg PO bid, or erythromycin, 500 mg or 12.5 mg/kg PO qid for 10 d; parenteral therapy with penicillin G or ceftriaxone recommended for CNS involvement

CNS, Central nervous system; ELISA, enzyme-linked immunosorbent assay; IFA, immunofluorescence assay; PCR, polymerase chain reaction.
Adapted from Diaz, J.H., 2019. Section on Ectoparasitic Diseases. Chapter 296. Ticks (Including Tick Paralysis). In: Bennett, J.E., Dolin, R., Blaser, M.J. (Eds.), *Mandell, Douglas and Bennett's Principles and Practice of Infectious Diseases*, Ninth Edition, Elsevier, Philadelphia. Elsevier publication.

Lyme borreliosis

Lyme disease, or Lyme borreliosis (LB), is now the most common tickborne infectious disease in the Northern Hemisphere and the most common arthropod-borne infectious disease in the United States and Europe (Yu et al., 2017; Yamanaka et al., 2020). In the United States, LB is caused by *Borrelia burgdorferi* sensu stricto, first identified as a novel bacterial spirochete in 1982, and transmitted to humans by *Ixodes* species hard ticks in regional pockets, specifically the Northeast *(I. scapularis),* upper Midwest *(I. scapularis),* and Pacific Coast *(I. pacificus)* (Figs. 10.2, 10.5 and 10.6) (Yu et al., 2017; Yamanaka et al., 2020).

Most cases of LB in Europe and northern Asia are caused by *Borrelia afzelii* and *Borrelia garinii.* Collectively, the three *Borrelia* species are often referred to as *B. burgdorferi* sensu lato (Yu et al., 2017). Ticks usually acquire *Borrelia* infections as larvae or nymphs by blood-feeding on small reservoir hosts, most commonly birds and rodents. *Borrelia* organisms are further maintained in nature as infected adult *Ixodes* ticks blood-feed on larger mammals, especially deer. Infected ixodid ticks transmit LB to humans during blood-feeding, and bites by nymphal ticks often go unnoticed.

Because *Borrelia* spirochetes must migrate from the tick's midgut to the salivary glands during blood-feeding, tick attachments for less than 24 h rarely result in LB in humans. After an incubation period of 1—2 weeks, the hallmark of spirochete transmission manifests as solitary erythema migrans, a maculopapular erythematous rash with a bull's-eye or target pattern, at the site of tick attachment (Fig. 10.9) (Yu et al., 2017; Schwartz, no date). Erythema migrans in LB results from the subcutaneous centrifugal movement of the spirochetes from the bite sites to the central circulation and target organs (Figs. 10.3 and 10.9) (Yu et al., 2017; Schwartz, no date), An erythema migrans-like rash not necessarily in a target pattern also occurs in STARI at the site of *A. americanum* (Lone Star tick) attachment, but the underlying mechanisms responsible for the rash in STARI are unclear (Schwartz, no date).

In a meta-analysis of 53 longitudinal studies of LB in the United States and Europe, Tibbles and Edlow (Schwartz, no date) reported that many patients did not recall a tick bite (74% in the United States and 36% in Europe). However, constitutional symptoms of low-grade fever (<39°C [102.2°F]) and headache were common, nausea and vomiting were rare, and a solitary erythema migrans lesion was the most common initial presentation (81% in the USA and 88% in Europe) (Schwartz, no date). If LB is recognized and treated early in the erythema migrans stage, cure rates will exceed 90%, and outcomes will be excellent (Table 10.1) (Yu et al., 2017; Schwartz, no date)

A total of 265,589 cases of LB were reported to the CDC during 2008—2015 with 208,834 cases confirmed and 66,755 probable (Yu et al., 2017). Most cases were reported from the highest incidence states in the Northeast, Mid-Atlantic, and Upper Midwest with the case counts remaining stable or falling in these states over the reporting period

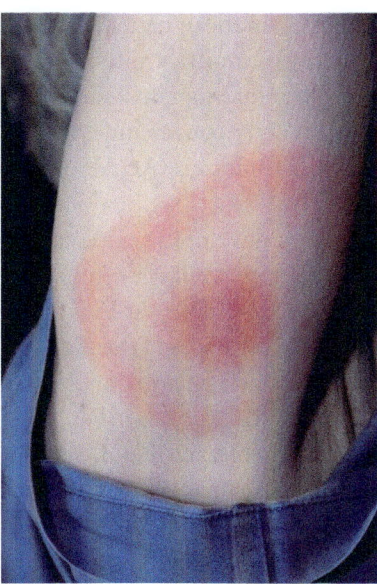

Figure 10.9 Erythema migrans, the characteristic bull's eye-pattern rash of Lyme disease or Lyme bor-reliosis (LB). Shown is the pathognomonic concentric red "bull's-eye" or target-shaped rash at the bite sites of *Borrelia burgdorferi*– or *B. lonestari*–infected ixodid ticks, tick vectors of Lyme disease and southern tick-associated rash illness (STARI), respectively, in endemic regions of the United States. *(From Public Health Image Library. Image 9875. Atlanta, GA: Centers for Disease Control and Prevention. CDC. Public Domain. No Permission needed.)*

(Yu et al., 2017). Case counts actually increased in states bordering high incidence states confirming a contiguous expansion of LB-endemic regions in the United States (Yu et al., 2017). In the high incidence states, the demographic characteristics of confirmed cases were similar to those described previously with greater incidences in males and bimodal age distribution peaks in children and older adults (Yu et al., 2017). In contrast, neighboring low incidence states reported greater incidences among females than males and among older adults (Yu et al., 2017). Although deaths from LB were rate, 1.5% developed carditis, and 12.5% had neurological manifestations, most commonly facial nerve palsies (8.4%) (Yu et al., 2017).

Europe reports fewer cases of LB per year, around 200,000, than the USA with most cases reported from forested regions in the Scandinavian and Baltic nations and western and central Europe. As noted, most cases of LB in Europe are caused by *B. afzelli* and *B. garinii*, which are not found in the United States, where *B. burgdorferi* causes most cases of LB. These strain differences in causative pathogens are responsible for the variations in the clinical presentations of LB in the United States and Europe.

Although erythema migrans remains the most common initial cutaneous manifestation of LB in the United States and Europe, American patients are less likely to recall a tick bite than European patients. American patients also report more concomitant systemic symptoms. Incubation periods from tick bite to lesions are shorter in the United States, and central clearing of erythema migrans lesions in less common in the United States. In addition, two additional cutaneous manifestations of LB, borrelial lymphocytoma and acrodermatitis chronica atrophicans (ACA), occur in European and not American cases (Fig. 10.10).

Borrelial lymphocytoma usually develops as an area of induration on the nipple in adults and on the ear lobe in children that enlarges to a solitary bluish-red nodule or plaque a few centimeters in diameter (Fig. 10.10). ACA is a later manifestation of European LB that usually occurs on the extensor surfaces of the distal extremities with an edematous area of reddish-blue discoloration which enlarges and, without treatment, can result in long-term atrophic changes months to years later (Fig. 10.10).

The most common neurologic manifestation of LB in the United States is facial nerve palsy, and the most common neurologic manifestation of LB in Europe is painful meningoradiculitis. Lyme arthritis is rare in Europe, but may develop in up to 60% of untreated American cases. Most cases of LB in the United States occur in males in high incidence states, and most cases in Europe occur in females (Yu et al., 2017). In the USA, this reflects differential exposure rates, but the reason for the European differences is not apparent.

Recommendations for diagnosis and treatment of LB with tetracycline–class antibiotics are similar in the United States and Europe (Yu et al., 2017; Hickling et al., 2018). A single 200-mg dose of doxycycline is recommended for post-tick bite exposure antimicrobial chemoprophylaxis in both the USA and Europe (Hickling et al., 2018).

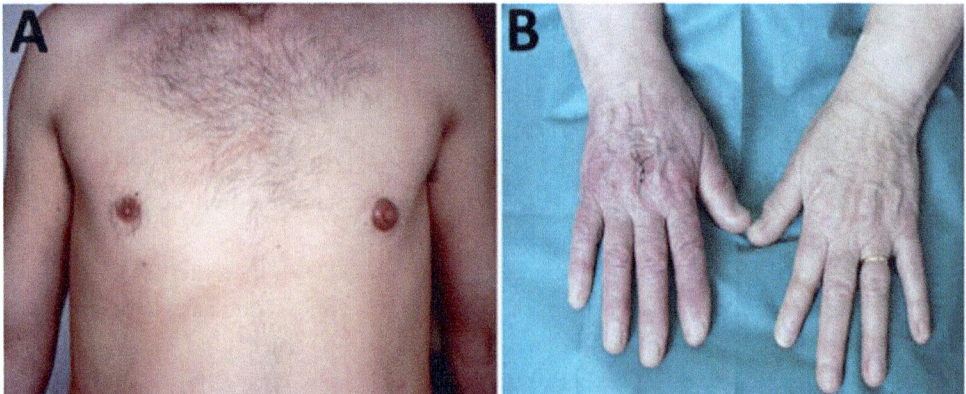

Figure 10.10 (A) A borrelial lymphocytoma on the left nipple in an adult with European Lyme borreliosis. Note the resolving erythema migrans rash on the chest. (B) Acrodermatitis chronica atrophicans on the extensor surfaces of the hands in an adult with European Lyme borreliosis. *(From Marques, A.R., Strle, F., Wormser, G.P., et al. 2021. Comparison of Lyme disease in the United States and Europe. Morb. Mort. Wkly. Rep. 27 (8), 1—9. CDC. Public Domain. No Permission needed.)*

In patients who previously had antibiotic-treated erythema migrans, reinfections with *B. burgdorferi* may occur in subsequent summers and will be again heralded by another erythema migrans lesion. Recent investigations by Nadelman and coworkers demonstrated that repeated episodes of erythema migrans in patients with previous appropriately treated early LB were due to reinfections and not to recurrences (Marques and et al., 2021; Nadelman et al., 2001).

Despite adequate antibiotic treatment of LB, persistent arthritis (now called postinfectious Lyme arthritis) may occur and was formerly referred to as chronic Lyme arthritis. The proliferative synovitis of postinfectious Lyme arthritis may extend for months to years and has been attributed to retained, nonviable spirochetal fragments (such as *B. burgdorferi* peptoglycan) and/or autoimmune responses to these antigens and not to recurrent LB (Tibbles and Edlow, 2007; Nadelman et al., 2001, 2012).

Unfortunately, some practitioners continue to diagnose patients who are suffering from a variety of generalized myofascial, arthritic, and neurologic pain conditions after tick bites as having "*chronic Lyme disease*" and have prescribed long courses of oral and intravenous antibiotics despite evidence demonstrating that such therapies provide no improvement and can cause harm (Nadelman et al., 2012).

In 2017, Marzec and coauthors reported a case series of five patients diagnosed with "*chronic Lyme disease*" who were then treated with protracted courses of antibiotics (Steere, 2012). The resulting complications from this unnecessary therapy included (1) septic shock from central venous catheter—associated bacteremia in two patients, with one fatality; (2) vertebral osteomyelitis in one patient; (3) intractable *Clostridioides difficile* (formerly *Clostridium difficile*) colitis in one patient who later died from complications of amyotrophic lateral sclerosis (ALS); and (4) a paraspinal abscess that required surgical drainage in the last case (Steere, 2012).

Although the concept of chronic LB has been dispelled by carefully conducted clinical studies, lingering and unconfirmed associations continue to be made between LB cases and subsequent deaths due to four neurodegenerative disorders: amyotrophic lateral sclerosis (ALS), Alzheimer disease (AD), multiple sclerosis (MS), and Parkinson disease (PD) (Arvikar and Steere, 2015). If such associations truly existed, then the geographic distributions of LB cases and deaths from these four neurodegenerative disorders would be anticipated to significantly overlap (Arvikar and Steere, 2015).

Forrester and coinvestigators compared LB incidence rates in each state from the National Notifiable Diseases Surveillance System during 2001—2010 with age-adjusted death rates for AD, ALS, MS, and PD obtained from the CDC Wide-Ranging Online Data for Epidemiologic Research (CDC WONDER) database over the same reporting period (Arvikar and Steere, 2015). LB incidence per US state was not correlated with rates of death due to ALS, MS, or PD. However, an inverse correlation was detected between LB and AD (Arvikar and Steere, 2015). The authors concluded that their failure to accurately confirm any positive correlations between the geographic distribution of LB and the geographic distribution of deaths due to AD, ALS, MS, and PD provided further evidence that LB was not associated with the development of these common neurodegenerative diseases in our aging population (Arvikar and Steere, 2015).

The Jarisch-Herxheimer reaction (JHR), an inflammatory cytokine-mediated reaction to dying spirochetes with a worsening of presenting symptoms, vasodilation, and myocardial dysfunction, may occur during initial antibiotic treatment for LB, but is even more common during antibiotic therapy for the tickborne relapsing fevers (TBRFs). There have been no reported deaths from JHR during antibiotic therapy for LB, and the very rare case fatalities from LB have been attributed to cardiac conduction disturbances from myocarditis in untreated cases.

Southern tick-associated rash illness (STARI)

First recognized in 1998, STARI manifests initially as erythema migrans, as in LB, but occurs in regions in which *B. burgdorferi* is not endemic and follows the prolonged attachment of blood-feeding Lone Star ticks *(A. americanum),* more abundant in the southeastern and south central United States (Fig. 10.3) (Vannier et al., 1997, 2015). Patients who are bitten by Lone Star ticks may develop LB-like erythema migrans rashes, which may or may not display target or bull's eye patterns. Patients may occasionally develop milder constitutional symptoms than in LB, including fever, headache, fatigue, and generalized myalgias (Vannier et al., 1997, 2015). However, unlike LB, STARI is not a reportable infectious disease and has no diagnostic serologic tests, such as enzyme-linked immunosorbent assays (ELISAs), immunofluorescence assays, and Western immunoblot assays (Kirkland et al., 1997).

Because distinguishing STARI from LB may be difficult, Wormser and coworkers (Feder et al., 2007) have recommended that the differential diagnosis relies on a combination of regional exposures, clinical presentations, serologic results, and potential for long-term sequelae based on their comparison of LB cases from New York and STARI cases from Missouri. The investigators noted that the timing of rash onset was shorter (6 days) in STARI compared with LB (10 days) and that STARI patients were less likely to be symptomatic than LB patients (Feder et al., 2007). In addition, the STARI rash was more often circular with central clearing than the LB target rash (Feder et al., 2007).

Because some patients have recovered from STARI without antibiotic treatment, and there have been no long-term sequelae reported in STARI cases as in LB cases, some have questioned whether antibiotic therapy is indicated in STARI. Most authorities, however, recommend antibiotic therapy for STARI with oral doxycycline preferred or amoxicillin if contraindicated. The same regimen is recommended to cover any missed diagnoses of LB classified as STARI with the potential for chronic arthritic and cardiac sequelae. However, there remains no conclusive evidence about treatment necessity or efficacy in STARI (Table 10.1) (Yu et al., 2017; Marques and et al., 2021; Nadelman et al., 2001).

Relapsing fevers

The tickborne relapsing fevers (TBRFs) comprise a worldwide group of serious bacterial infections caused by *Borrelia* spirochetes after painless, and usually unnoticed, bites by *Ornithodoros* species argasid or soft ticks (Fig. 10.11) (Marzec et al., 2017; Forrester et al., 2015; Wormser et al., 2005; Dworkin et al., 2002). *Ornithodoros* ticks prefer sheltered living in cabins, caves, crevices, woodpiles, and rodent burrows, and quickly abandon warm-blooded rodent hosts for egg-laying (Marzec et al., 2017; Wormser et al., 2005).

Transovarian transmission of the TBRF spirochetes occurs commonly among all species, and unlike LB-causing *Borrelia* species, TBRF spirochetes are already present in the salivary glands at the onset of blood-feeding and do not need time to migrate from the gut to the mouthparts (Marzec et al., 2017). The wild animal host reservoirs of TBRF are maintained in birds and several small mammals, most commonly rodents (Marzec et al., 2017). Adult soft ticks can live for as long as 10–15 years and can survive without blood meals for several years (Marzec et al., 2017).

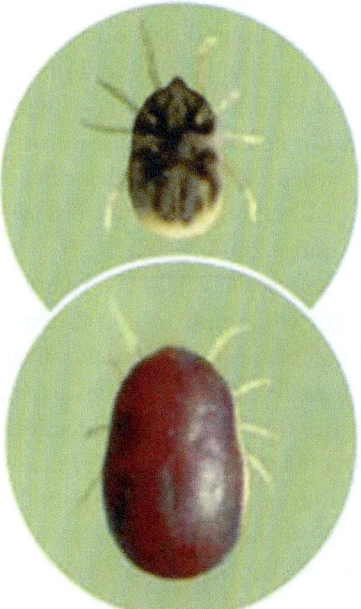

Figure 10.11 *Ornithodoros* species soft tick, before *(top)* and after *(bottom)* a blood meal. The *Ornithodoros* species of soft ticks include *Ornithodoros hermsii, O. parkeri,* and *O. turicatae.* They are widely distributed throughout the mountainous regions of the western half of the United States and southwestern Canada at elevations above 1500 m and transmit the spirochetes that cause tick-borne relapsing fever (*Borrelia hermsii, Borrelia parkeri,* and *Borrelia turicatae*). *(From Tickborne Diseases of the United States. Soft tick. Atlanta, GA: Centers for Disease Control and Prevention. https:// www.cdc.gov/ticks/tickbornediseases/tickID.html. CDC. Public Domain. No Permission needed.)*

The *Ornithodoros* species of soft ticks in the United States include *Ornithodoros hermsii, Ornithodoros parkeri,* and *Ornithodoros turicatae* (Fig. 10.11). *Ornithodoros hermsii* and *Ornithodoros turicatae* are widely distributed throughout the western half of the United States and southwestern Canada and transmit the spirochetes that cause TBRF (*Borrelia hermsii, Borrelia parkeri,* and *Borrelia turicatae*) during the spring through summer months (Marzec et al., 2017; Wormser et al., 2005). *Borrelia hermsii* transmitted by *Ornithodoros hermsii* soft ticks is the most commonly reported causative species of TBRF in high-elevation regions above 1500 m of the western United States. *Borrelia turicatae* transmitted by *Ornithodoros turicatae* soft ticks is the most commonly reported causative species of TBRF in low-elevation, arid regions of the southwestern United States (Marzec et al., 2017; Wormser et al., 2005).

Most cases of infection with *B. hermsii* have occurred in persons staying overnight in summer cabins and homes in mountainous regions of the western USA that are unoccupied during the winters and provide shelter to mice and soft ticks. Most cases of infection with *B. turicatae* have occurred in low-elevation dry regions among outdoor enthusiasts and cave explorers (Wormser et al., 2005).

Recently, a confirmed case of TBRF caused by *B. turicatae* was reported in an urban dweller from Austin, Texas, with a limited outdoor travel history. Local environmental sampling of rodent dens in a nearby public park identified *B. turicatae*-infected soft ticks (Acute respiratory distress syndrome in persons with tickborne relapsing fever—three states, 2004). Although typically considered a disease of outdoor enthusiasts living in primitive conditions, TBRF caused by *B. turicatae* has now emerged in densely populated urban areas of the Southwest (Acute respiratory distress syndrome in persons with tickborne relapsing fever—three states, 2004).

Unlike the ixodid ticks, *Ornithodoros* ticks feed very rapidly, usually for less than 30 minutes, and always at night while human hosts are asleep. The bites are painless as a result of local anesthetic-like chemicals in the tick saliva (or sialome). The bite site is marked after a few days by a small red to violaceous papule with a central eschar. One spirochete is sufficient to initiate TBRF, and the infection rate after a single bite by an infected tick is more than 50% (Marzec et al., 2017; Forrester et al., 2015). The incubation period from tick bite to onset of the first febrile episode is about 1 week with a range of 3—12 days (Marzec et al., 2017; Forrester et al., 2015; Wormser et al., 2005).

The clinical manifestations of TBRF are not affected by the species differences among the causative spirochetes. A case of TBRF is defined by the sudden onset of two or more episodes of high fever (up to 105°F, 40.6°C) spaced by afebrile periods of 4—14 days, with the first febrile episode lasting 3—6 days and the relapsing episodes lasting 1—3 days each. The first episode ends with a 15-to-30 minutes "crisis" with tachycardia, hypertension, hyperpyrexia (as high as 109.4°F, 43°C), and rigors, followed by diaphoresis and defervescence. All febrile episodes are accompanied by nausea, headache, neck stiffness, myalgia, and arthralgia. The relapsing febrile episodes result from the growth of new spirochete populations in the blood to replace those killed by phagocytic cells. Most patients have splenomegaly, and 10% will have hepatomegaly. Direct neurologic involvement is more common than in LB and may include cranial nerve neuritis (especially cranial nerves VII and VIII), radiculopathy, myelopathy, and, rarely, optic nerve inflammation with uveitis. Myocarditis is also more common than in LB; may be complicated by adult respiratory distress syndrome, pulmonary edema, and cardiomegaly; and is often fatal (Forrester et al., 2015).

Laboratory diagnostics include identifying the spirochetes microscopically on peripheral blood smears and detecting their nucleic acids in blood using PCR assays. Anemia, leukopenia, thrombocytopenia, hyperbilirubinemia, elevated aminotransferases and C-reactive protein levels, and prolonged prothrombin and partial thromboplastin times are common accompanying laboratory abnormalities (Marzec et al., 2017; Forrester et al., 2015; Wormser et al., 2005; Dworkin et al., 2002).

Treatment strategies include tetracycline (500 mg or 12.5 mg/kg PO four times daily), or doxycycline (100 mg PO twice daily), or erythromycin (500 mg or 12.5 mg/kg PO four times daily for 10 days) (Marzec et al., 2017; Forrester et al., 2015; Wormser et al., 2005; Dworkin et al., 2002). Parenteral therapy with penicillin G or ceftriaxone is recommended for central nervous system (CNS) involvement.

The JHR is much more common, although rarely fatal, during treatment of TBRF than during treatment of LB and occurs in 30%–40% of patients with TBRF (Wormser et al., 2005). In a small series of six cases of TBRF in persons visiting the White Mountains of southern Arizona during 2013–18, all patients responded promptly to doxycycline therapy, but two patients (30%) suffered JHRs in association with antimicrobial therapy (Wormser et al., 2005).

At present, no prophylactic strategies to reduce the severity of the JHR have proved beneficial or have been adequately tested in multiple clinical trials, including therapy with antipyretics, corticosteroids, or naloxone. For unknown reasons, antispirochetal therapy for TBRF with penicillin instead of tetracycline has a slightly lower risk of associated JHR (Wormser et al., 2005).

Rickettsioses

The family Rickettsiaceae contains two genera: the spotted fever (SF)-causing genus *Rickettsia* and the mite-transmitted, scrub typhus–causing genus *Orientia*. The rickettsiae may be further stratified clinically into the tickborne SF group and mouse mite–transmitted rickettsialpox caused by *Rickettsia akari*. The rickettsiae are obligate intracellular, Gram-negative bacteria that thrive in ixodid tick salivary glands and are transmitted during blood feeding. Once injected into the host, rickettsiae are initially distributed regionally through lymphatics, with some species causing marked regional lymphadenopathy, such as *Rickettsia slovaca*. Within 2–14 days (mean, 7 days), rickettsiae are disseminated hematogenously to vascular endothelial lining cells of target organs, including the CNS, lungs, and myocardium (Fig. 10.12).

Rickettsiae enter host endothelial cells in a Trojan horse—like manner by using their outer membrane proteins (OmpA and OmpB) to stimulate endocytosis. Once within phagosomes, rickettsiae escape to enter the cytosol or nucleus for rapid replication by binary fission, safe from host immune attack. The tickborne rickettsial diseases that cause SFs are compared in a descending order of clinical severity of infection by preferred tick vectors and wild animal reservoirs in Table 10.2.

Spotted fevers

The global epidemiology of the tickborne SF—causing rickettsiae has dramatically evolved since the transmission cycle of RMSF was first described by Ricketts in 1906. New strains and diseases have emerged, such as *R. slovaca*—associated lymphadenopathy. Several species have been identified as related and share a similar highly conserved genome including *Rickettsia africae, Rickettsia parkeri,* and *Rickettsia conorii* (Mafi et al., 2019). Many strains have demonstrated greater virulence and wider geographic distributions including *R. rickettsii, R. conorii,* and *R. australis* (Dworkin et al., 2002). Unanticipated new tick vectors have been discovered, such as the brown dog tick, *Rhipicephalus sanguineus,* for RMSF in the United States (Masters et al., 2008). Cluster outbreaks of tickborne rickettsioses have been reported in returning travelers, such as tick-bite fever caused by *R. africae* in returning African safari participants (Talagrand-Reboul et al., 2018; Bissett et al., 2018). Cluster outbreaks of rickettsioses have also been reported in neighborhoods and families, such as *R. japonica* outbreaks in Japan and China (Biggs

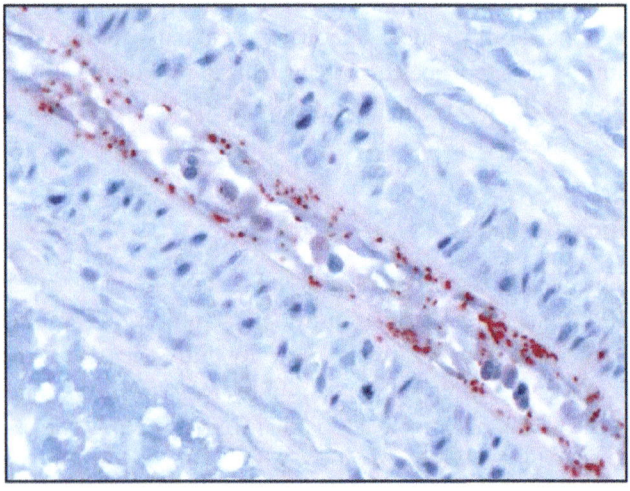

Figure 10.12 *Rickettsia rickettsii* tissue biopsy specimen, with immunohistochemical stain. Shown is an immunohistochemical stain of a tissue biopsy specimen demonstrating intracellular gram-negative *Rickettsia rickettsii* bacteria *(red)* within vascular endothelial lining cells. Infection with *R. rickettsia* causes the systemic vasculitis of Rocky Mountain spotted fever that manifests initially as petechial skin lesions and may progress without antirickettsial therapy to microvascular leakage and ischemic vasculopathy with gangrene and autoamputation of digits and limbs. *(From Biggs, H.M., Behravesh, C.B., Bradley, K.K., et al. 2016. Diagnosis and management of tickborne rickettsial diseases: Rocky Mountain spotted fever and other spotted fever group rickettsioses, ehrlichioses, and anaplasmosis—United States. MMWR Recomm. Rep. 65, 1—44. CDC. Public Domain. No Permission needed.)*

Table 10.2 Spotted fever group of tickborne rickettsioses.

Rickettsia species	Tickborne diseases	Geographic distribution	Tick vectors	Wild animal reservoirs (mammals)
R. rickettsii	Rocky Mountain spotted fever (SF), Brazilian SF	Continental United States, central America (Costa Rica, Mexico, Panama), south America (Argentina, Brazil)	*Amblyomma, Dermacentor, Rhipicephalus* spp.	Ungulates, rodents
R. conorii	Boutonneuse fever: Mediterranean SF, Israeli SF, Astrakhan SF, Indian tick typhus, Kenyan tick typhus	Mediterranean Basin, Africa, Middle East, Asia	*Rhipicephalus* spp.	Ungulates, rodents
R. sibirica	North Asian tick typhus (Siberian tick typhus)	Africa (Niger, Mali, South Africa), Asia (Russia, China, Mongolia, Pakistan, Kazakhstan, Kirgizia, Tajikistan), Europe (France)	*Dermacentor, Haemaphysalis, Hyalomma* spp.	Ungulates, rodents
R. japonica	Japanese SF	Japan and China	*Haemaphysalis* spp., *Ixodes ovatus*	Ungulates, rodents
R. australis	Queensland tick typhus	Eastern Australian seaboard from Cairns, Queensland, to Gipps island, Victoria	*Ixodes* spp., especially *I. holocyclus* and *I. tasmania*	Rodents, bandicoots, wombats, cattle, domestic dogs
R. honei / *R. honei subspecies marmionii*	Flinders island SF / Australian SF	Southern Australia, Thailand Cape York, Queensland	*Aponomma* spp. *Haemaphysalis novaeguineae*	Rodents / Similar to *R. australis*: Rodents, bandicoots, wombats, cattle, domestic dogs
R. africae and *R. parkeri*	African tick-bite fever	Sub-Saharan Africa, North America, South America, Caribbean	*Amblyomma* spp.	Rodents
R. 364D (*R. philipii* [proposed])	*R. 364D* "spotless" rickettsiosis with tick-bite eschar	California	*Dermacentor occidentalis*	Rodents, other small mammals
R. slovaca	Tickborne lymphadenopathy; *Dermacentor*-borne eschar, lymphadenopathy, or necrosis	Europe	*Dermacentor* spp.	Ungulates, rodents
R. aeschlimannii	Not named at present	Southern Europe, Africa	*Hyalomma* spp.	Ungulates, rodents

Adapted from Diaz, J.H., 2019. Section on Ectoparasitic Diseases. Chapter 296. Ticks (Including Tick Paralysis). In: Bennett, J.E., Dolin, R., Blaser, M.J. (Eds.), *Mandell, Douglas and Bennett's Principles and Practice of Infectious Diseases*, Ninth Edition, Elsevier, Philadelphia. Elsevier publication.

et al., 2016; Tsai et al., 2008; Mack and Ritz, 2019; Matsuura and Yokota, 2018; Lu et al., 2018).

The incidence rate for SF group rickettsioses in the United States increased from 1.7 cases per million person-years in 2000 to 14.3 cases per million person-years in 2012 (Ishizuka and Sugaya, 2022). This was likely due to a combination of improved diagnostic use in endemic areas, as well as an aging at-risk population with increasing immunosuppressive conditions, such as cancer, chemotherapy, biologics and corticosteroid therapy, and organ transplants (Ishizuka and Sugaya, 2022; Liu et al., 2014). SF group rickettsiosis cases were more frequently reported among males and persons of white race and non-Hispanic ethnicity (Ishizuka and Sugaya, 2022; Liu et al., 2014). The most common causative rickettsial species in the United States today include the highly pathogenic *R. rickettsii* and the less pathogenic species, *R. parkeri* and *Rickettsia* 364D (Figs. 10.8 and 10.13) (Liu et al., 2014).

Although all prior reported cases of *R. parkeri* rickettsiosis were described in the coastal Southeast US and linked to transmission by the Gulf Coast tick, *Amblyomma maculatum*, Herrick and coauthors described one confirmed and one probable case of *R. parkeri* rickettsiosis acquired in a mountainous region of Arizona, well outside of the distribution range of the Gulf Coast tick and likely transmitted by a newly recognized tick vector, *Amblyomma triste* (Fig. 10.13) (Liu et al., 2014).

The tickborne SF rickettsioses share many common presenting features, including: (1) incubation periods of about 1 week; (2) flu-like prodromes of fever, headache, myalgia, nausea, vomiting, and abdominal pain that can mimic acute appendicitis in RMSF; (3) spotty rashes within 3–5 days of fever onset (Fig. 10.14); and (4) necrotic eschars at tick-bite sites (Fig. 10.12B).

The tickborne rickettsial infections that can cause spotty rashes include *R. rickettsia*, causative agent of RMSF, *R. conorii*, causative agent of Mediterranean spotted fever (MSF), *R. australis*, causative agent of Queensland tick typhus (QTT), and the *R. africae*–*R. parkeri* complex, causative agent of African–North American tick-bite fever (Mafi et al., 2019; Qin et al., 2019; Drexler et al., 2016). The tickborne rickettsial infections that usually cause one or more necrotic eschars at tick-bite sites include *R. conorii*, *R. australis*, *R. africae*–*R. parkeri*, *R. helvetica*, *R. japonica*, *R. slovaca*, *R. aeschlimannii*, *R. honei*, and *R.* 364D (*R. philipii* [proposed]) (Mafi et al., 2019; Qin et al., 2019; Drexler et al., 2016). The SF rickettsioses may vary in severity from causing multisystem organ failure (RMSF, MSF) to painful regional lymphadenopathy (*R. africae*–*R. parkeri* complex, *R. slovaca*) to mild or subclinical disease (*R. aeschlimannii*) (Mafi et al., 2019; Qin et al., 2019; Drexler et al., 2016).

RMSF was until recently a rare and sporadically reported disease in the United States with most cases reported from the Mid-Atlantic states and not from the Rocky Mountain states (Herrick et al., 2016). Fatal cases of RMSF have now been reported along the United States–Mexico border with four case described during the period 2013–16

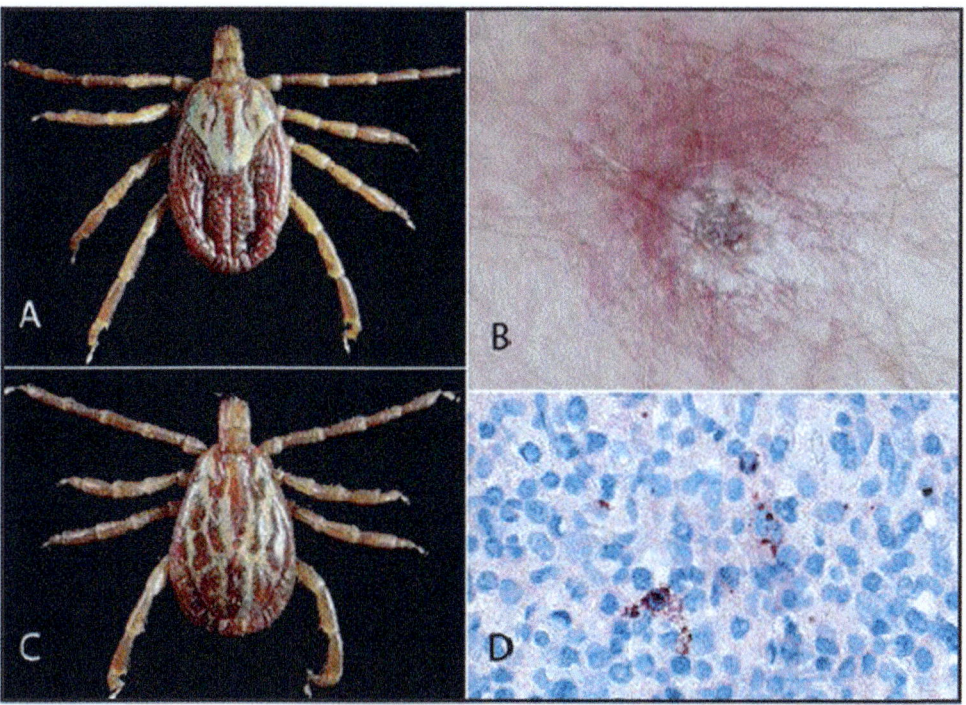

Figure 10.13 *Rickettsia parkeri* rickettsiosis, preferred tick vectors (A, C), eschar (B), and immunohistochemical stain of tissue biopsy (D). *Rickettsia parkeri* rickettsiosis is transmitted by female (A) and male (C) Gulf coast ticks (*Amblyomma maculatum*). Rickettsiosis is characterized by initial erythema, swelling, and itching at the bite site that ulcerates and then scabs over as an inoculation eschar (B). Patients often report fever, rash, and regional lymphadenopathy. Additional symptoms may include chills, myalgia, arthralgia, malaise, and headache. Laboratory diagnostics include immunohistochemical staining of eschar biopsy sites to demonstrate intracellular, gram-negative spotted fever group *Rickettsia* (D); growth of the organism in cell cultures from specimens; and nucleic acid speciation by quantitative polymerase chain reaction assays. Treatment is with oral doxycycline, 100 mg twice a day for a minimum of 10 days. *(From Straily, A., Feldpausch, A., Ulbrich, C., et al., 2016. Notes form the field: Rickettsia parkeri rickettsiosis—Georgia, 2012–14. MMWR Morb. Mortal. Wkly. Rep. 65, 718–719. CDC. Public Domain. No Permission needed.)*

(Herrick et al., 2016). In all cases, RMSF was contracted in northern Mexico, and all patients presented clinically to hospitals in the United States with nonspecific symptoms of fever, headache, nausea, vomiting, myalgia, maculopapular progressing to petechial rashes, and subsequent fatal cardiorespiratory failure. Investigators cautioned the need for heightened awareness of RMSF cases in nonendemic areas, such as the United States—Mexico border, northern Mexico, and southern Arizona (Herrick et al., 2016). Investigators attributed the increasing incidence of RMSF in these areas to expanding large animal host reservoirs of disease in dogs and transmission by regionally large

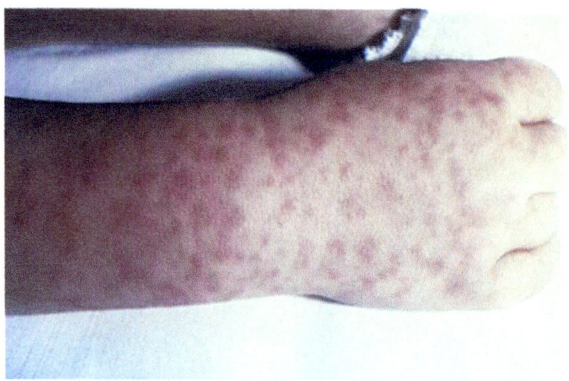

Figure 10.14 Characteristic initial distal maculopapular-petechial rash of Rocky Mountain spotted fever. This rash is shown on the dorsal aspect of a child's right hand and wrist. *(From Public Health Image Library. Image 1962. Atlanta, GA: Centers for Disease Control and Prevention. CDC. Public Domain. No Permission needed.)*

numbers of brown dog ticks, *Rhipicephalus sanguineus* (Masters et al., 2008; Herrick et al., 2016).

RMSF is a rapidly progressing and potentially fatal disease, especially if unrecognized and not treated immediately and without laboratory confirmation on first suspicion of disease with tetracycline-class antibiotics, such as doxycycline. The disease may prove fatal for patients who do not receive appropriate antibiotic therapy within the first 5 days of illness, and half of all deaths from RMSF occur within the first 8 days of illness (Mafi et al., 2019; Herrick et al., 2016).

After an average incubation period of 1 week, RMSF starts with a flu-like, febrile prodrome followed by a characteristic maculopapular evolving to petechial rash in 85%—90% of cases in 3—5 days (Mafi et al., 2019; Herrick et al., 2016). The pathognomonic rash starts distally on the wrists and ankles and then spreads centripetally up the limbs (Fig. 10.14).

The pathophysiologic mechanisms responsible for the petechial rashes and target organ system damage (CNS, lungs, heart) in the SF rickettsioses include vascular endothelial cell damage by microbial replication, vascular inflammation, and increased vascular permeability, which may result in hypovolemic shock, oliguric prerenal failure from acute tubular necrosis, cerebral edema, and noncardiogenic pulmonary edema (Fig. 10.12) (Mafi et al., 2019). Distal, digital skin necrosis and gangrene of the digits and limbs may occur in severe cases of RMSF and Queensland tick typhus (QTT) from hypoperfusion-related ischemia (Fig. 10.15) (Mafi et al., 2019; Drexler et al., 2016).

Cardiac vasculitis may manifest as myocarditis with intraventricular conduction blocks. Aside from petechial rash and thrombocytopenia, other hemorrhagic manifestations in RMSF and other SFs are rare (Mafi et al., 2019). CNS complications in RMSF and other severe SF infections may include ataxia, photophobia, transient deafness, focal neurologic deficits, meningismus, meningoencephalitis, seizures, and coma (Mafi et al., 2019). Pulmonary complications may include cough, alveolar infiltrates, interstitial

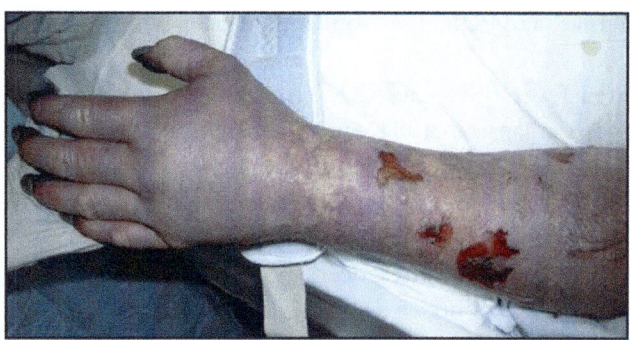

Figure 10.15 Digital ischemia with gangrene resulting from Rocky Mountain spotted fever. Gangrene of the terminal finger digits has developed in a patient with ischemic vasculopathy from late-stage Rocky mountain spotted fever caused by tick-transmitted infection with *Rickettsia rickettsii*. *(From Biggs, H.M., Behravesh, C.B., Bradley, K.K., et al., 2016. Diagnosis and management of tickborne rickettsial diseases: Rocky Mountain spotted fever and other spotted fever group rickettsioses, ehrlichioses, and anaplasmosis—United States. MMWR Recomm. Rep. 65, 1–44. CDC. Public Domain. No Permission needed.)*

pneumonitis, pleural effusions, pulmonary edema, and adult respiratory distress syndrome (Mafi et al., 2019).

Initially, Mediterranean Spotted Fever (MSF) caused by *R. conorii* was thought to be a more benign disease than RMSF. Severe cases of MSF with multiple eschars and multi-system disease similar to RMSF with CNS, renal, and pulmonary complications were first reported in 1981 and now appear to be increasing across Europe (Qin et al., 2019). QTT, African tick-bite fever, and *R. slovaca*—associated lymphadenopathy are generally milder diseases than RMSF and MSF (Qin et al., 2019; Drexler et al., 2016). However, severe cases of QTT with RMSF-like complications, including renal insufficiency, pulmonary infiltrates, and distal gangrene from ischemia, have been reported from Australia (Drexler et al., 2016).

Some SF rickettsial diseases may be "spotless," complicating early differential diagnosis, including RMSF in 10%–15% of cases. Several other SF infections may be spotless in up to 50% of cases, but still manifest typical rickettsial SF prodromes. The spotless SF group include *R. africae* that causes African tick-bite fever, *R. parkeri* that cause a disease similar to African tick bite fever in North America, and *R. slovaca* that causes painful regional lymphadenopathy. All of these SF infections can cause multiple necrotic eschars and regional lymphadenopathy without rashes.

A history of tick bites, eschars, and painful regional lymphadenopathy helps to establish the correct diagnosis, especially in the absence of adequate diagnostic laboratory services. The precise laboratory diagnosis of tickborne rickettsial SFs may be established by microbiologic isolation of the causative organisms from skin and eschar biopsy specimens or blood cultures, nonspecific immunofluorescence antibody tests that cross-react with many SF antigens, especially RMSF, other immunocytologic techniques to demonstrate intracellular rickettsiae, and PCR assay to identify and speciate rickettsial DNA or RNA (Mafi et al., 2019).

Japanese spotted fever (JSF) caused by *Rickettsia japonica* was first reported as an emerging rickettsiosis in Japan in 1984. Since then, the annual number of reported cases has increased threefold with most cases reported from Pacific sides of the southern islands of Japan and new cases reported from traditionally nonendemic areas (Biggs et al., 2016). Investigators attributed the increasing prevalence of JSF to increasing host animal reservoirs of *R. japonica* in capybaras, horses, deer, and wild boar (Biggs et al., 2016; Mack and Ritz, 2019). Investigators attributed a delay in the diagnosis of JSF in Japan to the absence of a known tick bite and a several day delay in the appearance of rash following a flu-like febrile prodrome (Biggs et al., 2016; Mack and Ritz, 2019). Fever, chills, myalgia, malaise, and a maculopapular progressing to petechial rash will typically follow within 1 week of a tick bite and be accompanied by significant laboratory abnormalities, especially elevated inflammatory biomarkers and thrombocytopenia. Investigators recommend PCR-confirmation of disease by eschar or skin biopsies, and immediate treatment of JSF with tetracycline-class antibiotics (Bissett et al., 2018; Mack and Ritz, 2019).

Today, human *R. japonica* infections have increased in nearby countries including China, South Korea, and the Philippines, with 16 cases reported from Zhejiang Province, China, in 2015, and 20 cases reported from Xinyang, China, during 2014—17 (Tsai et al., 2008; Matsuura and Yokota, 2018). Chinese investigators attributed the increasing prevalence of JSF in China to a wider spectrum of *R. japonica*-infected ticks from three genera, *Dermacentor*, *Haemaphysalis*, and *Ixodes*, and eight species of these ticks (Tsai et al., 2008; Matsuura and Yokota, 2018).

Rickettsialpox (see Chapter 6)
Q (Query) fever
Q (Query) fever was first described in Australia in 1935, and its causative organism, *Coxiella burnetii,* was isolated shortly thereafter (Qin et al., 2019). *C. burnetii* is a gram-negative, intracellular, spore-forming bacterium that is the sole species of its genus. *C. burnetii* is genetically related to *Legionella pneumophila* and, like *L. pneumophila, C. burnetii* is usually transmitted to humans by the inhalation of contaminated aerosols (Qin et al., 2019; Drexler et al., 2016). Q fever is a zoonosis with worldwide distribution and extensive domestic animal (cattle, sheep, goats, cats, dogs), wild animal (birds, rabbits, reptiles), and arthropod (ticks) reservoirs (Drexler et al., 2016). In most cases, humans are not infected by tick bites but by inhaling spores or bacteria in aerosols contaminated with infectious particles in dried animal feces, milk, or animal products of conception (Qin et al., 2019; Drexler et al., 2016; Herrick et al., 2016). Q fever may also be transmitted by ingestion of contaminated milk or cheese, by vertical transmission from mother to

fetus, by contaminated blood product transfusion, and even percutaneously by crushing infected ticks near breaks in the skin barrier (Qin et al., 2019).

C. burnetii is reactivated during pregnancy and multiplies extensively in the placenta, exposing abattoir workers, veterinarians, researchers (especially those working with parturient ewes), and domestic pet owners (especially of cats) to highly infectious aerosols during delivery (Qin et al., 2019; Drexler et al., 2016). Recently, several cases of Q fever were reported among US military personnel deployed to Iraq and Afghanistan and in travelers returning from Asia, Latin America, and sub-Saharan Africa (Herrick et al., 2016; Rovery et al., 2008). *C. burnetii* has long been considered a potential bioterrorism weapon for several reasons, including its environmental stability, spore-forming capability, ease of aerosolized dispersal, and high pathogenicity, with an ability to initiate infection with a single microorganism.

Over 3000 cases of acute Q fever presenting as pneumonia in most cases (62%) were reported from the Netherlands during the period 2007-09. Most of the patients were males, smokers, and adults 40–60 years old. Very few patients worked in agriculture (3.2%) or in meat-processing, including abattoirs (0.5%). Public health investigators determined that the Q fever epidemic was caused by the aerosolization of contaminated dust particles from commercial dairy goat farms located in densely populated areas that were experiencing waves of Q fever-induced abortions in infected goats. Strict veterinary infectious disease control measures on dairy goat and sheep farms halted the epidemic in 2010, but left many infected patients at increased risks of developing chronic Q fever endocarditis years later.

After an average 2-week incubation period (range, 2–29 days), Q fever may manifest as a wide variety of illnesses in humans, including: (1) acute Q fever, a self-limited febrile illness with severe headache, retro-orbital pain, and nonproductive cough; (2) Q fever pneumonia with consolidated opacities, pleural effusions, and hilar lymphadenopathy on chest radiographs; (3) Q fever granulomatous hepatitis, usually after ingestion of un-pasteurized contaminated milk; (4) CNS Q fever with protean manifestations ranging from aseptic meningoencephalitis and transient behavioral and sensory disturbances to cranial nerve palsies and hemifacial pain mimicking trigeminal neuralgia; and (5) chronic Q fever endocarditis, especially in predisposed patients with congenital valvulopathies, prosthetic heart valves, aortic aneurysms, or vascular grafts (Rovery et al., 2008; McBride et al., 2007). Patients who are immunocompromised by pregnancy, congenital immuno-deficiency disorders, cancer, HIV/AIDS, organ transplant antirejection therapy, renal dialysis, or prolonged corticosteroid therapy are at greater risk for acquiring more severe and chronic Q fever infections (Drexler et al., 2016; McBride et al., 2007).

Recent reports have recommended that clinicians should consider a diagnosis of Q fever in the absence of infected livestock exposure and should preoperatively screen patients undergoing elective cardiac valve surgery for Q fever (Rovery et al., 2008; McBride et al., 2007). In an analysis of two national surveillance systems for Q fever cases in the United States during the reporting period 2000-2012, CDC investigators noted that most cases (61%) did not report any livestock or slaughterhouse exposures, but a substantial proportion reported drinking raw milk (prevalence rate, 8.4%) (Rovery et al., 2008). The overall incidence rate of Q fever during the reporting period was 0.38 cases per million persons per year, with a hospitalization rate of 62% and a case fatality rate of 2.0% (Rovery et al., 2008). In 2015, Dutch investigators reported three cases of postoperatively diagnosed chronic Q fever endocarditis in patients requiring cardiac valve surgery (McBride et al., 2007). Earlier diagnosis and antimicrobial therapy might have prevented progressive valve dysfunction from chronic Q fever endocarditis in these cases and eliminated the need for cardiac valvuloplasty or replacement (McBride et al., 2007).

Because the isolation of *C. burnetii* requires Biosafety Level 3, most diagnostic laboratory strategies for Q fever rely on microscopic detection on Giemsa-stained smears of blood or sputum or tissue biopsies (liver, excised heart valves), on antibody detection by immunofluorescent assays, or on DNA detection by PCR assay (Qin et al., 2019; Herrick et al., 2016). The prognosis is usually excellent in the acute Q fever illnesses, and mortality is rare after appropriate antibiotic therapy with tetracyclines (doxycycline is preferred—100 mg PO twice daily for 14 days) or fluoroquinolones. Chronic Q fever endocarditis will require prolonged treatment with two antibiotics, either rifampin (300 mg PO twice daily) and ciprofloxacin (750 mg PO twice daily) for 3 years or doxycycline (100 mg PO twice daily) and hydroxychloroquine (200 mg PO three times daily) for at least 18 months. Such combined therapies will require close monitoring for drug toxicities, especially hepatotoxicity from rifampin and oculotoxicity from hydroxychloroquine. In addition, all patients with Q fever endocarditis should undergo screening transesophageal echocardiography for underlying valvulopathies and/or aortic aneurysms (McBride et al., 2007). Chronically infected heart valves and vascular grafts will require surgical replacement.

Tularemia

Tularemia, also known as rabbit fever or deer fly fever, was first described as a zoonosis in squirrels in Tulare County, California, in 1911. Its causative agent, *Francisella tularensis,* was later identified as a gram-negative coccobacillus by Edward Francis, M.D. (1872-1957) of the United States Public Health Service, during an investigation of deer fly fever in Utah in 1921.

Tularemia occurs in regional pockets worldwide, has a very large wild and domestic host animal reservoir, and is seasonally transmitted to humans by ixodid tick and deer fly bites and by contact with infected wild animals, especially rabbits and muskrats. The primary tick vector of tularemia in the United States is the American dog tick, *Dermacentor variabilis* (Fig. 10.16) (Ta et al., 2008; Dahlgren et al., 2015). Tick-transmitted tularemia is most commonly reported during the spring and summer worldwide (Dahlgren et al., 2015). Tularemia transmitted through contact with an infected animal occurs more often during the fall through hunting and trapping seasons, especially among male hunters who field-clean infected animal carcasses (Dahlgren et al., 2015).

F. tularensis is an extremely stable microorganism in nature, surviving in soil, water, and animal carcasses for months to years. In addition to fecal or vomit contamination of tick bites and direct inoculation of intact skin or mucosal surfaces when crushing ticks or skinning infected animals, tularemia may be transmitted by ingesting raw or under-cooked infected game or bush meats, drinking contaminated water, or inhaling aerosolized microorganisms (Ta et al., 2008; Dahlgren et al., 2015).

There are two biovars of *F. tularensis,* with biovar A (*F. tularensis* biogroup *tularensis*) causing 60%−90% of tularemia cases in North America and biovar B (*F. tularensis* biogroup *palearctica*) causing a milder disease throughout Europe and Asia. The presenting clinical manifestations of infection depend on the virulence of the biovars (A > B), route of entry of microorganisms, multisystem infections, and immunocompetency of infected hosts (Dahlgren et al., 2015).

The portal of entry of *F. tularensis* has historically been used to classify the clinical manifestations of tularemia, with untreated pneumonic tularemia having the highest CFRs of 30%−60% (Table 10.3) (Dahlgren et al., 2015). The differential diagnosis of ulceroglandular tularemia, the most common presentation, is extensive and includes other infected arthropod bites, bacterial and viral infections, and fungal diseases capable of causing skin ulcers with painful regional lymphadenopathy (Dahlgren et al., 2015).

Diagnosis of tularemia

Diagnostic procedures for tularemia include microscopic identification or culture in Biosafety Level 3 facilities of microorganisms from blood, sputum, gastric lavage fluid,

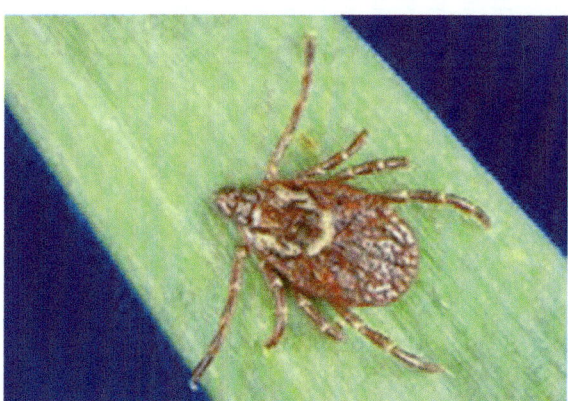

Figure 10.16 *Dermacentor variabilis,* the American dog tick, questing for a host. This female American dog tick is a vector of tick paralysis in the south-eastern United States and Pacific North-west and is a vector of Rocky Mountain spotted fever in addition to the Rocky mountain wood tick (*D. andersoni*) in the western United States. *(From Public Health Image Library. Image 170. Atlanta, GA: Centers for Disease Control and Prevention. CDC. Public Domain. No Permission needed.)*

Table 10.3 Clinical classification of tularemia based on the portal of entry.

Clinical classification of tularemia cases	Case definition by clinical presentation	Portals of entry of *Francisella tularensis*	Case frequency, United States (%)
Ulceroglandular	Malaise, fever, bite eschars or ulcers, painful regional lymphadenopathy	Tick or deer fly bite, or direct inoculation across intact dermis	80
Glandular	Malaise, fever, suppurative lymphadenopathy	Direct inoculation across intact dermis	15
Oropharyngeal	Malaise, fever, sore throat, dysphagia, painful cervical lymphadenopathy	Ingestion of raw or undercooked infected game or bush meats	<5
Oculoglandular	Malaise, fever, ocular infection, regional facial lymphadenopathy	Ocular inoculation of infectious fluids or animal danders or autoinoculation from bite eschar or ulcers	1
Typhoidal	Malaise, fever, abdominal pain, mesenteric lymphadenopathy; mimics typhoid fever	Ingestion of contaminated water	Rare
Pneumonic	Malaise, fever, pneumonia with multiple ill-defined infiltrates, hilar lymphadenopathy; mimics inhalational anthrax	Inhalation of contaminated aerosols, aerosolized bioweapon exposures, or hematogenous spreading from glandular or typhoidal infections	Rare, except on Martha's vineyard after aerosolized exposures during mechanized bush trimming and lawn mowing

Adapted from Diaz, J.H., 2019. Section on Ectoparasitic Diseases. Chapter 296. Ticks (Including Tick Paralysis). In: Bennett, J.E., Dolin, R., Blaser, M.J. (Eds.), *Mandell, Douglas and Bennett's Principles and Practice of Infectious Diseases*, Ninth Edition, Elsevier, Philadelphia. Elsevier publication.

lung biopsy, or lymph node aspirates (sensitivity, 10%—25%); acute and convalescent serology comparing antibody titers (sensitivity, >85%); direct immunofluorescence antibody testing; and antigen detection by PCR (sensitivity, 50%—73%) (Dahlgren et al., 2015). Frequently accompanying laboratory abnormalities in tularemia include significant elevations in the erythrocyte sedimentation rate and C-reactive protein; significant leukocytosis (>10,000/μL), often with normal differential counts; and thrombocytosis (Dahlgren et al., 2015).

Treatment of tularemia

The recommended treatment strategies for tularemia have evolved considerably from historical treatments with painful intramuscular injections of streptomycin to oral therapy with the aminoglycosides or fluoroquinolones, which are effective in 86% of cases and may result in resolution of ulcers within 72 hours (Dahlgren et al., 2015). Most cases in adults, including pneumonic tularemia, may be managed with fluoroquinolones alone (ciprofloxacin, 400 mg IV or 500 mg PO twice daily for 7—14 days, or levofloxacin, 500 mg IV or PO twice daily for 7—14 days), with aminoglycosides (gentamicin or amikacin, 3—5 mg/kg/day for 10—14 days) reserved for pediatric infections and widely disseminated systemic infections (Dahlgren et al., 2015). Relapse rates are highest with oral tetracyclines, including doxycycline, and chloramphenicol, which may still be indicated for cases with CNS dissemination despite its potential for bone marrow toxicity.

Anaplasmosis and the ehrlichioses

The human ehrlichioses and anaplasmosis (formerly known as human monocytic and human granulocytic ehrlichiosis respectively) are classic examples of emerging tickborne infectious diseases. Since 1986, four new tickborne bacterial species have been identified and classified into a new family, Anaplasmataceae. The four genera of Anaplasmataceae comprise obligate, intracellular, gram-negative bacteria, closely related genetically to the family Rickettsiaceae.

The Anaplasmataceae include two genera that are synergistic parasites of flatworms (*Neorickettsia sennetsu*) and filarial worms (*Wolbachia* spp.), and two genera that are tickborne bacterial infections of many mammals, including humans, *Ehrlichia* and *Anaplasma* (Figs. 10.17 and 10.18). Like rickettsiae, the Anaplasmataceae attach to molecular ligands on phagocytic cells to gain Trojan horse—like entry into leukocytes and then trick intracellular phagosomes into releasing them into the cytosol for immune evasion and replication (Figs. 10.17 and 10.18).

The Anaplasmataceae are now endemic in the United States and have preferred geographic distributions, tick vectors, and wild and domestic animal reservoirs. They spread from the infected tick's gut to its salivary glands, are inoculated over 24—36 h into the host's dermis, and cause subclinical to severe and potentially fatal infections

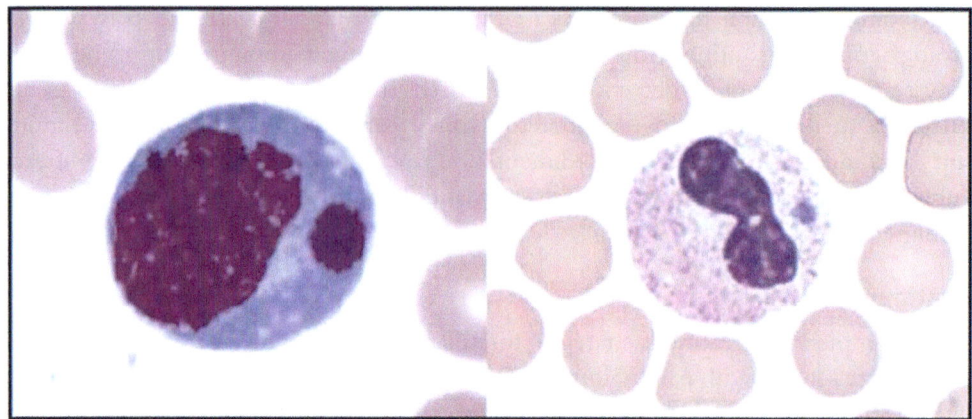

Figure 10.17 Intracellular morulae in ehrlichiosis, Wright-stained peripheral blood smears that demonstrate an intramonocytic morula characteristic of ehrlichiosis caused by *Ehrlichia chaffeensis* *(left)* and an intragranulocytic morula associated with either ehrlichiosis caused by *Ehrlichia ewingii* or anaplasmosis caused by *Anaplasma phagocytophillum (right)*. *(From Biggs, H.M., Behravesh, C.B., Bradley, K.K., et al., 2016. Diagnosis and management of tickborne rickettsial diseases: Rocky Mountain spotted fever and other spotted fever group rickettsioses, ehrlichioses, and anaplasmosis—United States. MMWR Recomm. Rep. 65, 1—44. Photos courtesy J. Stephen Dumler, M.D., University of Maryland, and Bobbi S. Pritt, MD, Mayo Clinic. CDC. Public Domain. No Permission needed.)*

Figure 10.18 *Ehrlichia chaffeensis* morula *(arrowhead)* within a monocyte (peripheral blood smear, Wright stain, ×1000). This finding is diagnostic of ehrlichiosis caused by *Ehrlichia chaffeensis*. *(From Safdar, N., Love, R.B., Maki, D.G., 2002. Severe Ehrlichia chaffeensis infection in a lung transplant recipient: a review of ehrlichiosis in the immunocompromised patient. Emerg. Infect. Dis. 8, 320—323. CDC. Public Domain. No Permission needed.)*

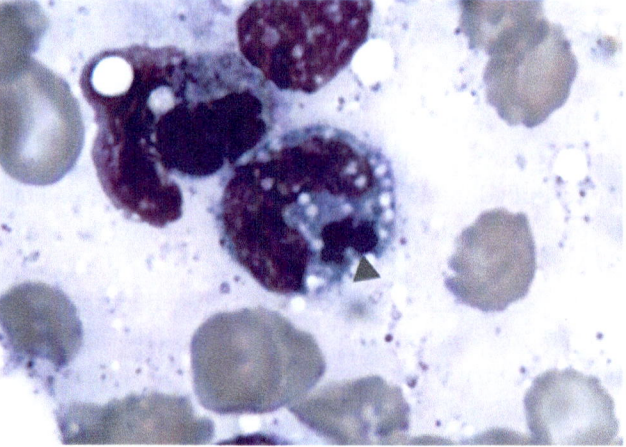

within 1—4 weeks, especially in young children and in elderly and immunocompromised adults. Because transovarian transmission in ticks has not been observed, the major host reservoirs of the Anaplasmataceae in nature are in wild and domestic animals.

Although the presenting clinical manifestations are similar among Anaplasmataceae infections, the potential multisystem complications and resulting CFRs from these diseases are ultimately determined by the age and immunocompetence of human hosts, with subclinical infections more common in children and potentially fatal infections in the elderly. The human Anaplasmataceae are resistant to fluoroquinolones, but remain susceptible to tetracycline-class antibiotics, which are now recommended for children as well as for adults. Because there are no vaccines for the tickborne ehrlichioses and anaplasmosis, the best preventive measures are tick avoidance and control, insect repellants, and rapid removal of blood-feeding ticks by 36 hours or less.

Anaplasmosis

Anaplasmosis is a rapidly emerging tickborne disease that occurs worldwide with highest incidence in North America (Dijkstra et al., 2012; Nelson et al., 2001; Feldman et al., 2001). Anaplasmosis is caused by obligate intracellular bacteria, *Anaplasma phagocytophilum*, which infect granulocytes, principally neutrophils, and cause an asymptomatic or nonspecific febrile illness within 5—21 days (average 7—14 days) after a tick bite (Dijkstra et al., 2012; Nelson et al., 2001; Feldman et al., 2001). Although primarily tickborne, anaplasmosis may also be transmitted by blood product transfusion, by congenital transmission, and by percutaneous or inhalational transmission while butchering an infected host animal, most commonly, a deer (Feldman et al., 2001).

Anaplasmosis occurs in the same regions as Lyme borreliosis and is transmitted by the same vector, the blacklegged tick (*Ixodes scapularis*), with the highest incidence rates in the Northeast (Connecticut, New York, Rhode Island, and Vermont) and in the Upper Midwest (Minnesota and Wisconsin) (Dijkstra et al., 2012; Nelson et al., 2001). The nationwide case counts for anaplasmosis increased over 16-fold from 348 cases in 2000 to 5762 cases in 2017 with Minnesota reporting the highest annual incidence rate and New York the second highest annual incidence rate (Dijkstra et al., 2012; Nelson et al., 2001). These findings most likely reflected improved diagnostic use in endemic regions, and an aging at-risk population with increasing immunosuppressive conditions, such as cancer, chemotherapy, and organ transplants. Since 2015, anaplasmosis has consistently surpassed babesiosis as the second most common tickborne disease after Lyme borreliosis in New York and accounted for 11% of tickborne disease there in 2018 (Dijkstra et al., 2012; Nelson et al., 2001).

The host animal reservoirs for anaplasmosis vary locally, but are primarily confined to rodents including white-footed mice, eastern chipmunks, northern short-tailed shrews, and eastern gray squirrels (Dijkstra et al., 2012; Nelson et al., 2001; Feldman et al., 2001). Since the bacteria are passed transstadially from infected host animals to nymphs to adults and not by transovarian transmission from females to eggs, larvae cannot transmit anaplasmosis.

Symptomatic patients with anaplasmosis will present within an average incubation period of 7—14 days after a blacklegged tick bite with fever, chills, headache, malaise, myalgia, and arthralgia, especially during the summer months (Dijkstra et al., 2012;

Nelson et al., 2001; Feldman et al., 2001). Less common presenting manifestations include stiff neck, nausea, vomiting, diarrhea, and cough (Dijkstra et al., 2012; Nelson et al., 2001; Feldman et al., 2001). Laboratory abnormalities are common and include anemia, leukopenia, thrombocytopenia, and elevated creatinine and hepatic transaminase levels (Keesing et al., 2014; Russell et al., 2021). Severe illness with septic shock, disseminated intravascular coagulation, and cardiorespiratory failure is rare, but more common in patients over 50 years of age and in immunocompromised patients undergoing cancer chemotherapy or organ transplant (Nelder et al., 2019; Kim et al., 2017). Most cases of anaplasmosis, especially in young persons, are asymptomatic. Symptomatic cases respond rapidly to outpatient treatment with oral doxycycline, 17%–56% of patients are hospitalized for treatment, and about 1% of cases are fatal (Nelson et al., 2001; Nelder et al., 2019).

Laboratory diagnostic strategies for anaplasmosis include isolation of *A. phagocytophilum* in blood cultures, microscopic identification of pathognomonic morulae within neutrophils on Giemsa-stained blood smears, positive serologic results by seroconversion or high titer of antibodies, and PCR detection of pathogen DNA in the buffy coat of centrifuged blood (Keesing et al., 2014; Russell et al., 2021; Nelder et al., 2019). Among these tests, blood smears, serology, and PCR are most recommended with the highest sensitivity (0.74) and specificity (1.0) for PCR assays compared to blood smears (sensitivity 0.21, specificity 1.0) and seroconversion (sensitivity 0.32, specificity 0.97) (Keesing et al., 2014; Russell et al., 2021; Nelder et al., 2019).

In a 2017 case report, Korean investigators were the first to demonstrate that crust tissue at tick bite eschar sites remained PCR-positive for *A. phagocytophilum* for up to 6 days after starting doxycycline therapy (Russell et al., 2021). This important observation suggested that crust tissue at eschar sites could be used for early diagnosis even after patients had been started on antibiotics (Russell et al., 2021).

Both anaplasmosis and ehrlichiosis been transmitted by blood transfusions and organ transplants with fatal cases reported (Nelder et al., 2019; Hansmann et al., 2019; Kim et al., 2017).

Ehrlichioses

The human ehrlichioses are a group of potentially fatal tickborne infectious diseases in the United States caused by three related species of obligate, intracellular bacteria, *Ehrlichia chaffeensis*, *E. ewingii*, and *E. muris eauclairensis* (Kemperman et al., 2008). During the reporting period 2008-2012, 4613 cases of *E. chaffeensis* infections were reported for an incidence rate (IR) of 3.2 cases per million person-years (PY) (Goel et al., 2018). The hospitalization rate (HR) was 57%; the case fatality rate (CFR) was 1%; and children less than 5 years of age had the highest CFRs of 4% (Goel et al., 2018). During the same period, 55 cases of *E. ewingii* infection were reported for a national IR of 0.04 cases per million PY with an HR of 77% and no deaths (Goel et al., 2018). Investigators confirmed that the overall IR for ehrlichiosis infections had increased fourfold in the United States between 2000 and 2012; most cases occurred in immunocompetent persons; and children under 5 years of age had increased CFRs relative to older patients (Goel et al., 2018). Investigators attributed the increasing incidences of reported infections to improved diagnostic use in endemic regions, and to an aging, at-risk population with more immunosuppressive conditions and more outdoor exposures in highly endemic areas.

Ehrlichiosis is most commonly reported from the southeastern and midwestern United States with most cases in the spring through the summer months (Kemperman et al., 2008; Goel et al., 2018; Mowla et al., 2021; Dumler et al., 2007; Heitman et al., 2016). The principal host animal reservoirs for ehrlichiosis are white-tailed deer. Both transstadial and transovarian transmission occur in the tick vectors of ehrlichiosis. *E. chaffeensis* and *E. ewingii* are primarily transmitted by the lone star tick (*Amblyomma americanum*), and *E. muris eauclairensis* is primarily transmitted by the eastern blacklegged tick (*Ixodes scapularis*) (Kemperman et al., 2008; Goel et al., 2018; Mowla et al., 2021; Dumler et al., 2007; Heitman et al., 2016).

Symptomatic infections occur 5—14 days after tick bites and are characterized by early manifestations of nonspecific flu-like symptoms with fever, chills, headache, malaise, weakness, myalgia, and nausea (Kemperman et al., 2008; Goel et al., 2018; Mowla et al., 2021; Dumler et al., 2007; Heitman et al., 2016; Pritt et al., 2011). A rash will occur in 60% of children and 30% of adults. In untreated infections, progression of disease may be complicated by brain abscess and intracerebral hemorrhage, septic shock, rhabdomyolysis, hepatorenal and cardiorespiratory failure. The disease is more common in adults than children, with a predominance in older men during June and July, most likely from seasonal occupational exposures (Kemperman et al., 2008; Goel et al., 2018). Other risk factors for ehrlichiosis include the extremes of age, immunosuppression of any type, and any delay in diagnosis (Kemperman et al., 2008; Heitman et al., 2016). About half of all cases require hospitalization, 7% require critical care, and the CFR for *E. chaffeensis*-caused ehrlichiosis is 0.3% (Kemperman et al., 2008; Goel et al., 2018; Mowla et al., 2021; Dumler et al., 2007; Heitman et al., 2016). Early laboratory abnormalities include may include anemia, leukopenia, thrombocytopenia, hyponatremia, and elevated hepatic transaminases, and, less commonly, lactic acidosis and coagulopathies (Kemperman et al., 2008).

Like anaplasmosis, diagnostic strategies for ehrlichiosis include isolation of *Ehrlichia* species in blood cultures, microscopic identification of pathognomonic Maltese cross-shaped inclusions or morulae within monocytes on Giemsa-stained blood smears, positive serologic results by seroconversion or high titer of antibodies, and PCR detection of pathogen DNA in the buffy coat of centrifuged blood. Like anaplasmosis, treatment is with tetracycline-class antibiotics, with doxycycline preferred (Kemperman et al., 2008; Goel et al., 2018; Mowla et al., 2021; Dumler et al., 2007).

Prevention and control of tickborne diseases

A number of strategies can be used in the prevention and control of tickborne infectious diseases and paralytic poisonings, including immunization, personal protective measures, landscape management, and wildlife management (Pritt et al., 2011; Boyce et al., 2016).

In 1998, the FDA approved a new recombinant Lyme disease vaccine which reduced LB infections in 80% of vaccinated adults (Overmiller and Bitter, 2021). In 2002, the manufacturer withdrew the vaccine from the market in response to increasing media coverage of unconfirmed possible vaccine adverse effects; these reports resulted in potential liability for the manufacturer and to declining sales, leading to the economic decision to retreat from the market (Overmiller and Bitter, 2021).

Immunization strategies to prevent tickborne infectious diseases have proved far more effective in Europe and Asia than in the United States, where neurologic complications from TBEVs are second only to Japanese encephalitis virus as causes of permanent paraparesis. Current immunization programs for tickborne viral diseases now provide primary prevention of TBEV-Eu in Europe, TBEV-Sib in Russia and the Middle East, TBEV-FE in China and the Far East, and CCHF in Bulgaria. A canine antitoxin for *I. holocyclus*—induced tick paralysis has been used to reverse tick paralysis in animals and humans in Australia.

In 2021, the FDA approved the first tickborne encephalitis vaccine, TICOVAC, that has been administered for over 20 years in Europe. Today, two new vaccines for LB are under development (Eisen, 2020). One is a multivalent protein-subunit vaccine that targets the outer surface protein of *Borrelia* species causing LB. The other vaccine is a monoclonal antibody designed for pre-exposure prophylaxis for LB (Eisen, 2020).

In addition to immunization, antibiotic therapy after presumed ixodid tick bites with erythema migrans has been recommended as a prophylactic therapeutic strategy for the primary prevention of some tickborne infections. A randomized clinical trial found that a single 200-mg dose of doxycycline administered within 72 hours of a tick bite was 87% effective in preventing Lyme borreliosis (Eisen, 2020).

Finally, because most tickborne infectious diseases may also be transmitted by blood product transfusions, screening blood product donors in high seroprevalence areas for Lyme borreliosis and other borrelioses, babesiosis, ehrlichioses, and anaplasmosis would eliminate transfusion-transmitted cases. Physicians are encouraged to order leukocyte-reduced blood components for blood product transfusions to potentially reduce the risks for ehrlichiosis and anaplasmosis, especially in regions that are highly endemic for leukocytotropic tickborne infectious diseases.

Personal protective measures to prevent tick-transmitted diseases include wearing appropriate clothing, using insect repellents, and performing regular tick checks. Wearing long pants tucked into socks, long-sleeved shirts, and light-colored clothing can help keep ticks off the skin and make them easier to spot on clothing. Impregnating clothing with permethrin, routinely performed by the military on maneuvers, is a highly effective repellent against ticks and other insects. The topical application of insect repellents containing 20%–50% formulations of *N,N*-diethyl-meta-toluamide (DEET) or 7%–15% picaridin directly on the skin is another effective and recommended measure.

Most patients with Lyme borreliosis, TBRF, babesiosis, ehrlichioses, and anaplasmosis will not recall tick bites because these diseases are often transmitted by diminutive nymphal ticks. Nevertheless, tick localization and removal as soon as possible, preferably within 36 hours, remain recommended strategies to prevent the rickettsial and viral ixodid tickborne diseases and to reverse tick paralysis. Ticks should always be removed with fine-tipped forceps (or tweezers), not fingers (because squashing ticks can transmit several tickborne diseases across dermal barriers or create infectious aerosols), and in contiguity with their feeding mouthparts, rather than burning ticks with spent matches or painting embedded ticks with adhesives or nail polishes.

References

Acute respiratory distress syndrome in persons with tickborne relapsing fever—three states. Centers for Disease Control and Prevention 56 (41), 2004, 1073.

Arvikar, S.L., Steere, A.C., 2015. Diagnosis and treatment of lyme arthritis. Infectious Disease Clinics of North America 29 (2), 269–280. https://doi.org/10.1016/j.idc.2015.02.004.

Biggs, H.M., Behravesh, C.B., Bradley, K.K., Dahlgren, F.S., Drexler, N.A., Dumler, J.S., Folk, S.M., Kato, C.Y., Lash, R.R., Levin, M.L., Massung, R.F., Nadelman, R.B., Nicholson, W.L., Paddock, C.D., Pritt, B.S., Traeger, M.S., 2016. Diagnosis and management of tickborne rickettsial diseases: Rocky Mountain spotted fever and other spotted fever group rickettsioses, ehrlichioses, and anaplasmosis — United States. MMWR. Recommendations and Reports 65 (2), 1–44. https://doi.org/10.15585/mmwr.rr6502a1.

Bissett, J.D., Ledet, S., Krishnavajhala, A., Armstrong, B.A., Klioueva, A., Sexton, C., Replogle, A., Schriefer, M.E., Lopez, J.E., 2018. Detection of tickborne relapsing fever Spirochete, Austin, Texas, USA. Emerging Infectious Diseases 24 (11), 2003–2009. https://doi.org/10.3201/eid2411.172033.

Blanton, L., Keith, B., Brzezinski, W., 2008. Southern tick-associated rash illness: erythema migrans is not always lyme disease. Southern Medical Journal 101 (7), 759–760. https://doi.org/10.1097/SMJ.0b013e31817a8b3f.

Boyce, R.M., Sanfilippo, A.M., Boulos, J.M., 2016. Ehrlichia infections. Emerging Infectious Diseases 24 (11), 2087–2089.

Dahlgren, F.S., McQuiston, J.H., Massung, R.F., Anderson, A.D., 2015. Q fever in the United States: summary of case reports from two national surveillance systems, 2000-2012. The American Journal of Tropical Medicine and Hygiene 92 (2), 247–255. https://doi.org/10.4269/ajtmh.14-0503.

Demma, L.J., Traeger, M.S., Nicholson, W.L., Paddock, C.D., Blau, D.M., Eremeeva, M.E., Dasch, G.A., Levin, M.L., Singleton, J., Zaki, S.R., Cheek, J.E., Swerdlow, D.L., McQuiston, J.H., 2005. Rocky Mountain spotted fever from an unexpected tick vector in Arizona. New England Journal of Medicine 353 (6), 587–594. https://doi.org/10.1056/NEJMoa050043.

Dijkstra, F., van der Hoek, W., Wijers, N., Schimmer, B., Rietveld, A., Wijkmans, C.J., Vellema, P., Schneeberger, P.M., 2012. The 2007–2010 Q fever epidemic in The Netherlands: characteristics of notified acute Q fever patients and the association with dairy goat farming. FEMS Immunology and Medical Microbiology 64 (1), 3–12. https://doi.org/10.1111/j.1574-695x.2011.00876.x.

Drexler, N.A., Dahlgren, F.S., Heitman, K.N., Massung, R.F., Paddock, C.D., Behravesh, C.B., 2016. National surveillance of spotted fever group rickettsioses in the United States, 2008-2012. The American Journal of Tropical Medicine and Hygiene 94 (1), 26–34. https://doi.org/10.4269/ajtmh.15-0472.

Dumler, J.S., Madigan, J.E., Pusterla, N., Bakken, J.S., 2007. Ehrlichioses in humans: epidemiology, clinical presentation, diagnosis, and treatment. Clinical Infectious Diseases 45 (1), S45—S51. https://doi.org/10.1086/518146.

Dworkin, M.S., Schoemaker, P.C., Fritz, C.L., 2002. The epidemiology of tickborne relapsing fever in the United States. The American Journal of Tropical Medicine and Hygiene 54 (6), 289—293.

Eisen, L., 2020. Stemming the rising tide of human-biting ticks and tickborne diseases, United States. Emerging Infectious Diseases 26 (4), 641—647. https://doi.org/10.3201/eid2604.191629.

Feder, H.M., Johnson, B.J.B., O'Connell, S., Shapiro, E.D., Steere, A.C., Wormser, G.P., 2007. A critical appraisal of "chronic lyme disease". New England Journal of Medicine 357 (14), 1422—1430. https://doi.org/10.1056/nejmra072023.

Feldman, K.A., Enscore, R.E., Lathrop, S.L., Matyas, B.T., McGuill, M., Schriefer, M.E., Stiles-Enos, D., Dennis, D.T., Petersen, L.R., Hayes, E.B., 2001. An outbreak of primary pneumonic tularemia on Martha's vineyard. New England Journal of Medicine 345 (22), 1601—1606. https://doi.org/10.1056/NEJMoa011374.

Forrester, J.D., Kugeler, K.J., Perea, A.E., Pastula, D.M., Mead, P.S., 2015. No geographic correlation between lyme disease and death due to 4 neurodegenerative disorders, United States, 2001—2010. Emerging Infectious Diseases 21 (11), 2036—2039. https://doi.org/10.3201/eid2111.150778.

Goel, R., Westblade, L.F., Kessler, D.A., Sfeir, M., Slavinski, S., Backenson, B., Gebhardt, L., Kane, K., Laurence, J., Scherr, D., Bussel, J., Dumler, J.S., Cushing, M.M., Vasovic, L.V., 2018. Death from transfusion-transmitted anaplasmosis, New York, USA, 2017. Emerging Infectious Diseases 24 (8), 1548—1550. https://doi.org/10.3201/eid2408.172048.

Hansmann, Y., Jaulhac, B., Kieffer, P., Martinot, M., Wurtz, E., Dukic, R., Boess, G., Michel, A., Strady, C., Sagez, J.F., Lefebvre, N., Talagrand-Reboul, E., Argemi, X., De Martino, S., 2019. Value of PCR, serology, and blood smears for human granulocytic anaplasmosis diagnosis, France. Emerging Infectious Diseases 25 (5), 996—998. https://doi.org/10.3201/eid2505.171751.

Heitman, N., Scott Dahlgren, F., Drexler, N.A., Massung, R.F., Behravesh, C.B., 2016. Increasing incidence of ehrlichiosis in the United States: a summary of national surveillance of ehrlichia chaffeensis and ehrlichia ewingii infections in the United States, 2008-2012. The American Journal of Tropical Medicine and Hygiene 94 (1), 52—60. https://doi.org/10.4269/ajtmh.15-0540.

Herrick, K.L., Pena, S.A., Yaglom, H.D., Layton, B.J., Moors, A., Loftis, A.D., Condit, M.E., Singleton, J., Kato, C.Y., Denison, A.M., Ng, D., Mertins, J.W., Paddock, C.D., 2016. Rickettsia parkeri rickettsiosis, Arizona, USA. Emerging Infectious Diseases 22 (5), 780—785. https://doi.org/10.3201/eid2205.151824.

Hickling, G.J., Kelly, J.R., Auckland, L.D., Hamer, S.A., 2018. Increasing prevalence of borrelia burgdorferi sensu stricto—Infected blacklegged ticks in Tennessee valley, Tennessee, USA. Emerging Infectious Diseases 24 (9), 1713—1716. https://doi.org/10.3201/eid2409.180343.

Ishizuka, K., Sugaya, M., 2022. Japanese spotted fever. New England Journal of Medicine 387 (5). https://doi.org/10.1056/NEJMicm2119475.

Keesing, F., McHenry, D.J., Hersh, M., Tibbetts, M., Brunner, J.L., Killilea, M., LoGiudice, K., Schmidt, K.A., Ostfeld, R.S., 2014. Prevalence of human-Active and variant 1 strains of the tickborne pathogen Anaplasma phagocytophilum in hosts and forests of Eastern North America. The American Journal of Tropical Medicine and Hygiene 91 (2), 302—309. https://doi.org/10.4269/ajtmh.13-0525.

Kemperman, M., Neitzel, D., Jensen, K., Gorlin, J., Perry, E., Myers, T., Miley, T., McQuiston, J., Eremeeva, M.E., Nicholson, W., Singleton, J., Adjemian, J., 2008. Anaplasma phagocytophilum transmitted through blood transfusion - Minnesota, 2007. Morbidity and Mortality Weekly Report 57 (42), 1145—1148.

Kim, C.M., Kim, S.W., Kim, D.M., Yoon, N.R., Jha, P., Jang, S.J., Ahn, Y.J., Lim, D., Lee, S.H., Hwang, S.D., Lee, Y.S., 2017. Case report: polymerase chain reaction testing of tick bite site samples for the diagnosis of human granulocytic anaplasmosis. The American Journal of Tropical Medicine and Hygiene 97 (2), 403—406. https://doi.org/10.4269/ajtmh.16-0570.

Kirkland, K.B., Klimko, T.B., Meriwether, R.A., Schriefer, M., Levin, M., Levine, J., Mac Kenzie, W.R., Dennis, D.T., 1997. Erythema migrans-like rash illness at a camp in North Carolina: a new tick-borne disease? Archives of Internal Medicine 157 (22), 2635—2641. https://doi.org/10.1001/archinte. 157.22.2635.

Krause, P.J., Narasimhan, S., Wormser, G.P., Rollend, L., Fikrig, E., Lepore, T., Barbour, A., Fish, D., 2013. Human Borrelia miyamotoi infection in the United States. New England Journal of Medicine 368 (3), 291—293. https://doi.org/10.1056/NEJMc1215469.

Liu, Y., Zhang, X.P., Liu, H., Wu, H.Y., Zhou, D.A., Tian, Y., 2014. Prognostic predictors for non-small cell lung cancer patients with brain metastasis after radiotherapy. Chinese Journal of Cancer Prevention and Treatment 21 (21), 1719—1722.

Lu, Q., Yu, J., Yu, L., Zhang, Y., Chen, Y., Lin, M., Fang, X., 2018. Rickettsia japonica infections in humans, Zhejiang Province, China, 2015. Emerging Infectious Diseases 24 (11), 2077—2079. https://doi.org/10.3201/eid2411.170044.

Mack, I., Ritz, N., 2019. African tick-bite fever. New England Journal of Medicine 380 (10). https://doi.org/10.1056/NEJMicm1810093.

Mafi, N., Yaglom, H.D., Levy, C., Taylor, A., O'grad, C., Venkat, H., Komatsu, K.K., Roller, B., Seville, M.T., Kusne, S., Po, J.L., Thorn, S., Ampel, N.M., 2019. Tick-borne relapsing fever in the white mountains, Arizona, USA, 2013—2018. Emerging Infectious Diseases 25 (4), 649—653. https://doi.org/10.3201/eid2504.181369.

Marques, et al., 2021. Computer Communications 1—9.

Marzec, N.S., Nelson, C., Waldron, P.R., Blackburn, B.G., Hosain, S., Greenhow, T., Green, G.M., Lomen-Hoerth, C., Golden, M., Mead, P.S., 2017. Serious bacterial infections acquired during treatment of patients given a diagnosis of chronic Lyme Disease — United States. Morbidity and Mortality Weekly Report 66 (23), 607—609. https://doi.org/10.15585/mmwr.mm6623a3.

Masters, E.J., Grigery, C.N., Masters, R.W., 2008. STARI, or Masters disease-tick-vectored Lyme-like illness. Infectious Disease Clinics of North America 22 (2), 361.

Matsuura, H., Yokota, K., 2018. Case report: family cluster of Japanese spotted fever. The American Journal of Tropical Medicine and Hygiene 98 (3), 835—837. https://doi.org/10.4269/ajtmh.17-0199.

McBride, W.J.H., Hanson, J.P., Miller, R., Wenck, D., 2007. Severe spotted fever group rickettsiosis, Australia. Emerging Infectious Diseases 13 (11), 1742—1744. https://doi.org/10.3201/eid1311.070099.

Mowla, S.J., Drexler, N.A., Cherry, C.C., Annambholta, P.D., Kracalik, I.T., Basavaraju, S.V., 2021. Ehrlichiosis and anaplasmosis among transfusion and transplant recipients in the United States. Emerging Infectious Diseases 27 (11), 2768—2775. https://doi.org/10.3201/eid2711.211127.

Nadelman, R.B., Nowakowski, J., Fish, D., Falco, R.C., Freeman, K., McKenna, D., Welch, P., Marcus, R., Agüero-Rosenfeld, M.E., Dennis, D.T., Wormser, G.P., 2001. Prophylaxis with single-dose doxycycline for the prevention of lyme disease after an Ixodes scapularis tick bite. New England Journal of Medicine 345 (2), 79—84. https://doi.org/10.1056/NEJM200107123450201.

Nadelman, R.B., Hanincová, K., Mukherjee, P., Liveris, D., Nowakowski, J., McKenna, D., Brisson, D., Cooper, D., Bittker, S., Madison, G., Holmgren, D., Schwartz, I., Wormser, G.P., 2012. Differentiation of reinfection from relapse in recurrent Lyme disease. New England Journal of Medicine 367 (20), 1883—1890. https://doi.org/10.1056/NEJMoa1114362.

Nelder, M.P., Russell, C.B., Lindsay, L.R., Dibernardo, A., Brandon, N.C., Pritchard, J., Johnson, S., Cronin, K., Patel, S.N., 2019. Recent emergence of Anaplasma phagocytophilum in Ontario, Canada: early serological and entomological indicators. The American Journal of Tropical Medicine and Hygiene 101 (6), 1249—1258. https://doi.org/10.4269/ajtmh.19-0166.

Nelson, C., Kugeler, K., Petersen, J., 2001. Tularemia—United States. Morbidity & Mortality Weekly Report 62 (47), 963—966.

Otsuki, Y., Kobayashi, H., Arai, Y., Inoue, N., Matsubayashi, T., Koide, M., Yamakawa, M., 2020. A patient with 22q11.2 deletion syndrome presenting with systemic skin rash and dermatopathic lymphadenitis of unusual histology. American Journal of Case Reports 21, 1—6. https://doi.org/10.12659/AJCR.924961.

Overmiller, A.C., Bitter, C.C., 2021. Rhabdomyolysis and multisystem organ failure due to fulminant ehrlichiosis infection. Wilderness and Environmental Medicine 32 (2), 226—229. https://doi.org/10.1016/j.wem.2021.01.009.

Pritt, B.S., Sloan, L.M., Hoang Johnson, D.K., Munderloh, U.G., Paskewitz, S.M., McElroy, K.M., McFadden, J.D., Binnicker, M.J., Neitzel, D.F., Liu, G., Nicholson, W.L., Nelson, C.M., Franson, J.J., Martin, S.A., Cunningham, S.A., Steward, C.R., Bogumill, K., Bjorgaard, M.E., Davis, J.P., McQuiston, J.H., Warshauer, D.M., Wilhelm, M.P., Patel, R., Trivedi, V.A., Eremeeva, M.E., 2011. Emergence of a new pathogenic Ehrlichia species, Wisconsin and Minnesota, 2009. New England Journal of Medicine 365 (5), 422—429. https://doi.org/10.1056/NEJMoa1010493.

Qin, X.R., Han, H.J., Han, F.J., Zhao, F.M., Zhang, Z.T., Xue, Z.F., Ma, D.Q., Qi, R., Zhao, M., Wang, L.J., Zhao, L., Yu, H., Liu, J.W., Yu, X.J., 2019. Rickettsia japonica and novel rickettsia species in ticks, China. Emerging Infectious Diseases 25 (5), 992—995. https://doi.org/10.3201/eid2505.171745.

Rovery, C., Brouqui, P., Raoult, D., 2008. Questions on mediterranean spotted fever a century after its discovery. Emerging Infectious Diseases 14 (9), 1360—1367. https://doi.org/10.3201/eid1409.071133.

Russell, A., Prusinski, M., Sommer, J., O'Connor, C., White, J., Falco, R., Kokas, J., Vinci, V., Gall, W., Tober, K., Haight, J., Oliver, J.A., Meehan, L., Sporn, L.A., Brisson, D., Backenson, P.B., 2021. Epidemiology and spatial emergence of anaplasmosis, New York, USA, 2010–2018. Emerging Infectious Diseases 27 (8), 2154—2162. https://doi.org/10.3201/eid208.210133.

Schwartz, Journal of Dynamic Systems, Measurement and Control, Transactions of the ASME 1—12.

Steere, A.C., 2012. Reinfection versus relapse in lyme disease. New England Journal of Medicine 367 (20), 1950—1951. https://doi.org/10.1056/NEJMe1211361.

Ta, T.H., Jiménez, B., Navarro, M., Meije, Y., González, F.J., Lopez-Velez, R., 2008. Q fever in returned febrile travelers. Journal of Travel Medicine 15 (2), 126—129. https://doi.org/10.1111/j.1708-8305.2008.00191.x.

Talagrand-Reboul, E., Boyer, P.H., Bergström, S., Vial, L., Boulanger, N., 2018. Relapsing fevers: neglected tick-borne diseases. Frontiers in Cellular and Infection Microbiology 8. https://doi.org/10.3389/fcimb.2018.00098.

Tibbles, C.D., Edlow, J.A., 2007. Does this patient have erythema migrans? JAMA 297 (23), 2617—2627. https://doi.org/10.1001/jama.297.23.2617.

Tsai, Y.S., Wu, Y.H., Kao, P.T., Lin, Y.C., 2008. African tick bite fever. Journal of the Formosan Medical Association 107 (1), 73—76. https://doi.org/10.1016/S0929-6646(08)60011-X.

Vannier, E.G., Diuk-Wasser, M.A., Mamoun, C.B., Krause, P.J., Kirkland, K.B., Klimko, T.B., Meriweather, R.A., 1997. Diagnosis and management of tickborne rickettsial diseases: Rocky Mountain spotted fever and other spotted fever group rickettsioses, ehrlichioses, and anaplasmosis-United States. A practical guide for health professionals. Overmiller AC, Bitter CC. Rhabdomyolysis and Multisystem Organ Failure Due to Fulminant Ehrlichiosis Infection 29, 1763—1773. https://doi.org/10.3389/fcimb.2018.00098.

Vannier, E.G., Diuk-Wasser, M.A., Ben Mamoun, C., Krause, P.J., 2015. Babesiosis. Infectious Disease Clinics of North America 29 (2), 357—370. https://doi.org/10.1016/j.idc.2015.02.008.

Varela, A.S., Luttrell, M.P., Howerth, E.W., Moore, V.A., Davidson, W.R., Stallknecht, D.E., Little, S.E., 2004. First culture isolation of Borrelia lonestari, putative agent of southern tick-associated rash illness. Journal of Clinical Microbiology 42 (3), 1163—1169. https://doi.org/10.1128/JCM.42.3.1163-1169.2004.

Wormser, G.P., Masters, E., Nowakowski, J., McKenna, D., Holmgren, D., Ma, K., Ihde, L., Cavaliere, L.F., Nadelman, R.B., 2005. Prospective clinical evaluation of patients from Missouri and New York with erythema migrans-like skin lesions. Clinical Infectious Diseases 41 (7), 958—965. https://doi.org/10.1086/432935.

Yamanaka, A., Kirino, Y., Fujimoto, S., Ueda, N., Himeji, D., Miura, M., Sudaryatma, P.E., Sato, Y., Tanaka, H., Mekata, H., Okabayashi, T., 2020. Direct transmission of severe fever with thrombocytopenia syndrome virus from domestic cat to veterinary personnel. Emerging Infectious Diseases 26 (12), 2994—2998. https://doi.org/10.3201/EID2612.191513.

Yu, P., Tian, H., Li, S., Huang, S., Chowell, G., Brownstein, J.S., Tian, H., Wei, J., Xu, B., Zhou, S., Han, Z., Lv, W., Yang, J., Wang, J., 2017. Severe fever with thrombocytopenia syndrome virus in humans, domesticated animals, ticks, and mosquitoes, shaanxi Province, China. The American Journal of Tropical Medicine and Hygiene 96 (6), 1346—1349. https://doi.org/10.4269/ajtmh.16-0333.

CHAPTER 11

Babesiosis

History

The first *Babesia* species was identified as a cause of hemolytic anemia in cattle in 1888 by Victor Babes, M.D. (1854–1926), a Romanian microbiologist, who was awarded the Nobel Prize in Medicine in 1924 for his investigations (Gray et al., 1997). The zoonotic disease was later named in his honor. Further research in the transmission of babesiosis in animals conducted by Smith and Kilbourne between 1889 and 1893 firmly established the transmission of a pathogen by a tick vector (Gray et al., 1997). The first human case of babesiosis was reported in 1957 (Gray et al., 1997).

Vectors, reservoirs, and regional distributions

Babesia protozoans may be mistaken for intraerythrocytic malaria parasites, such as *Plasmodium falciparum*, during diagnostic light microscopy. The primary tick vector for the *Babesia* parasite is the black-legged tick, *Ixodes scapularis*. The black-legged tick is the same preferred tick vector for Lyme borreliosis, ehrlichiosis, and anaplasmosis and is capable of transmitting coinfections of these diseases along with babesiosis (Gray et al., 1997; Gray and Herwaldt, 2011; Ingram and Crook, 2005).

The primary zoonotic reservoirs for the parasite are in white-footed mice and rabbits, which develop inapparent infections and remain highly parasitemic and capable of infecting blood-feeding ticks for life (Gray et al., 1997; Gray and Herwaldt, 2011; Ingram and Crook, 2005).

The range of distribution of babesiosis mirrors the distributions of the vector and host animals and is now expanding in the Northeast, particularly in the New England states, especially Connecticut. Like other tick-borne infectious diseases, babesiosis occurs in a seasonal pattern with most cases reported during late spring, summer, and early fall, when people are active outdoors (Gray et al., 1997).

Microbiology

Although there are over 100 species of *Babesia*, most of which infect animals, especially cattle, only a few species and their variants cause most disease in the United States including: (1) *Babesia microti*, which is responsible for the majority cases in the United States, especially in the Northeast and Upper Midwest; (2) *Babesia duncani* (and its variants

Ectoparasitic Diseases
ISBN 978-0-443-26724-6,
https://doi.org/10.1016/B978-0-443-26724-6.00011-4

WA-1 and CA1 through CA-4), which is responsible for sporadic cases in the West; (3) *Babesia divergens*, which is responsible for sporadic cases scattered across the country,; and (4) an unnamed variant strain designated MO-1 that also causes sporadic cases in the Midwest (Gray et al., 1997; Ingram and Crook, 2005) (Table 11.1). The *B. microti* strain is most common species transmitted by blood transfusion in the United States (Gray and Herwaldt, 2011; Ingram and Crook, 2005). Despite species and regional differences, transmission modes and clinical manifestations are similar.

Epidemiology

In addition to tick bite transmission, babesiosis may also be transmitted by blood transfusion and congenitally (Ingram and Crook, 2005; Gibbons et al., 2021; Goethert and Telford, 2003). During the reporting period 2011—15, the CDC was notified of 7612 cases of babesiosis among residents in 27 states with 6277 confirmed (82.5%) and 1335 probable (17.5%) cases. Most of the cases (94.5%) occurred in seven states (Connecticut, Massachusetts, Minnesota, New Jersey, New York, Rhode Island, and Wisconsin) with only two other (contiguous) states reporting more than 100 cases over 5 years, Maine (152 cases) and New Hampshire (149 cases) (Gray et al., 1997).

The median age of case-patients with complete clinical information was 63 years (range 1—99 years), with 57.9% over 60 years of age, and less than 1% under a year of age (Gray et al., 1997). Most (>70%) cases occurred during June through August in the Northeast and Upper Midwest (Gray et al., 1997). About half (46.9%) of the patients were hospitalized, especially patients who were 80 years of age and older and asplenic patients (Gray et al., 1997). There were 51 cases of babesiosis among recipients of blood transfusions (Gray et al., 1997). Asplenic patients of all ages are particularly predisposed to babesiosis after bites by *Babesia*-carrying ixodid ticks (Gray et al., 1997).

The incidence of babesiosis has now increased nearly five times in some New England states with Connecticut reporting an incidence of 2 cases per 100,000 persons in 2011 and nine cases per 100,000 persons in 2019 (New et al., 1997). Although *B. microti* is the predominant species causing babesiosis in the United States today, more than 100 species of *Babesia* are now known to cause babesiosis in animals and humans (New et al., 1997).

Risk factors for babesiosis

(New et al., 1997; Herwaldt et al., 1997) Parasitemia may persist for up to 2 years in these cases, especially in asplenic patients, despite prolonged antimicrobial therapy, and may result in potentially fatal complications including hemolytic anemia, thrombocytopenia, elevated transaminases, jaundice, renal failure, acute adult respiratory distress syndrome, shock, and multiorgan failure (Kjemtrup et al., 2002). Relapses requiring retreatment with antimalarial-type antibiotics can occur in high-risk cases in immunocompromised

Table 11.1 Causal agents and clinical manifestations of babesiosis.

BABESIA species	Geographic distribution	Tick vectors	Animal reservoirs	Epidemiology	Clinical manifestations
B. divergens	United Kingdom, Western Europe, Eastern Europe, Sweden, Russia; not reported in United States	*Ixodes ricinus*	Cattle, reindeer	Incubation 1–4 wk occurs during summer months in cattle-raising regions Targets splenectomized or immunocompromised patients primarily	Fulminant course with high case-fatality rate fever, rigors, headache, myalgia, jaundice, hemoglobinuria, hemolytic anemia, acute renal failure, multiorgan failure
B. microti	Parallels the US Northeast endemic regions for *Borrelia burgdorferi*, especially the islands off New York, Massachusetts, Connecticut, and Rhode Island and focal areas in Connecticut, New Jersey, Wisconsin, and Minnesota	Deer ticks: *Ixodes scapularis*	White-footed mouse (*Peromyscus leucopus*)	Incubation 1–4 wk after tick bites or 4–9 wk after blood transfusions transmission primarily by nymphal ticks Targets older, not necessarily immunocompromised patients; particularly severe in those immunocompromised by HIV infection, advanced age, coinfections with *Borrelia burgdorferi* Seasonality parallels tick nymph activity; 80% of cases occur May –August	Often asymptomatic in young, healthy patients self-limited influenza-like febrile illness with onset of anorexia, malaise, lethargy, followed in 1 wk by high fever, diaphoresis, myalgias; mild splenomegaly, rarely hepatomegaly later hemolysis, hemolytic anemia, thrombocytopenia, jaundice, acute renal failure, especially in the splenectomized, elderly, or immunocompromised complications include ARDS and DIC case-fatality rate: 5%

Continued

Table 11.1 Causal agents and clinical manifestations of babesiosis.—cont'd

BABESIA species	Geographic distribution	Tick vectors	Animal reservoirs	Epidemiology	Clinical manifestations
MO-1 (a relative or subspecies of *B. divergens*)	Rural Missouri and Kentucky	*Ixodes dentatus* (rabbit tick)	Rabbits, birds	Incubation 1–4 wk after tick bites spring to autumn seasonality Targets splenectomized patients, like *B. divergens*	Same as above: Often asymptomatic, except in the splenectomized, who will develop high parasitemias and multiorgan failure
WA-1 (a relative or subspecies of *B. gibsoni*)	Rural Washington state	Ixodid ticks, including *Ixodes dentatus*	Unknown; wild canids and ungulates suspected	Incubation 1–4 wk Targets the splenectomized, elderly, immunocompromised, premature infants May be transmitted by blood transfusion	Same as above: Often asymptomatic, except in the splenectomized, who will develop high parasitemias and multiorgan failure
CA-1, CA-2, etc. (relatives or subspecies of mule deer and bighorn sheep *Babesia* species)	US Pacific Coast, primarily rural and semirural areas of California	Ixodid ticks	Unknown; mule deer and bighorn sheep suspected	Incubation 1–4 wk Targets the splenectomized, elderly, immunocompromised, and premature infants	Same as above: Often asymptomatic, except in the splenectomized, who will develop high parasitemias and multiorgan failure

ARDS, Acute respiratory distress syndrome; *DIC*, disseminated intravascular coagulation; *HIV*, human immunodeficiency virus.
Adapted from Diaz JH: Section on Ectoparasitic Diseases. Chapter 296. Ticks (Including Tick Paralysis). In Bennett JE, Dolin R, Blaser MJ, Eds. *Mandell, Douglas and Bennett's Principles and Practice of Infectious Diseases*, Ninth Edition, Elsevier, Philadelphia, 2019. Elsevier publication.

and asplenic persons, and reinfections requiring retreatment can occur after new ixodid tick bites (Herwaldt et al., 1997; Kjemtrup et al., 2002; Locke et al., 2011).

Clinical manifestations

Although most persons with babesiosis experience short-term influenza-like illnesses, elderly persons with chronic diseases and the immunocompromised can suffer prolonged disease characterized by hematologic and neurologic manifestations and multiorgan failure. Babesiosis may result in asymptomatic parasitemia in immunocompetent persons, who can still transmit the disease congenitally or by blood transfusion or organ transplant due to a prolonged parasitemia of up to 1 year, even after antimicrobial therapy (Kjemtrup et al., 2002). In symptomatic cases, the clinical manifestations of babesiosis include nonspecific, influenza-like symptoms of fever, fatigue, malaise, diaphoresis, and myalgia, usually of a gradual onset one to 2 weeks after a noticed tick bite (Gray et al., 1997; New et al., 1997). Most infections are either self-limited or cured with a 7—10 day course of recommended antimicrobial agents.

Autoimmune hemolytic anemia in babesiosis

Although the most common clinical presentation of babesiosis is a febrile viral-like illness with laboratory evidence of nonimmune hemolytic anemia and thrombocytopenia, investigators reported six cases of autoimmune hemolytic anemia among 86 patients treated for babesiosis at their institution over a 7.5-year period (Tompkins et al., 2017). All six patients were asplenic ($P < 0.0001$) and demonstrated positive direct antiglobulin tests for immunoglobulin G and complement complex 3, which confirmed production of autoantibodies against erythrocytes (Tompkins et al., 2017).

Unlike the non-immune-mediated hemolysis, which characterizes most cases of babesiosis and resolves after appropriate antimicrobial therapy, autoimmune hemolysis continues to cause hemolysis in babesiosis patients posttreatment and requires immunosuppressive therapy with corticosteroids and/or monoclonal antibodies, such as rituximab (anti-CD20 monoclonal antibody) (Tompkins et al., 2017). The investigators recommended that asplenic and immunosuppressed patients with worsening or recrudescent hemolytic anemia after treatment for babesiosis be evaluated for prolonged autoimmune hemolytic anemia and potential immunosuppressive therapy (Tompkins et al., 2017).

Neurologic effects

In addition to hematologic effects, babesiosis frequently causes neurologic effects in persons affected including altered state of consciousness, headache, syncope, neuropathy, and retinal nerve infarcts (New et al., 1997). In 2023, Locke and coinvestigators reported the results of their retrospective medical record review of the neurologic complications in 163 patients with confirmed (by microscopy or PCR) babesiosis admitted to the

Yale—New Haven Connecticut Hospital during the reporting period 2011—2021 (New et al., 1997). More than half of the patients experienced one or more neurologic complications including headache, confusion/delirium, and impaired consciousness (New et al., 1997). Neurologic symptoms were associated with high parasitemia, renal failure, and diabetes mellitus (New et al., 1997).

Laboratory Diagnosis

Diagnostic strategies for babesiosis include the demonstration of characteristic intraerythrocytic and extraerythrocytic organisms on Giemsa-stained thin smears and subinoculation of human blood samples into hamsters for suspected *B. microti* infections or into gerbils for suspected *B. divergens* infections (Fig. 11.1). (Gray et al., 1997; Gray and Herwaldt, 2011) Other diagnostic tests, usually only available at reference laboratories, that are especially useful when microscopic methods fail in low parasitemias, include indirect immunofluorescence antibody testing for specific immunoglobulin M antibodies in acute infections and PCR-based assays to detect *Babesia* DNA and species-specific DNA sequences (Gray et al., 1997; Gray and Herwaldt, 2011).

In highly parasitemic cases of babesiosis, stained peripheral blood smears such as this one may demonstrate the characteristic intraerythrocytic ring forms of *Babesia* that microscopically resemble the intraerythrocytic ring forms of malaria.

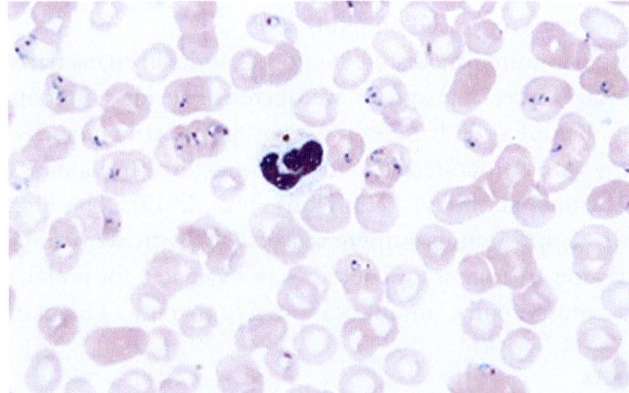

Figure 11.1 Intraerythrocytic *Babesia* species in a peripheral blood smear. (Thin blood smear, Giemsa stain, ×1000). Intraerythrocytic *Babesia* species in a peripheral blood smear. (Thin blood smear, Giemsa stain, ×1000). Note the vacuolated intraerythrocytic ring forms that resemble *Plasmodium* species trophozoites and the clumped extraerythrocytic forms. *(From DPDx Image Library. Babesiosis Image Library: Babesia sp. in thin blood smears stained with Giemsa, Fig. A. Atlanta, GA: Centers for Disease Control and Prevention. http://www.cdc.gov/dpdx/babesiosis/index.html)*

Therapy

Quinine (650 mg PO three times daily) and clindamycin (1.2 g IV twice daily or 600 mg PO three times daily), continued for 1 week until parasitemias diminish, are recommended to treat uncomplicated babesiosis caused by all species (Gray et al., 1997; Gray and Herwaldt, 2011; Locke et al., 2011). Quinine and clindamycin are preferred therapies for severe *B. microti* infections, especially in older adults and asplenic or immunosuppressed individuals (Herwaldt et al., 1997). For non-life-threatening *B. microti* infections, a 2-week course of oral atovaquone (750 mg twice daily) and azithromycin (500 mg on day 1, followed by 250–600 mg/day for 1 week) cleared parasitemias as effectively as quinine and clindamycin, with fewer side effects (Gray et al., 1997; Gray and Herwaldt, 2011; Herwaldt et al., 1997; Kjemtrup et al., 2002).

Treating coinfections

For coinfections with *Borrelia burgdorferi*, patients should be treated specifically for Lyme borreliosis with doxycycline (200 mg PO twice daily for 2 weeks) and with antimalarial-type agents for babesiosis (Gray et al., 1997).

Prevention and control

A number of strategies can be used in the prevention and control of tick-borne infectious diseases, such as babesiosis, including immunization, personal protective measures, landscape management, and wildlife management. Although some vaccines are available for some tick-borne viruses, there is no vaccine for babesiosis. Since babesiosis is caused by a protozoan, there is no antibiotic chemoprophylaxis for babesiosis after tick bites.

Screening banked blood for babesiosis

Since babesiosis may also be transmitted by blood product transfusions, screening blood product donors in high seroprevalence areas for would eliminate transfusion-transmitted cases (Krause et al., 1998).

Personal protective measures

Personal protective measures to prevent tick-transmitted diseases include wearing appropriate clothing, using insect repellents, and performing regular tick checks. Wearing long pants tucked into socks, long-sleeved shirts, and light-colored clothing can help keep ticks off the skin and make them easier to spot on clothing. Impregnating clothing with permethrin, routinely performed by the military on maneuvers, is a highly effective repellent against ticks and other insects. The topical application of insect repellents containing 20%–50% formulations of *N,N*-diethyl-meta-toluamide (DEET) or 7%–15% picaridin directly on the skin is another effective and recommended measure.

Removing ticks

Most patients with babesiosis will not recall tick bites, especially bites by diminutive nymphal ticks. Nevertheless, tick localization and removal as soon as possible, preferably within 36 h, remain recommended strategies to prevent the rickettsial and viral ixodid tick-borne diseases and to reverse tick paralysis. Ticks should always be removed with fine-tipped forceps (or tweezers), not fingers (because squashing ticks can transmit several tick-borne diseases across dermal barriers or create infectious aerosols), and in contiguity with their feeding mouthparts, rather than burning ticks with spent matches or painting embedded ticks with adhesives or nail polishes.

References

Gibbons, M.D., Mendoza, D.P., Waheed, A., Barshak, M.B., Villalba, J.A., 2021. Case 14-2021: a 64-year-old woman with fever and pancytopenia. New England Journal of Medicine 384 (19), 1849–1857. https://doi.org/10.1056/NEJMcpc2100275, 15334406.

Goethert, H.K., Telford, S.R., 2003. Enzootic transmission of Babesia divergens among cottontail rabbits on Nantucket Island, Massachusetts. The American Journal of Tropical Medicine and Hygiene 69 (5), 455–460. https://doi.org/10.4269/ajtmh.2003.69.455, 00029637.

Gray, E.B., Herwaldt, B.L., 2011. Babesiosis surveillance—United States. Morbidity & Mortality Weekly Report 68 (6), 1–11.

Gray, E.B., Herwaldt, B.;, Ingram, D., Crook, T., Gibbons, M.D., Mendoza, D.P., Waheed, A., 1997. Risk factors for severe infection, hospitalization, and prolonged antimicrobial therapy in patients with babesiosis. Goethert HK, Telford SR III 68, 2236–2245.

Herwaldt, B.L., Kjemtrup, A.M., Conrad, P.A., Barnes, R.C., Wilson, M., McCarthy, M.G., Sayers, M.H., Eberhard, M.L., 1997. Transfusion-transmitted babesiosis in Washington state: first reported case caused by a WA1-type parasite. Journal of Infectious Diseases 175 (5), 1259–1262. https://doi.org/10.1086/593812, 00221899.

Ingram, D., Crook, T., 2005. Rise in babesiosis cases. Emerging Infectious Diseases 26 (8), 1703–1709.

Kjemtrup, A.M., Lee, B., Fritz, C.L., Evans, C., Chervenak, M., Conrad, P.A., 2002. Investigation of transfusion transmission of a WA1-type babesial parasite to a premature infant in California. Transfusion 42 (11), 1482–1487. https://doi.org/10.1046/j.1537-2995.2002.00245.x, 00411132.

Krause, P.J., Spielman, A., Telford, S.R., Sikand, V.K., McKay, K., Christianson, D., Pollack, R.J., Brassard, P., Magera, J., Ryan, R., Persing, D.H., 1998. Persistent parasitemia after acute babesiosis. New England Journal of Medicine 339 (3), 160–165. https://doi.org/10.1056/NEJM199807163390304, 00284793.

Locke, Bryan, O., Zubair, J., et al., 2011. Neurologic complications of babesiosis. Emerging Infectious Diseases 29 (6), 1127–1135.

New, D.L., Quinn, J.B., Qureshi, M.Z., Sigler, S.J., 1997. Vertically transmitted babesiosis [2]. The Journal of Pediatrics 131 (1 I), 163–164. https://doi.org/10.1016/S0022-3476(97)70143-4, 00223476.

Tompkins, J., Schotthoefer, A.M., Fritsche, T.R., Mareedu, N., Hall, M.C., Frost, H.M., 2017. Risk factors for severe infection, hospitalization, and prolonged antimicrobial therapy in patients with babesiosis. The American Journal of Tropical Medicine and Hygiene 97 (4), 1218–1225. https://doi.org/10.4269/ajtmh.17-0146.

CHAPTER 12

Tick-transmitted viral diseases

Introduction

The tickborne viral infections are caused primarily by flaviviruses (family Flaviviridae) and may be divided into two separate clinical presentations, each with preferred tick vectors and wild animal reservoirs: (1) the viral encephalitides (Table 12.1) and (2) the viral hemorrhagic fevers (Table 12.2). The tickborne viral infections share several common clinical and epidemiologic characteristics, including incubation periods of approximately 1 week; biphasic illnesses separated by symptom-free periods, beginning with flu-like viremic stages and ending with CNS or hemorrhagic manifestations; nonspecific serodiagnosis by comparing acute and convalescent sera for increased antibody titers or by hemagglutination inhibition; specific serodiagnosis by ELISA and antigen detection from blood or cerebrospinal fluid (CSF) by reverse-transcriptase PCR; no specific treatments other than supportive therapy; and significantly increased postinfection morbidity (Varnaite et al., 2022).

Epidemiology

Tickborne encephalitis viruses (TBEV) are regionally endemic in Europe and Asia and cause acute febrile neurologic disease, which often results in hospitalization. TBEVs are transmitted to animals and humans by bites of infected *Ixodes* species ticks, but can also be transmitted by ingestion, breastfeeding, blood transfusion, solid organ transplantation, and the slaughtering of viremic animals. The risks for TBEV among American travelers in low. Risk factors for TBEV include prolonged outdoor activities of any type in rural endemic areas during the main TBEV transmission season of April through November, age 60 years and older, and laboratory workers.

From 2010 to 2020, diagnostic testing at the Centers for Disease Control and Prevention (CDC) identified only six patients with TBEV (Hills et al., 2022). Cases occurred in children and adults, and all cases were males (Hills et al., 2022). All case-patients had traveled to various countries in Europe or to Russia, and all engaged in outdoor activities, including camping, hiking, trail running, and working outdoors (Hills et al., 2022). Three cases reported visiting friends and relatives, and remaining patients were vacationers (Hills et al., 2022). Patients were diagnosed with either meningitis (n = 2) or encephalitis (n = 4). All patients were hospitalized for supportive care and no patients died (Hills et al., 2022).

Ectoparasitic Diseases
ISBN 978-0-443-26724-6,
https://doi.org/10.1016/B978-0-443-26724-6.00012-6

Table 12.1 Representative tickborne encephalitis viruses.

Virus name	Family taxonomy	Geographic distribution	Tick vectors	Wild animal reservoirs
Alongshan virus (ALSV)	Flaviviridae	China, Europe (Finland, France, Russia, Switzerland)	Ixodid ticks, *Ixodes ricinus* in Europe	Domestic animals, cattle, sheep
Central European tickborne encephalitis virus (TBEV-Eu)	Flaviviridae	Europe, except Iberian Peninsula	Ixodid ticks, especially *Dermacentor marginatus*, *Ixodes persulcatus*, and *Ixodes ricinus*	Mammals: Especially rodents, including hedgehogs, wood mice, and voles; also, deer and other ungulates, birds, and domestic livestock, especially goats
Deer tick virus	Flaviviridae	US New England states (Connecticut, Massachusetts, New York)	*Ixodes scapularis*	Deer
Far Eastern TBEV (TBEV-FE)	Flaviviridae	Eastern Russia, China to far eastern Japan	*I. persulcatus*	Mammals: Rodents, including hedgehogs, wood mice, voles; also, birds, deer, other ungulates, and domestic livestock, especially goats
Langat virus	Flaviviridae	Malaysia	Ixodid ticks	Mammals: Monkeys, rodents
Louping ill virus	Flaviviridae	United States, Scotland	Ixodid ticks	Sheep
Powassan encephalitis virus	Flaviviridae	Canada, US Northeast, far eastern Russia	*Ixodes* spp., particularly *I. scapularis*, *I. cookei*; *Dermacentor andersoni*	Mammals: Rodents, skunks, and other medium-sized mammals, especially woodchucks

	Family	Geography	Tick vector	Host
Siberian (Russian) spring-summer TBEV (TBEV-Sib)	Flaviviridae	Russia	*Ixodes* spp., particularly *I. persulcatus, I. ricinus*	Mammals: Rodents, including hedgehogs, wood mice, voles; also, birds, deer, other ungulates, and domestic livestock, especially goats
Turkish sheep encephalitis virus	Flaviviridae	Turkey	Ixodid ticks	Sheep
Bhanja virus	Bunyaviridae	Eastern Europe, Russia, central and West Africa	*Dermacentor* spp.; *Haemaphysalis intermedia*	Cattle, sheep, goats, hedgehogs
Antu virus	Nairoviridae	China, Korea	*Dermacentor silvarum*	Rodents, livestock
Songling virus	Nairoviridae	China, Korea	*Dermacentor silvarum*	Rodents, livestock

Adapted from Diaz, J.H., 2019. Section on Ectoparasitic Diseases. Chapter 296. Ticks (Including Tick Paralysis). In: Bennett, J.E., Dolin, R., Blaser, M.J. (Eds.), *Mandell, Douglas and Bennett's Principles and Practice of Infectious Diseases*, Ninth ed. Elsevier, Philadelphia. Elsevier publication.

Table 12.2 Representative tickborne hemorrhagic fever viruses.

Virus name	Family taxonomy	Geographic distribution	Tick vectors	Wild animal reservoirs
Alkhurma hemorrhagic fever virus	Flaviviridae	Saudi Arabia	*Ornithodoros savignyi* (suspected)	Camels, sheep
Omsk hemorrhagic fever virus	Flaviviridae	Western Siberia	*Dermacentor reticulatus*, *Ixodes apronophorus*	Mammals: Rodents, especially muskrats, water voles
Kyasanur Forest disease	Flaviviridae	Western India	*Haemaphysalis spinigera*	Mammals: Especially monkeys, domestic livestock (cattle, goats, sheep), rodents, insectivores
Heartland virus	Bunyaviridae	Missouri, Kansas, Tennessee	*Amblyomma americanum*	Mammals: Rodents, skunks, other medium-sized mammals
Crimean–Congo hemorrhagic fever virus	Bunyaviridae	Asia, Eastern Europe, Africa, Middle East	*Hyalomma marginatum*, *Hyalomma anatolicum*	Mammals: Many domestic animals (buffalo, camels, cattle, goats, sheep), rabbits, rodents (hedgehogs), birds
Severe fever with thrombocytopenia virus	Bunyaviridae	China (mostly), Japan, Korea	*Haemaphysalis* spp., especially *H. longicornis* > *H. concinna*	Primarily domestic animals, especially goats
Bourbon virus	Orthomyxoviridae	Missouri, Kansas, Oklahoma	Unknown	Unknown

Adapted from Diaz, J.H., 2019. Section on Ectoparasitic Diseases. Chapter 296. Ticks (Including Tick Paralysis). In: Bennett, J.E., Dolin, R., Blaser, M.J. (Eds.), *Mandell, Douglas and Bennett's Principles and Practice of Infectious Diseases*, Ninth ed. Elsevier, Philadelphia. Elsevier publication.

The TBEV vaccine is recommended for all high-risk travelers, such as elderly persons age 60 years and older, who engage in prolonged outdoor activities of any type in rural endemic areas during the main TBEV transmission season of April through November (Centers for Disease Control and Prevention, 2023).

Tickborne viral encephalitides

From a global distribution perspective, the tickborne encephalitis viruses (TBEVs) are separated into the Old World (Eastern Hemisphere) and New World (Western Hemisphere) strains, with the Old World strains having significantly higher case fatality rates (CFRs) (20%—40%) and permanent neurologic morbidity rates (28%—30%) than the New World strains (CFR, 10%—15%; morbidity rate, <10%) (Varnaite et al., 2022). In most cases of tickborne infectious diseases, the CFRs are calculated as the number of deaths among the more severe diagnosed cases and do not include the less severe probable and subclinical cases in the denominators, which would make the CFRs significantly smaller.

Although additional Old World flaviviral strains have now been discovered in sheep reservoirs, the most common Old World TBEVs have been further stratified regionally into three major subtypes: European or central European (TBEV-Eu), Siberian or Russian spring-summer (TBEV-Sib), and Far Eastern (TBEV-FE; see Table 12.1). Except for the Old World TBEVs with sheep reservoirs, all the TBEVs are transmitted by the injection of infected saliva from viremic ixodid ticks. During blood feeding, viruses in tick saliva increase up to 10-fold and render early removal of the feeding tick ineffective in preventing disease. The preferred wild animal reservoirs for TBEVs include rodents, insectivores, medium-sized mammals, deer and other ungulates, birds, and, less often, domestic animals (Table 12.1) (Hills et al., 2022).

New World TBEVs: Powassan encephalitis

Powassan encephalitis, first isolated in 1958, typifies a New World TBEV with a confined regional distribution in the New England states (especially Connecticut, Maine, Massachusetts, New York, and Vermont), Minnesota, and Eastern Canada; several tick vectors, primarily *Ixodes* species; an extensive wild animal reservoir in rodents and medium-sized mammals, especially woodchucks and skunks; and seasonal occurrences (CDC, 1999; Cumbie et al., 2021). Cases occur from May to December and peak during June—September, when ticks are most active (CDC, 1999). Patients with Powassan encephalitis present with somnolence, headache, confusion, high fever, weakness, ataxia, and CSF lymphocytosis (CDC, 1999). Transient improvement may be followed by neurologic deterioration, evidence of cerebral ischemia or demyelination on magnetic resonance imaging (MRI) or computerized tomography (CT), and slow recovery, often with permanent deficits including memory loss, weakness, ophthalmoplegia, and lower extremity paraparesis (CDC, 1999).

Unlike the Old World TBEVs, Powassan encephalitis is uncommon, with only 31 confirmed cases reported by the CDC from 1958 to 2001 (Cumbie et al., 2021). Because there is no vaccine or specific therapy for Powassan encephalitis, the best means of prevention is protection from tick bites. Since 2008, Powassan encephalitis cases historically confined to the Northeastern United States and Canada have been increasingly confirmed further westward in Minnesota and Wisconsin, with fatal cases reported in the elderly (Cumbie et al., 2021).

Powassan virus (POWV) disease can be transmitted to humans by blood-feeding ixodid ticks in as little as 15 minutes and mimics other arthropod-borne viral encephalitidies, such as La Crosse encephalitis and West Nile virus neuroinvasive disease, in clinical presentation (Cumbie et al., 2021). The CFR can be as high as 10% among the more severe confirmed cases and permanent neurologic sequelae are common (Cumbie et al., 2021). Therefore, clinicians should include POWV in their differential diagnosis of encephalitis in endemic regions, such as New England and Minnesota, during the mosquito-borne encephalitis season and also obtain serologic tests for POWV on CSF samples (POWV-specific neutralizing immunoglobulin M antibody titers) (Cumbie et al., 2021). Unlike the prolonged attachment time required for the transmission of Lyme borreliosis, the short attachment time required for transmission of POWV underscores the critical importance of personal protective measures, such as insect repellents and clothing, in preventing tick-transmitted viruses (Cumbie et al., 2021).

The deer tick virus is closely related to Powassan virus and is also transmitted by ixodid ticks in the same endemic regions of New England (Tavakoli et al., 2009). It also causes a meningoencephalitis syndrome with a high CFR (Tavakoli et al., 2009).

Old World TBEVs

The Old World TBEVs remain common causes of permanent neurologic morbidity from Scandinavia to eastern Japan, with more than 10,000 cases reported per year, a third of which result in permanent neurologic deficits. In addition to tick bites, the Old World TBEVs may occasionally be transmitted by ingestion of unpasteurized milk products from viremic livestock (especially goats), breastfeeding, and by inoculation during slaughter of viremic animals.

Old World TBEV is typically biphasic in over 70% of cases, with an initial febrile flu-like presentation followed by a 1-week (range, 1−21 days) symptom-free interval. This honeymoon or recovery period is followed by meningoencephalitis with CSF pleocytosis, with or without myelitis, and a poliomyelitis-like flaccid paralysis that targets the arms, neck, and shoulders. MRI and electroencephalographic abnormalities are common, but nonspecific. Other acute neurologic complications may include altered consciousness, seizure activity, cranial nerve palsies, and an often-fatal bulbar syndrome with cardiorespiratory failure. Because no specific treatments other than supportive therapy exist, tick avoidance and immunization remain the best preventive measures. Effective vaccines have now been developed for the three subtypes of Old World TBEVs, and some have been shown to even provide cross-protection among the subtypes in experimentally infected animals. The US Food and Drug Administration approved a TBEV vaccine, *Ticovac*, in July 2021 for persons 1 year of age and older traveling to endemic areas of Europe and Asia (Centers for Disease Control and Prevention, 2023).

Emerging tickborne flaviviruses: China 2017, Switzerland 2021–22

In 2017, a new flavivirus causing TBE and transmitted by ixodid ticks, the Alongshan virus (ALSV), was first detected in patients in China who presented with histories of tick bites and symptoms of TBE, but negative molecular diagnostics for all known strains of Old World TBE-causing flaviviruses (Bao et al., 2011; Wang et al., 2019; Varnaite et al., 1999, 2022). This new ASLV flaviviruses has segmented genomes with four segments of positive sense, single-stranded RNA (ssRNA), when all other Old World strains of flaviviruses had nonsegmented, ssRNA genomes.

During 2021–22, ASLV flaviviruses with four-segmented genomes were isolated from a pool of 60 adult male *Ixodes ricinus* ticks collected in Switzerland and determined by sequence analysis at amino acid levels to demonstrate high similarities to proteins sequenced from other European ASLV strains in ixodid ticks from France, Finland, and Russia (Kuivanen et al., 2019; Stegmüller et al., 2022).

These recent discoveries have the following global public health implications. (1) New strains of TBE-causing Alongshan flaviviruses are now circulating in ixodid tick vectors in China and throughout Europe, adding to an expanding list of emerging, unanticipated tickborne infectious diseases. (2) These new viral strains differ genotypically from the Old World strains of TBE-causing flaviviruses in Asia and Europe with nonsegmented genomes and will pose new, additional human health threats. (3) The existing vaccines in Asia, Europe, and the USA developed for the Old World strains of TBE-causing flaviviruses will not fully protect patients from encephalitis caused by the ASLV flaviviruses in Asia and Europe even by inducing cross-reacting antibodies. (4) The continuing genomic sequencing work with the ASLV flaviviruses will lead researchers to conduct epidemiological investigations to determine the true prevalence of ASLV carriage by ixodid ticks and the prevalence of ASLV infections in humans. (5) This work will also enable researchers to identify the protein subunits needed to manufacture new, polyvalent vaccines designed to protect populations from an increasing geographic distribution of TBE-causing flaviviruses.

Hemorrhagic fever viruses

The tickborne hemorrhagic fever (TBHF) viruses are maintained in nature in extensive wild and domestic animal reservoirs and are transmitted by infected ixodid tick bites, squashing infected ticks creating infective aerosols, direct contact with blood or tissues from infected animals or humans, and nosocomial spread among medical personnel. TBHFs are usually caused by either flaviviruses or bunyaviruses, which are distributed throughout eastern Europe, Africa, and Asia. A previously unidentified tickborne thogotovirus (family Orthomyxoviridae) was described in the United States in 2014 in a healthy man in eastern Kansas and later named Bourbon virus after the patient's county of residence.

The TBHFs are characterized clinically by biphasic illnesses that present initially as febrile flu-like symptoms and end as hepatomegaly with liver failure and hemorrhagic manifestations (petechiae, purpura, subconjunctival and pharyngeal hemorrhage, thrombocytopenia, cerebral hemorrhage, intrapulmonary hemorrhage, disseminated intravascular coagulation) separated by a few afebrile days. CFRs range from 10% to over 50%, with most deaths occurring within 5—14 days of symptom onset during hemorrhagic stages (Conger et al., 2015) (Ergönül et al., 2018). Diagnoses may be confirmed by immunologic techniques, such as antibody increases in paired sera and ELISA, and by molecular techniques, such as real-time PCR (Conger et al., 2015).

All patients with TBHFs should be placed in isolation with strict universal precautions, including personal protective equipment. Strict universal precautions should also be practiced by all medical personnel because nosocomial transmission has been reported, most likely by the generation of infectious aerosols during bag-valve-mask ventilation, endotracheal intubation, and bronchoscopy (Ergönül et al., 2018).

Although ribavirin can inhibit Crimean-Congo hemorrhagic fever (CCHF) virus replication in animal models, it has not been tested in clinical trials in humans with CCHF. Nevertheless, if TBHF is suspected in the tropics and laboratory confirmation is unavailable, intravenously administered ribavirin (30 mg/kg initially, followed by 16 mg/kg four times daily for 4 days, and then 8 mg/kg three times daily for 6 days) is recommended for severe cases, and oral ribavirin is recommended for high-risk contacts (Ergönül et al., 2018).

In a systematic review and meta-analysis of postexposure prophylaxis (PEP) for CCHF virus (CCHFV) among healthcare workers, investigators reported that PEP with ribavirin significantly reduced the odds of infection (OR 0.01, 95% CI 0—0.03), and ribavirin use within 48 h after symptom onset significantly reduced the odds of death (OR 0.03, 95% CI 0—0.58) (Ergönül et al., 2018). The investigators recommended that ribavirin be considered for PEP and early treatment for healthcare workers at high risk of CCHFV infection (Ergönül et al., 2018).

A mouse brain—derived CCHF vaccine has been developed in Bulgaria, but is not available elsewhere. In the absence of a universal vaccine, the best preventive measures for the TBHFs are tick avoidance and control, rapid burial of dead animals, and personal protective equipment for abattoir workers and medical personnel.

Another novel, tick-transmitted phlebovirus (family Bunyaviridae), the severe fever with thrombocytopenia syndrome virus was first described in 2009 in China, and has now been detected in *Haemaphysalis* species ticks in Japan and Korea (Varnaite et al., 1999; Wang et al., 2019; Yu et al., 2017). Severe fever with thrombocytopenia syndrome virus is transmitted by at least two species of *Haemaphysalis* species ticks in Asia, *H longicornis* and *H concinna* (Yu et al., 2017).

Domestic animals, especially goats, serve as the zoonotic reservoirs for the severe fever with thrombocytopenia syndrome virus in China (Yu et al., 2017). Central and eastern China report the greatest number of cases with over 2500 reported since 2010 (Varnaite et al., 1999; Wang et al., 2019). The disease presents with a sudden onset of high fever, abdominal pain, nausea, vomiting, leukocytopenia, thrombocytopenia, and hemorrhage. There are no specific drug treatments for severe fever with thrombocytopenia syndrome virus disease. The median case-fatality rate is 7%.

H. longicornis, the Asian long-horned tick, is native to eastern China, Japan, the Russian Far East, and Korea (Yu et al., 2017). It is an introduced, and now established, exotic species in Australia, New Zealand, several island nations in the western Pacific, and the United States (Yu et al., 2017).

The initial US detection of *H. longicornis* outside of imported animal quarantine was on a sheep in New Jersey in August 2017 (Yu et al., 2017). By the spring of 2018, the tick was again detected at the same site in New Jersey, and later, in other counties in New Jersey, in seven other states in the eastern United States, and in northwestern Arkansas (Yu et al., 2017). The animal hosts included six species of domestic animals, six species of wildlife, and humans (Yu et al., 2017). At present, there is no evidence that *H longicornis* has transmitted any pathogens to humans, domestic animals, or wildlife in the United States. *H longicornis* is, however, capable of transmitting several pathogens including bacteria (*Rickettsia, Borrelia, Ehrlichia, Anaplasma,* and *Theileria* spp), viruses (Bourbon, Heartland, and severe fever with thrombocytopenia syndrome viruses), and, probably, parasites (*Babesia* spp) (Yu et al., 2017; Bao et al., 2011).

Coltiviruses

The tickborne coltiviruses of the family Reoviridae are all double-stranded RNA viruses of the genus *Coltivirus* and include Colorado tick fever virus (CTFV), which is endemic in the United States and Canadian Rocky Mountain regions; the California tick fever virus of rabbits (CTFV-Ca), and the Salmon River virus (SRV) of Idaho, serotypes of the CTFVs; and the European Eyach virus (EYAV). The ixodid or hard ticks are the only vectors of the coltiviruses, with *Dermacentor* ticks (mainly *D. andersoni*) being the principal vectors of CTFV and SRV in the Rocky Mountains and *Ixodes* ticks (*I. ricinus, I. ventalloi*) being the only vectors of EYAV throughout Europe.

Among the coltiviruses, CTFV has the widest host animal range, which includes squirrels, other rodents, rabbits, porcupines, marmots, deer, elk, sheep, and coyotes. The remaining coltiviruses have fewer, more specific wild animal hosts, including the black-tailed jackrabbit (*Lepus californicus*) for CTFV-Ca and the European rabbit (*Oryctolagus cunniculus*) for EYAV. The coltiviruses are maintained in nature by ixodid ticks that blood-feed on wild animal hosts with prolonged viremias and then pass coltiviruses transstadially but not transovarially. Infected nymphs hibernate over winter, and previously infected nymphs and newly infected adults then transmit coltiviruses to human dead-end hosts during spring-summer blood-feeding. CTFV has also been transmitted by blood transfusion and congenitally.

Both CTFV and SRV can cause biphasic to triphasic febrile illnesses that mimic mild cases of RMSF without rash. Leukopenia and thrombocytopenia are common laboratory manifestations of coltivirus infections and are strong indicators for the diagnosis. Complications are rare but may include meningoencephalitis, orchitis, hemorrhagic fever, pericarditis, and myocarditis. EYAV infections are more often complicated by CNS manifestations than American strain coltivirus infections. The most common differential diagnoses for the tickborne coltiviruses are other tickborne febrile diseases, most commonly RMSF in North America, which may be distinguished from CTFV and SRV infections by its characteristic rash and leukocytosis.

Serologic diagnostic methods to detect anticoltivirus antibodies include complement fixation test, seroneutralization assay, immunofluorescence assay, ELISA, and Western immunoblot assay. The most specific and confirmatory laboratory diagnostic methods include reverse-transcriptase PCR assays to identify CTFV RNA (or the RNA of its cross-reacting serotypes, CTFV-Ca and SRV) or the isolation of coltiviruses after intracerebral inoculation of infected human blood into suckling mice. Treatment of all tickborne coltivirus infections is entirely supportive, and long-term complications are rare in uncomplicated cases.

References

Bao, C.J., Guo, X.L., Qi, X., Hu, J.L., Zhou, M.H., Varma, J.K., Cui, L.B., Yang, H.T., Jiao, Y.J., Klena, J.D., Li, L.X., Tao, W.Y., Li, X., Chen, Y., Zhu, Z., Xu, K., Shen, A.H., Wu, T., Peng, H.Y., Li, Z.F., Shan, J., Shi, Z.Y., Wang, H., 2011. A family cluster of infections by a newly recognized bunyavirus in Eastern China, 2007: further evidence of person-to-person transmission. Clinical Infectious Diseases 53 (12), 1208–1214. https://doi.org/10.1093/cid/cir732.

CDC, 1999. Outbreak of Powassan encephalitis—Maine and Vermont. MMWR Morbidity and Mortality Weekly Report 50 (35), 761.

Centers for Disease Control and Prevention, 2023. Tick-borne Encephalitis Vaccine: Recommendations of the Advisory Committee on Immunization Practices, vol 75, pp. 1—29.

Conger, N.G., Paolino, K.M., Osborn, E.C., Rusnak, J.M., Günther, S., Pool, J., Rollin, P.E., Allan, P.F., Schmidt-Chanasit, J., Rieger, T., Kortepeter, M.G., 2015. Health care response to CCHF in US soldier and nosocomial transmission to health care providers, Germany, 2009. Emerging Infectious Diseases 21 (1), 23—31. https://doi.org/10.3201/eid2101.141413.

Cumbie, A.N., Whitlow, A.M., Eastwood, G., 2021. First evidence of Powassan virus (Flaviviridae) in Ixodes scapularis in Appalachian Virginia, USA. The American Journal of Tropical Medicine and Hygiene 106 (3), 905—908. https://doi.org/10.4269/ajtmh.21-0825.

Ergönül, Ö., Keske, Ş., Çeldir, M.G., Kara, İ.A., Pshenichnaya, N., Abuova, G., Blumberg, L., Gönen, M., 2018. Systematic review and meta-analysis of postexposure prophylaxis for Crimean-Congo hemorrhagic fever virus among healthcare workers. Emerging Infectious Diseases 24 (9), 1642—1648. https://doi.org/10.3201/eid2409.171709.

Hills, S.L., Broussard, K.R., Broyhill, J.C., Shastry, L.G., Cossaboom, C.M., White, J.L., Machesky, K.D., Kosoy, O., Girone, K., Klena, J.D., Backenson, B.P., Gould, C.V., Lind, L., Hieronimus, A., Gaines, D.N., Wong, S.J., Choi, M.J., Laven, J.J., Staples, J.E., Fischer, M., 2022. Tick-borne encephalitis among US travellers, 2010—20. Journal of Travel Medicine 29 (2). https://doi.org/10.1093/jtm/taab167.

Kuivanen, S., Levanov, L., Kareinen, L., Sironen, T., Jääskeläinen, A.J., Plyusnin, I., Zakham, F., Emmerich, P., Schmidt-Chanasit, J., Hepojoki, J., Smura, T., Vapalahti, O., 2019. Detection of novel tick-borne pathogen, alongshan virus, in Ixodes ricinus ticks, south-eastern Finland, 2019. Euro Surveillance 24 (27). https://doi.org/10.2807/1560-7917.ES.2019.24.27.1900394.

Stegmüller, S., Fraefel, C., Kubacki, J., 2022. Complete genome sequence of alongshan virus sequenced from Ixodes ricinus ticks collected in Switzerland. Zenodo 6. https://doi.org/10.5281/zenodo.7403328.

Tavakoli, N.P., Wang, H., Dupuis, M., Hull, R., Ebel, G.D., Gilmore, E.J., Faust, P.L., 2009. Fatal case of deer tick virus encephalitis. New England Journal of Medicine 360 (20), 2099—2107. https://doi.org/10.1056/NEJMoa0806326.

Varnaite, R., Gredmark-Russ, S., Klingstrom, J., Hills, S.L., Broussard, K.R., Broyhill, J.C., 1999. A family cluster of infections by a newly recognized Bunyavirus in eastern China, 2007: further evidence of person-to-person transmission. Centers for Disease Control and Prevention. Tick-borne encephalitis vaccine: Recommendations of the Advisory Committee on Immunization Practices 28, 1673—1679. https://doi.org/10.1093/jtm/taab167.

Varnaite, R., Gredmark-Russ, S., Klingstrom, J., 2022. Deaths from tick-borne encephalitis, Sweden. Emerging Infectious Diseases 28 (7), 1471—1474. https://doi.org/10.3201/eid2807.220010.

Wang, Z.D., Wang, B., Wei, F., Han, S.Z., Zhang, L., Yang, Z.T., Yan, Y., Lv, X.L., Li, L., Wang, S.C., Song, M.X., Zhang, H.J., Huang, S.J., Chen, J., Huang, F.Q., Li, S., Liu, H.H., Hong, J., Jin, Y.L., Wang, W., Zhou, J.Y., Liu, Q., 2019. A new segmented virus associated with human febrile illness in China. New England Journal of Medicine 380 (22), 2116—2125. https://doi.org/10.1056/NEJMoa1805068.

Yu, P., Tian, H., Li, S., Huang, S., Chowell, G., Brownstein, J.S., Tian, H., Wei, J., Xu, B., Zhou, S., Han, Z., Lv, W., Yang, J., Wang, J., 2017. Severe fever with thrombocytopenia syndrome virus in humans, Domesticated animals, ticks, and Mosquitoes, Shaanxi Province, China. The American Journal of Tropical Medicine and Hygiene 96 (6), 1346—1349. https://doi.org/10.4269/ajtmh.16-0333.

CHAPTER 13

The tick sialome, tick-transmitted coinfections, and tick paralysis

The tick sialome

The combinations of bioactive compounds in the tick salivary complex or sialome act synergistically to secure initial and sustained tick attachment, permit immediate and prolonged blood-feeding, disarm host humoral and cellular immunity, and assure pathogen transmission for infection and paralyzing chemical transmission for paralysis. Investigators have now identified many immunomodulatory compounds in the tick sialome that are family-specific, and even species-specific, as a result of the different tick blood-feeding behaviors (Ali et al., 1912).

Ixodid or hard ticks attach firmly to the host and feed for days as compared to argasid or soft ticks which attach to and release from hosts repeatedly and blood-feed for minutes to hours (Ali et al., 1912). This is particularly relevant for the ixodid ticks that can cause tick paralysis and will continue to inject paralytic substances into the victim until removed.

The chemical constituents of the tick sialome

The bioactive compounds in the tick sialome may be divided into proteinaceous and nonproteinaceous chemicals with different roles in maintaining blood-feeding and promoting pathogen transmission (Ali et al., 1912). The proteinaceous compounds in the tick sialome include cement cone proteins, protease inhibitors, anticoagulant proteins, antiplatelet activators, antiplatelet aggregators, complement inhibitors, and cytokine and chemokine inhibitors (Ali et al., 1912). The cement cone proteins are of two types and include those that promote initial tick−host attachment and those that secure prolonged tick−host attachment (Ali et al., 1912). The protease inhibitors suppress immediate, local coagulation responses by inhibiting specific extrinsic and intrinsic coagulation cascade elements including thrombin, plasmin, kallikrein, and activated factors V, X, and XII (Ali et al., 1912). Anticoagulant proteins have been intensely studied and include Om44 and TAI with Om44 preventing leukocyte and platelet adhesion to interior vessel walls, and TAI blocking platelet adhesion to collagen (Ali et al., 1912). The antiplatelet aggregators inhibit cathepsins, chymase, elastase, papain, and tryptase (Ali et al., 1912). The antiplatelet aggregators inhibit or bind ADP, serotonin, and thromboxane. The complement inhibitors disassociate the C3 and C5 complement complexes,

Ectoparasitic Diseases
ISBN 978-0-443-26724-6
https://doi.org/10.1016/B978-0-443-26724-6.00013-8

and the cytokine and chemokine inhibitors prevent the migration of leukocytes to the bite site by inactivating both cytokines and chemokines (Ali et al., 1912).

The nonproteinaceous compounds in the tick sialome include PGE2, prostacyclin, purine nucleoside adenine, fatty acids, endocannabinoids, noncoding RNAs, and micro-RNAs (Ali et al., 1912). All of these chemicals act synergistically to modulate the host responses to tick attachment and blood-feeding (Ali et al., 1912). In summary, the chemicals in the tick sialome can effectively secure tick attachment and release for short or prolonged periods, permit chelicera insertion without notice or pain, maintain anticoagulation as long as required for blood-feeding and egg laying, and inactivate host humoral and cellular responses to ectoparasitism (Ali et al., 1912).

Tick-transmitted coinfections

Ticks may be asymptomatically coinfected with several pathogens that can be simultaneously transmitted to human hosts during blood feeding (Ali et al., 1912; Ali et al., 2022; Belongia, 2002; Krause et al., 1996; Schwartz et al., 1997; Nadelman et al., 1997). In 1996, Krause and coworkers initially reported increased duration and severity of illness in patients coinfected with the Lyme disease spirochete, *Borrelia burgdorferi,* and *Babesia microti,* the protozoan agent of babesiosis (Krause et al., 1996). In 1997, Schwartz and coinvestigators in the eastern United States first identified coinfections in ixodid ticks with *B. burgdorferi* and *Anaplasma phagocytophilum*, the bacterial agent of anaplasmosis (Schwartz et al., 1997). In 1997, Nadelman and coauthors reported the first human case of concurrent Lyme borreliosis and anaplasmosis in the United States (Nadelman et al., 1997).

To date, most tickborne coinfections have been reported from geographic areas with overlapping endemic ranges of infected ticks capable of transmitting multiple pathogens during blood-feeding (Krause et al., 1996). The eastern black-legged or deer tick, *Ixodes scapularis* (Fig. 13.1), has been implicated most often by transmitting Lyme borreliosis and babesiosis in a northeastern coastal band extending from New Jersey north to New Hampshire (Ali et al., 1912; Schwartz et al., 1997; Nadelman et al., 1997). *I. scapularis* has also cotransmitted Lyme disease and anaplasmosis in an upper Midwest geographic band extending from Wisconsin across Minnesota to Canada, another endemic region of overlapping tick-transmitted infectious diseases (Fig. 13.1) (Ali et al., 1912; Schwartz et al., 1997; Nadelman et al., 1997).

In summary, the ability of ixodid ticks to be coinfected with multiple pathogens and to transmit coinfections to humans during prolonged blood-feeding has now been demonstrated in the United States. The immunologic confirmation of tickborne coinfections by rising antibody titers in paired serum samples and/or by nucleic acid determinations using PCR requires a substantial time period and may only be available in state and federal reference laboratories (Krause et al., 1996).

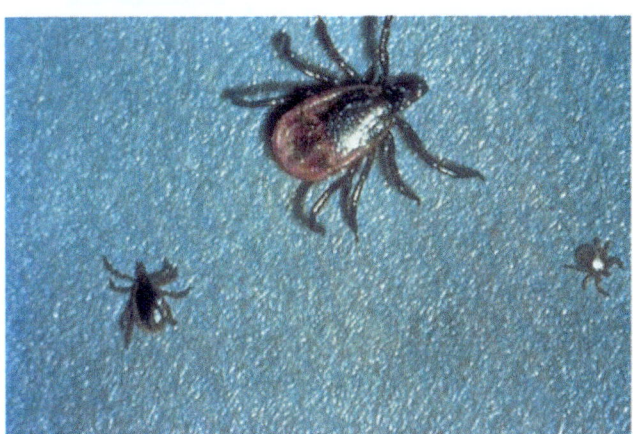

Figure 13.1 *Ixodes scapularis,* the eastern black-legged tick. Shown are the adult female and two smaller nymphs below. These are common arthropod vectors of babesiosis and Lyme disease, especially the diminutive nymphs, whose bites are most often unnoticed. *(From Public Health Image Library. Image 1205. Atlanta, GA: Centers for Disease Control and Prevention.)*

Decision tree models of tick-transmitted coinfections

Some critical tickborne infections, such as RMSF, LB-associated meningoencephalitis, and babesiosis with massive splenomegaly, may require immediate, empirical intravenous antibiotic management prior to confirmatory laboratory diagnoses (Krause et al., 1996). In such cases, Diaz has recommended the generation of probability-based decision tree models to expose potential coinfections based on (1) the regional distributions and prevalence rates of potentially coinfected tick vectors; (2) tick identification by experts; and (3) any cutaneous presenting manifestations of tick bites, such as eschars or erythema migrans, if present (Fig. 13.2) (Diaz, 2016). Clinicians should suspect tickborne coinfections in returning travelers and all patients with clinical and immunologic evidence of multiple infecting agents, especially in cases of unusual presentation or severity, prolonged duration, or nonresponse to single (typically doxycycline) antibiotic therapy (Ali et al., 1912; Schwartz et al., 1997; Nadelman et al., 1997).

Tick paralysis

First described in 1912 in Australia, Canada, and the United States, tick paralysis is a rare, regional, and seasonal cause of acute ataxia and ascending paralysis with an incubation period of 4–7 days after gravid female tick attachment and blood-feeding (Brown et al., 2016; Diaz, 2016; Swanson et al., 2006). Although 43 species of ticks have been implicated in tick paralysis cases worldwide, most cases occur in the United States and Canadian Pacific Northwest (Washington State and British Columbia) and in Australia (Temple, 1912; Todd, 1912). In the US Pacific Northwest, tick paralysis is caused by the American dog tick (*Dermacentor variabilis*) or the Rocky Mountain wood tick

a)

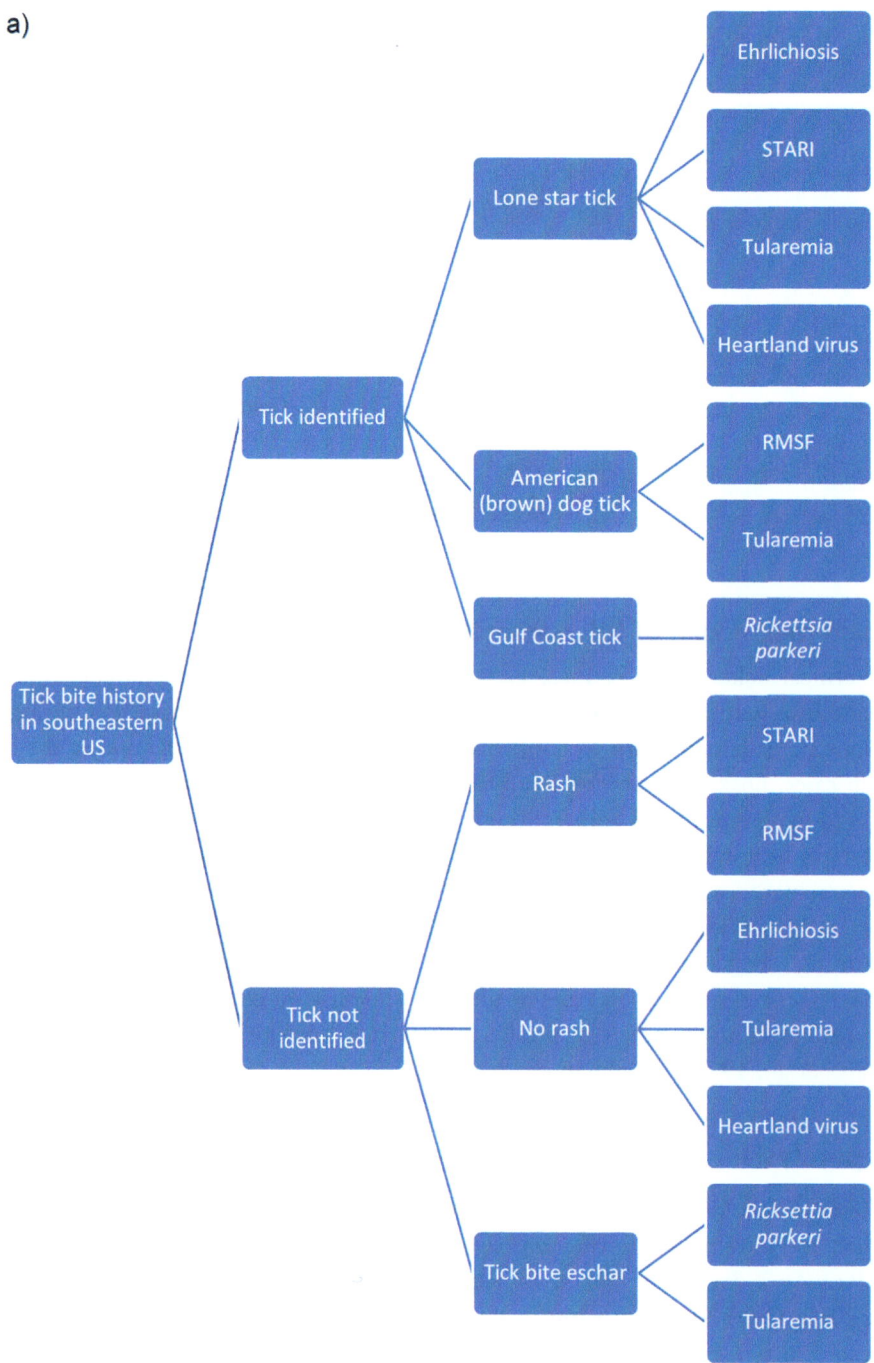

Figure 13.2 A hypothetical probability-based decision tree model for predicting tickborne infections and coinfections in the northeastern United States. (RMSF, *Rocky Mountain spotted fever.*) (a) This sample hypothetical decision tree illustrates the method for analyzing decision tree models of potential tickborne infections and coinfections in the northeastern United States. Predictions: Based on solution of the decision tree, the most common tickborne infections in this region will be Lyme disease transmitted by an Eastern black-legged (deer) tick, with an expected incidence rate of 21% (10,125/48,143); followed by anaplasmosis transmitted by the same tick, with an incidence rate of less than 1% (510/48,143); and followed by babesiosis transmitted by the same tick, with an incidence rate of less than 1% (213/48,143).

b)

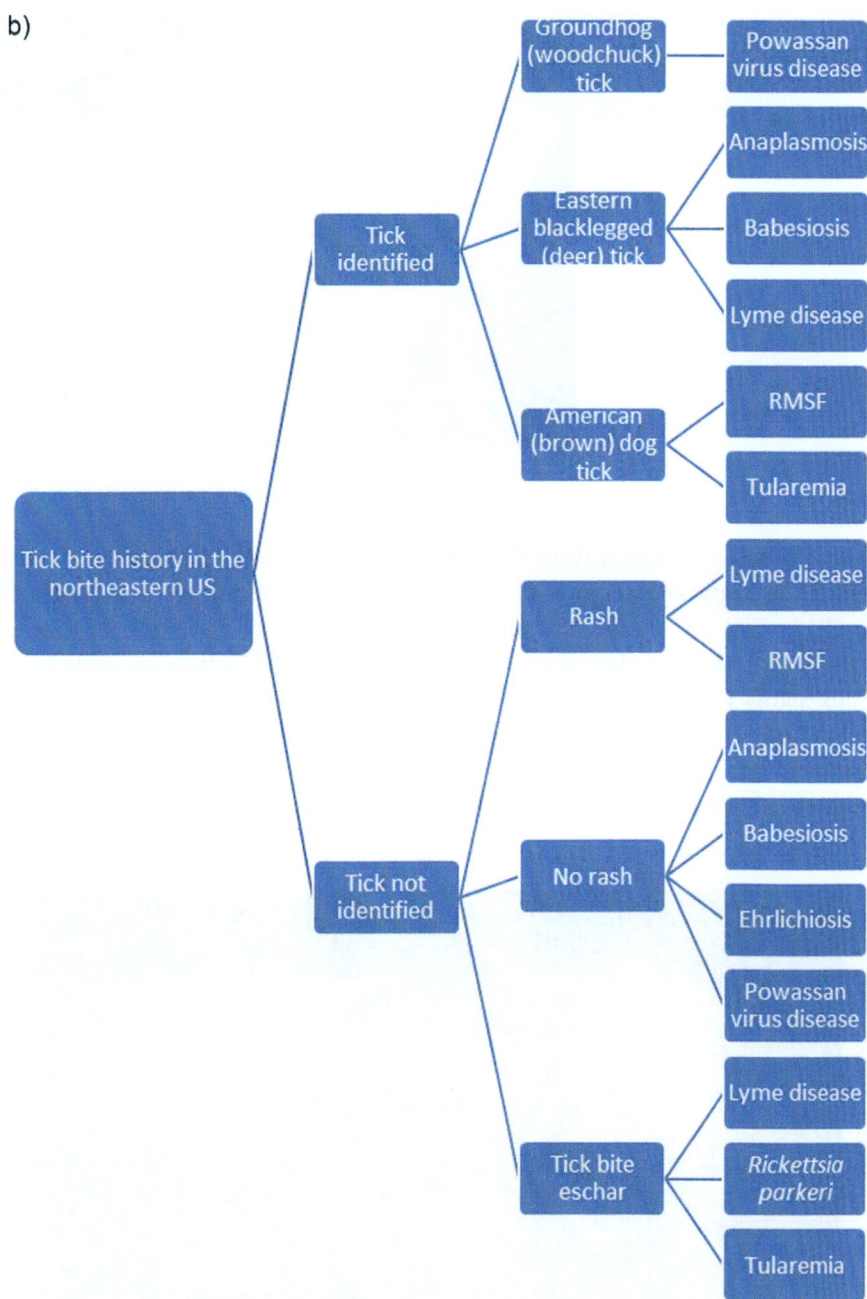

Figure 13.2, Cont'd. (b) This sample hypothetical decision tree illustrates the method for analyzing decision tree models of potential tickborne infections and coinfections in the southeastern United States. Decision trees are solved from right to left. (1) The first and largest entry on the far right is the outcome of confirmed number of cases by the CDC for the given year (2015 was used here). (2) Distributions of tick vectors are expressed as a percent or as probabilities. (3) The sum of probabilities for any set of possibilities must equal 1.0. (4) Multiply from right to left to solve for the greatest expected values. The calculations for expected values are shown in the outcomes boxes on the right. *(Source: Author. No copyright permission required).*

Figure 13.3 *Dermacentor variabilis,* the American dog tick, questing for a host. *(From Public Health Image Library. Image 170. Atlanta, GA: Centers for Disease Control and Prevention.)*

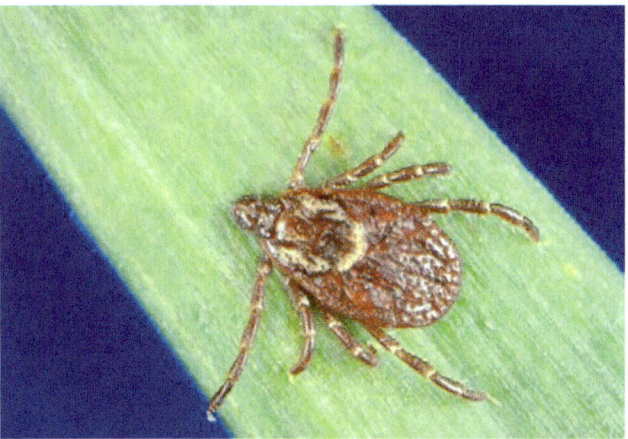

(*Dermacentor andersoni*) during April through June, when *Dermacentor* ticks emerge from hibernation to mate and to seek blood meals (Figs. 13.3 and 13.4) (Temple, 1912; Todd, 1912; Cleland, 1912). The mechanism of neurotoxic paralysis in *Dermacentor* tick paralysis is unknown, but neuroelectrophysiologic studies have suggested that sodium flux across axonal membranes is blocked at the nodes of Ranvier, leaving neuromuscular transmission unimpeded (Dworkin et al., 1999; Diaz, 2010).

The female American dog tick is a vector of tick paralysis in the southeastern United States and Pacific Northwest and is a vector of Rocky Mountain spotted fever in addition

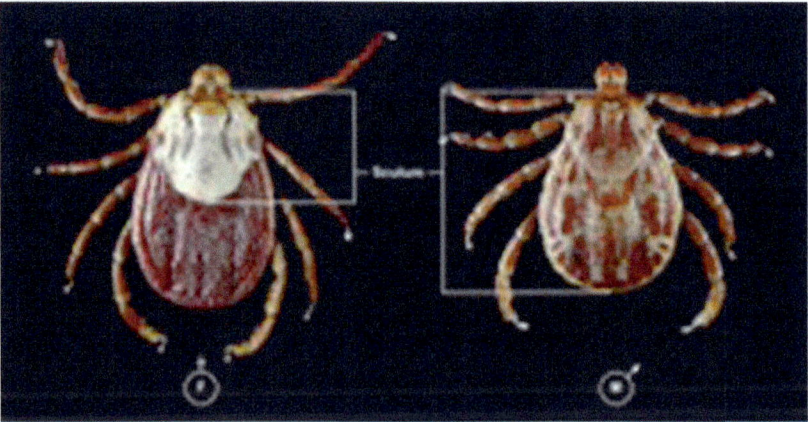

Figure 13.4 Female ***Dermacentor andersoni***, the Rocky Mountain wood tick, questing for a host. *(From Biggs, H.M., Behravesh, C.B., Bradley, K.K., et al., 2016. Diagnosis and management of tickborne rickettsial diseases: Rocky Mountain spotted fever and other spotted fever group rickettsioses, ehrlichioses, and anaplasmosis—United States. MMWR Recomm. Rep. 65, 1—44.)*

to the Rocky Mountain wood tick (*D. andersoni*) in the western United States. In the US Pacific Northwest, tick paralysis is caused by the American dog tick (*D. variabilis*) or the Rocky Mountain wood tick (*D. andersoni*) during April through June, when Dermacentor ticks emerge from hibernation to mate and to seek blood meals.

The Rocky Mountain wood tick is the preferred tick vector for *Rickettsia rickettsii*, the causative rickettsial agent of Rocky Mountain spotted fever in the US Rocky Mountains and the Canadian southwest. In the US Pacific Northwest, tick paralysis is caused by the American dog tick (*D. variabilis*) or the Rocky Mountain wood tick (*D. andersoni*) during April through June, when *Dermacentor* ticks emerge from hibernation to mate and to seek blood meals.

In Australia, the marsupial ixodid tick, *Ixodes holocyclus,* can cause a more severe form of ascending neuromuscular paralysis by producing a botulinum-like neurotoxin that blocks neuromuscular transmission by inhibiting the presynaptic release of acetylcholine (Grattan-Smith et al., 1997).

Most cases of tick paralysis in North America have occurred sporadically in young girls with long hair concealing ticks feeding on the scalp or neck (Schwartz et al., 1997; Pape et al., 2006; Swift and Ignacio, 1975). However, a four-patient cluster of *Dermacentor* tick paralysis, including a 6-year-old girl with a tick on her hairline and three adults with ticks on the neck ($n = 1$) and back ($n = 2$), was reported from Colorado in 2006 (Cleland, 1912).

The differential diagnosis of tick paralysis

Although botulism causes a descending neuromuscular paralysis with a preserved sensorium, tick paralysis, Guillain-Barré syndrome, acute poliomyelitis, and spinal cord tumors may all cause acute ascending paralysis with preserved mental status and must be differentiated from each other (Table 13.1) (Todd, 1912). Because poliomyelitis has been nearly eradicated by vaccination worldwide, tick paralysis is frequently misdiagnosed as Guillain-Barré syndrome, and the correct diagnosis is made accidently by finding an engorged, usually female, tick on the scalp, head, or neck during hair combing or when applying electroencephalographic electrodes (Todd, 1912; Pape et al., 2006; Swift and Ignacio, 1975).

Before 1954, postmortem examinations of persons who died suddenly of unexplained paralytic illnesses demonstrated attached ticks on their heads and necks (Todd, 1912; Dworkin et al., 1999). In a review of Canadian tick paralysis cases in the 1950s before the widespread availability of mechanical ventilation in intensive care units, Rose (Dworkin et al., 1999) reported a CFR of 10%—12% without tick removal. In a review of 33 tick paralysis cases in Washington State over the period 1946—66, Dworkin (Dworkin et al., 1999) and 12 reported a CFR of up to 10%, with most deaths occurring in the 1940s. In a 60-year metaanalysis of confirmed tick paralysis cases in the United States,

Table 13.1 Clinical differential diagnosis of tick paralysis versus ascending neuromuscular paralysis with preserved sensorium.

Presenting clinical features	Tick paralysis	Guillain-Barré syndrome	Cervical spinal cord lesion	Poliomyelitis	Acute flaccid myelitis (enterovirus-D68)
Onset of ascending paralysis	Acute, rapid, within 24–48 hours	Slower onset, days to weeks	Abrupt to gradual	Days to weeks	Acute, rapid, within 24–48 hours
Ataxia	Present	Absent	Absent	Absent	Present
Deep tendon reflexes	Hyporeflexia progressing to areflexia	Hyporeflexia progressing to areflexia	Variable	Hyporeflexia progressing to areflexia	Hyporeflexia progressing to areflexia
Babinski sign	Absent	Absent	Present	Absent	Absent
Sensory loss	None	Mild	Present	None	Variable
Meningeal signs	Absent	Rarely present	Absent	Present	Variable
Fever	Absent	Rarely present	Absent	Present	Present in prodrome
CSF findings					
Protein levels (mg/dL)	Normal	High ($\geq$40)	Normal to high	High	High
White cells (per mm (Ali et al., 1912))	<10	<10	>10	>10	>10
Differential counts	Normal	<10 mononuclear cells/mm (Ali et al., 1912)	Variable	Lymphocytosis	Leukocytosis>5 wbcs/mm (Ali et al., 1912)
Nerve conduction studies	↑ Latency in distal motor nerves ↓ Nerve conduction velocity ↓ Amplitude of motor and sensory nerve action potentials	Similar	Similar	Similar	Similar

	Rapid, ≤24 hours after tick removal	Weeks to months	Variable	Months to years	Days to weeks
Time to neurologic recovery					
Permanent neurologic deficits	None after tick removal	Permanent paresis possible	Permanent paresis possible	Permanent paresis possible	Often incomplete neurological recovery, especially in most affected extremities.

This table compares the clinical differential diagnosis of tick paralysis versus ascending neuromuscular paralysis with preserved sensorium. Although botulism causes a descending neuromuscular paralysis with a preserved sensorium, tick paralysis, Guillain-Barré syndrome, acute poliomyelitis, and spinal cord tumors may all cause acute ascending paralysis with preserved mental status and must be differentiated from each other.

Adapted from Diaz, J.H., 2019. Section on Ectoparasitic Diseases. Chapter 296. Ticks (Including Tick Paralysis). In: Bennett JE, Dolin R, Blaser MJ, (Eds), Ninth Edition. Elsevier, Philadelphia. Elsevier publication.

Diaz (Diaz, 2010) reported a CFR of 6% in the first 30 years, a seasonal pattern of case clusters in children and adults in both urban and rural locations, and a significant increase in initial misdiagnoses of tick paralysis as Guillain-Barré syndrome in more recently reported cases. In addition, the misdiagnoses of tick paralysis cases as Guillain-Barré syndrome often directed unnecessary therapies, such as central venous plasmapheresis with immunoglobulin G, and delayed correct diagnosis and treatment by tick removal (Diaz, 2010, 2016). In all cases of delayed diagnosis, the diagnosis of tick paralysis was later established when attached ticks were discovered either by caregivers or by cranial neuroimaging studies.[104] The CFR from tick paralysis has steadily declined over the past 60 years, with almost all deaths in Canada and the United States reported in the 1940s and 1950s (Temple, 1912; Todd, 1912). In summary, attentive history taking about outdoor exposures during tick questing seasons in endemic regions is recommended in all cases of acute-onset flaccid paralysis to reduce delayed and missed diagnoses of tick paralysis.

The treatment of *Dermacentor* tick paralysis simply requires removing the tick with fine-tipped forceps (or tweezers) to restore neuromuscular function within 24 hours (Todd, 1912; Cleland, 1912). Although *I. holocyclus* tick paralysis is also treated by tick removal, transient neuromuscular deterioration may occur for 24–48 hours after tick removal (Grattan-Smith et al., 1997). The administration of *I. holocyclus* antitoxin before tick removal and prolonged observation for hypoventilation are recommended (Grattan-Smith et al., 1997).

References

Ali, A., Zeb, I., Alouffi, A., 1912. Diaz JH. A 60-year meta-analysis of tick paralysis in the United States: a predictable, preventable, and often misdiagnosed poisoning. Host Immune Responses to Salivary Components-A Critical Factor in Tick-Host Interactions 12, 175–176. https://doi.org/10.3389/foimb.2022.809052.BelongiaEA.

Ali, A., Zeb, I., Alouffi, A., Zahid, H., Almutairi, M.M., Ayed Alshammari, F., Alrouji, M., Termignoni, C., Vaz, I.da S., Tanaka, T., 2022. Host immune responses to salivary components - a critical facet of tick-host interactions. Frontiers in Cellular and Infection Microbiology 12. https://doi.org/10.3389/fcimb.2022.809052.

Belongia, E.A., 2002. Epidemiology and impact of coinfections acquired from Ixodes ticks. Vector Borne and Zoonotic Diseases 2 (4), 265–273. https://doi.org/10.1089/153036602321653851.

Brown, t a, Allman, R., Herwaldt, B.L., 2016. Reference laboratory investigation of patients with clinically diagnosed Lyme disease and babesiosis—Indiana. Morbidity & Mortality Weekly Report 67 (41), 1160–1161.

Cleland, J.B., 1912. Injuries and diseases of man in Australia attributable to animals (except insects). Australas Medical Gaz 32, 295.

Diaz, J.H., 2010. A 60-year meta-analysis of tick paralysis in the United States: a predictable, preventable, and often misdiagnosed poisoning. Journal of Medical Toxicology 6 (1), 15–21. https://doi.org/10.1007/s13181-010-0028-3.

Diaz, J.H., 2016. Tickborne coinfections in the United States. Journal of the Louisiana State Medical Society: Official Organ of the Louisiana State Medical Society 168 (2), 44–53.

Dworkin, M.S., Shoemaker, P.C., Anderson, D.E., 1999. Tick paralysis: 33 human cases in Washington State, 1946-1996. Clinical Infectious Diseases 29 (6), 1435—1439. https://doi.org/10.1086/313502.

Grattan-Smith, P.J., Morris, J.G., Johnston, H.M., Yiannikas, C., Malik, R., Russell, R., Ouvrier, R.A., 1997. Clinical and neurophysiological features of tick paralysis. Brain 120 (11), 1975—1987. https://doi.org/10.1093/brain/120.11.1975.

Krause, P.J., Telford, S.R., Spielman, A., Sikand, V., Ryan, R., Christianson, D., Burke, G., Brassard, P., Pollack, R., Peck, J., Persing, D.H., 1996. Concurrent Lyme disease and babesiosis: evidence for increased severity and duration of illness. JAMA 275 (21), 1657—1660. https://doi.org/10.1001/jama.275.21.1657.

Nadelman, R.B., Horowitz, H.W., Hsieh, T.C., Wu, J.M., Aguero-Rosenfeld, M.E., Schwartz, I., Nowakowski, J., Varde, S., Wormser, G.P., 1997. Simultaneous human granulocytic ehrlichiosis and lyme borreliosis. New England Journal of Medicine 337 (1), 27—30. https://doi.org/10.1056/NEJM199707033370105.

Pape, W.J., Gershman, K., Bamberg, W.M., 2006. Cluster of tick paralysis cases - Colorado, 2006. Morbidity and Mortality Weekly Report 55 (34), 933—935.

Schwartz, I., Fish, D., Daniels, T.J., 1997. Prevalence of the rickettsial agent of human granulocytic ehrlichiosis in ticks from a hyperendemic focus of lyme disease [1]. New England Journal of Medicine 337 (1), 49—50. https://doi.org/10.1056/NEJM199707033370111.

Swanson, S.J., Neitzel, D., Reed, K.D., Belongia, E.A., 2006. Coinfections acquired from Ixodes ticks. Clinical Microbiology Reviews 19 (4), 708—727. https://doi.org/10.1128/CMR.00011-06.

Swift, T.R., Ignacio, O.J., 1975. Tick paralysis: electrophysiologic studies. Neurology 25 (12), 1130—1133. https://doi.org/10.1212/wnl.25.12.1130.

Temple, I.U., 1912. Acute ascending paralysis, or tick paralysis. Medical Sentinel 20, 507—514.

Todd, J.L., 1912. Tick bite in British Columbia. Canadian Medical Association Journal 2, 1118.

CHAPTER 14

Red meat allergies after tick bites

Introduction

Immunoglobulin E (IgE)-mediated allergic reactions to tick bites were first described in Australia in the 1980s following paralysis tick (*Ixodes holocyclus*) bites (Gauci et al., 1989). These reactions were characterized by urticaria and angioedema more often than by anaphylaxis. In 2007, 25 patients who lived in a paralysis tick-endemic region near Sydney, Australia, developed red meat allergies after paralysis tick bites that presented as anaphylaxis or combinations of urticaria, angioedema, and anaphylaxis (Nunen et al., 2007). An immunological cross-reaction between arthropod-injected and foodborne antigens was suspected (Nunen et al., 2007). The sensitizing antigen in these and later tick bite-linked red meat allergy cases worldwide was subsequently identified as galactose-alpha-1,3-galactose (α-gal) (Commins et al., 2009, 2011; Van Nunen et al., 2009; Commins and Platts-Mills, 2013a).

Alpha-gal is an oligosaccharide constituent of all nonprimate, mammalian red meat that structurally resembles human blood group antigen B (Commins et al., 2009, 2011; Van Nunen et al., 2009; Commins and Platts-Mills, 2013a). Ticks obtain α-gal sugars while feeding on host animals and inject small amounts of α-gal into the human circulation during blood-feeding sensitizing high-risk persons to α-gal in red meats including beef, pork, lamb, goat, rabbit, horse, kangaroo, and all other wild game meats (Commins et al., 2009, 2011; Van Nunen et al., 2009; Commins and Platts-Mills, 2013a).

Epidemiology

Since 2007, over 200 cases of mammalian meat allergy have been reported following hard tick (Family Ixodidae) bites from every continent except Antarctica (van Nunen, 2014). Experts agree that most cases are underreported, especially in Australia and the United States, and in developing nations (van Nunen, 2014; Commins and Platts-Mills, 2013b). In an allergy and immunology practice in a paralysis tick endemic area outside of Sydney, Australia, Van Nunen reported diagnosing two patients per week with red meat allergy, often presenting as anaphylaxis, following tick bites (van Nunen, 2014). The 0.12% prevalence of red meat anaphylaxis after paralysis tick bites in the region exceeded the 0.10% prevalence of peanut-mediated anaphylaxis (van Nunen, 2014). Van Nunen proposed that the increasing prevalence of red meat allergy after tick bites

Ectoparasitic Diseases
ISBN 978-0-443-26724-6
https://doi.org/10.1016/B978-0-443-26724-6.00014-X

Figure 14.1 *Amblyomma ameri-canum*, the North American lone star tick (female), is a common cause of tick bites throughout the southeastern United States and the only currently recognized vector of red meat allergy after tick bites, also known as the alpha-gal syndrome. Note the white mark on the dorsal scutum of this adult female that resembles the Texas lone star. *(United States Centers for Disease Control and Prevention, Atlanta, Georgia, USA. Public domain, no copyright permission required. Available at: https://www.cdc.gov/dpdx/ticks/index.html).*

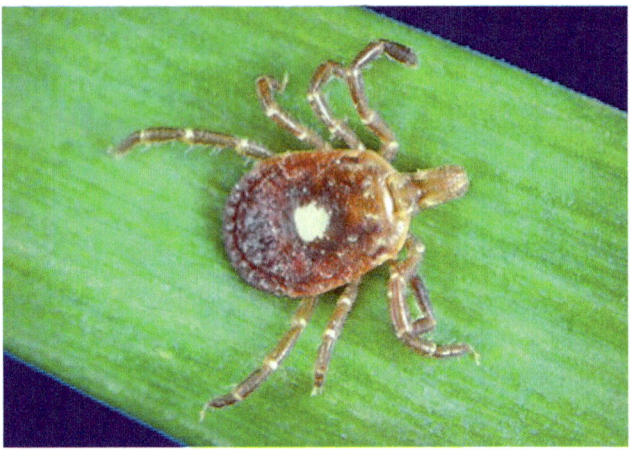

in Australia was the result of an increasing number of zoonotic reservoir hosts for ticks, especially bandicoots and other small mammals (van Nunen, 2014).

In the United States, Commins and Platts–Mills reported a seroprevalence in excess of 1000 persons with red meat allergy after tick bites and estimated that over 5000 persons have similar, but undiagnosed, conditions in the Southeast United States, where the Lone Star tick (*Amblyomma americanum*) is the predominant regional tick biting species (Fig. 14.1). (Commins and Platts–Mills, 2013c) Similar to the Australian experience, US investigators proposed that the increasing prevalence of red meat allergy after tick bites in the United States was the result of an increase in the white-tailed deer population, the preferred zoonotic reservoir hosts for Lone Star ticks in the southeastern United States (Fig. 14.2) (James et al., 2011)

As noted, cases of red meat allergy following tick bites have now been reported from six of seven continents with the exception of Antarctica. In most cases, only one predominant regional tick species has been the responsible vector of red meat allergy, now known as the α-gal syndrome.

At present, there is only one other case in which a second tick species in the same region was confirmed to have transmitted α-gal to humans during blood feeding (Kwak et al., 2018). Although the paralysis tick is responsible for most (95%) of the tick bites in Australia, Kwak et al. reported a recent case of mammalian meat allergy following multiple bites by another Australian tick species, *Ixodes (Endopalpiger) australiensis*, which was identified by an expert (Table 14.1) (Kwak et al., 2018).

Geographic distribution

In 2023, Thompson and coinvestigators reported the results of a retrospective descriptive analysis of the geographic distribution of all reference laboratory-confirmed case of the

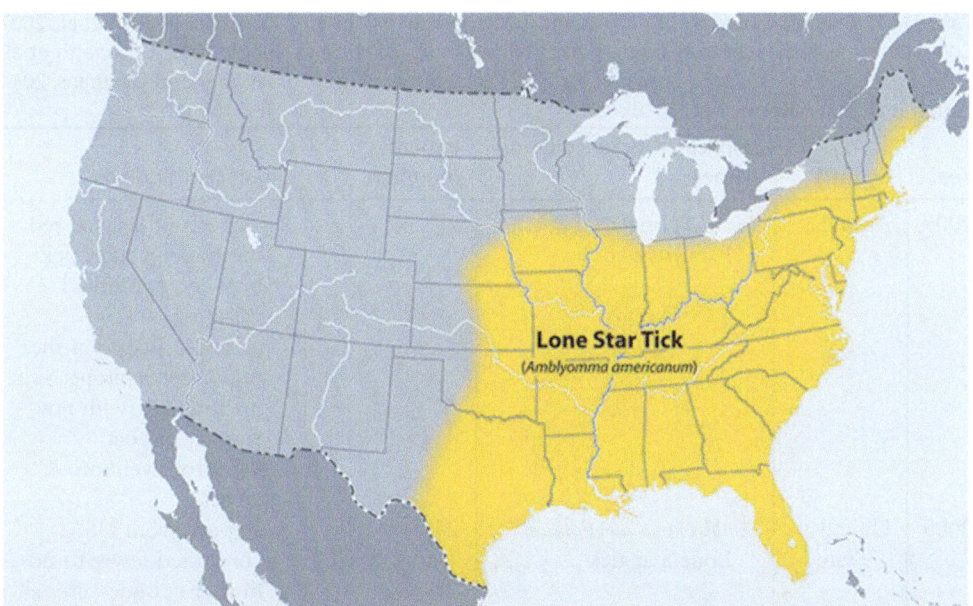

Figure 14.2 Geographic distribution range of ***Amblyomma americanum***, the North American lone star tick, throughout the southeastern United States and extending north along the Atlantic Coast to New England. *(United States Centers for Disease Control and Prevention, Atlanta, Georgia, USA. Public domain, no copyright permission required. Available at https://www.cdc.gov/ticks.geographic_distribution.html).*

alpha-gal-syndrome in the United States over the reporting period, 2017—2022 (Thompson et al., 2023). A total of 357,119 tests for alpha-gal-syndrome from 295,400 persons were submitted to a single reference laboratory responsible for nearly all testing in the United States (Thompson et al., 2023). Positive test results were reported in 90,018 persons or 30.5% of persons tested for alpha-gal-syndrome (Thompson et al., 2023). The number of persons with positive test results increased from 13,371 persons in 2017 to 18,885 persons in 2022 (Thompson et al., 2023). Among 233,521 persons for who census tract geographic data were available, cases predominantly occurred in counties within the southern, mid-Atlantic, and midwestern United States Census Bureau regions (Fig. 14.3) (Thompson et al., 2023)

Immunology

Medical oncologists engaged in early clinical trials of cetuximab in several southeastern states during the period, 2004—07, described hypersensitivity reactions, including fatal anaphylaxis, within 5—10 min of intravenous infusion (Chung et al., 2008). Cetuximab is a monoclonal antibody drug developed in mouse cell lines and designed to target the epidermal growth factor receptor in metastatic colorectal and head and neck cancers (Commins and Platts-Mills, 2013c).

Table 14.1 Selected global reports of red meat allergy after tick bites: 2007–2018 (Nunen et al., 2007; Commins et al., 2009; Van Nunen et al., 2009; Nuñez et al., 2011; Sekiya et al., 2012; Caponetto et al., 2013; Hamsten et al., 2013a; Morisset et al., 2013; Hamsten et al., 2013b; Wickner and Commins, 2014; Carter et al., 2018; Kwak et al., 2018).

Year	Country	Implicated ticks (common names)	Patients (number)	Significant findings
2007	Australia	*Ixodes holocyclus* Paralysis tick	25	1st reports of delayed red meat allergy after tick bites. 1st confirmed galactose-α-1,3-galactose (α-gal) as the responsible epitope. Skin prick tests + with raw extracts of goat kangaroo, venison, & rabbit.
2009	United States	*Amblyomma americanum* Lone Star tick	24	1st reports from USA; confirmed fewer to no further episodes after all red meat avoidance.
2009	Australia	*Ixodes holocyclus* Paralysis tick	25	Confirmed delayed onset allergic reactions; described + intradermal cetuximab skin tests. (Cetuximab is a monoclonal antibody anticancer chemotherapeutic drug produced in mouse cell lines that can causes anaphylaxis in patients sensitized to α-gal by milk or gelatin allergies or by tick bites.)
2011	Spain	*Ixodes ricinus* Sheep tick	5	1st reports from Europe; described + cetuximab skin prick tests.
2012	Japan	Tick not identified	1	1st report from Asia; described delayed onset anaphylaxis with oral pork ingestion test.
2013	Germany	*Ixodes ricinus* Sheep tick	21	Confirmed co-existing gelatin (animal collagen from rendered cattle hoofs & bones & pigskin) allergies as risk factors for anaphylaxis after tick bites.

Table 14.1 Selected global reports of red meat allergy after tick bites: 2007—2018 (Nunen et al., 2007; Commins et al., 2009; Van Nunen et al., 2009; Nuñez et al., 2011; Sekiya et al., 2012; Caponetto et al., 2013; Hamsten et al., 2013a; Morisset et al., 2013; Hamsten et al., 2013b; Wickner and Commins, 2014; Carter et al., 2018; Kwak et al., 2018).—cont'd

Year	Country	Implicated ticks (common names)	Patients (number)	Significant findings
2013	Sweden	*Ixodes ricinus* Sheep tick	5	1st reports from Scandinavia.
2013	France	*Ixodes ricinus* Sheep tick	1	Described cow's milk product allergy (cheese & yogurt) following tick bite.
2013	Sweden	*Ixodes ricinus* Sheep tick	39	Described moose meat allergies after tick bites.
2014	Panama	*Amblyomma cajennense* Cayenne tick	4	1st reports from Central America & 1st report of another species in the Americas capable of causing red meat allergies.
2017	United States	*Amblyomma americanum* Lone Star tick	6	Described male gender and co-existing systemic mastocytosis as risk factors for red meat allergies after tick bites.
2018	Australia	*Ixodes (Endopalpiger) australiensis*		1st report of the association of red meat allergy following a tick bite from a novel, second tick species in the same country. Until then, all regional red meat allergies followed bites by a single tick species.

When Karl Landsteiner identified the four major blood group antigens in 1900—01, he also discovered that humans possessed additional antigen group B-like antibodies to oligosaccharide epitopes found on nonprimate mammalian red blood cells (Steinke et al., 2015). Later immunologists identified this epitope as galactose-alpha-1,3-galactose, or α-gal, and classified the normal human antibodies to α-gal as IgG immuno-globulins (Steinke et al., 2015). Although all meat-eating primates, including man, possess IgG antibodies to red meat, the circulating concentration of these serum antibodies is typically low (<1% of circulating immunoglobulins), and red meat allergies are rare ($\leq$3% of foodborne allergies) (Chung et al., 2008).

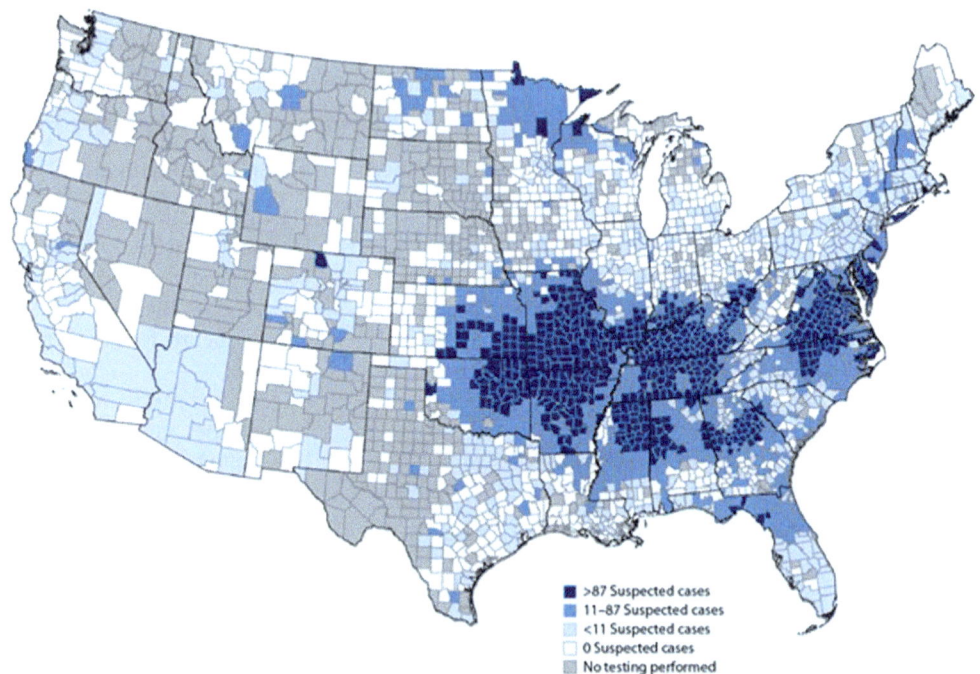

>87 Suspected cases
11–87 Suspected cases
<11 Suspected cases
0 Suspected cases
No testing performed

Figure 14.3 The geographic distribution of suspected alpha-gal-syndrome cases per one million population per year—United States, 2017–2022. Most cases have been confined to a mid-eastern band that runs from the Mississippi River to the coastal Atlantic states. *(Thompson JM, Carpenter A, Kersh GJ et al. Geographic distribution of suspected alpha-gal-syndrome cases —United States, 2017–2022. MMWR Morb Mort Wkly Rep 2023;72(30):815–20. United States Centers for Disease Control and Prevention, Atlanta, Georgia, USA. Public domain, no copyright permission required. Available at https://www.cdc.gov/mmwr/volumes/72/wr/mm7230a2.htm#F1_down).*

Red meat allergies, however, have been reported following antigenic sensitization to α-gal in meat by cow's milk, yogurt, and cheese; by exposures to oral or intravenous bovine and porcine albumin preparations; and by prior allergic reactions to foods containing bovine and/or porcine-derived gelatin (Steinke et al., 2015; Commins and Platts-Mills, 2013a; Mullins et al., 2012).

Gelatin is a manufactured mammalian meat product composed of hydrolyzed collagen processed from cattle bones, cow hides, and pig skins (Mullins et al., 2012). The sensitizing allergen in all of these exposures is galactose–alpha-1,3-galactose (α-gal) (Steinke et al., 2015; Commins and Platts-Mills, 2013a; Mullins et al., 2012).

Since cetuximab is a chimeric mouse-human monoclonal antibody, it contains the murine epitope α-gal which can sensitize certain at-risk humans with high concentrations of preexisting antibodies to α-gal to cetuximab-mediated allergic reactions (Chung et al., 2008). Later investigations determined that these preexisting antibodies were IgE antibodies, not IgG antibodies, specific for nonprimate α-gal (Commins and Platts-Mills, 2013a; Mullins et al., 2012; Rispens et al., 2013). The next question that investigators faced was why did the patients who experienced cetuximab allergic reactions have preexisting IgE antibodies to α-gal in the first place? (Steinke et al., 2015).

In 2009, Commins et al. reported a series of 24 patients from the southeastern United States who experienced delayed symptoms of urticaria, angioedema, or anaphylaxis 3—6 h after eating beef, pork, or lamb, and all were intradermal skin test positive to meat extracts and not to chicken extracts (Commins et al., 2009). Subsequent radioaller-gosorbent testing (RAST) detected IgE antibodies specific for α-gal and confirmed α-gal in red meat as the responsible allergen in all 24 patients, many of whom reported prior tick bites and resided in the same states as patients with cetuximab allergies (Arkansas, Missouri, Tennessee, Virginia, and North Carolina) (Commins et al., 2009; Steinke et al., 2015; O'Neil et al., 2007; Mariotte et al., 2011).

In 2009, Van Nunen et al. also described an association between paralysis tick bites and delayed, IgE-mediated mammalian meat allergies in Australia, and suggested that α-gal was once again the responsible epitope as in cetuximab allergy (Van Nunen et al., 2009). As in the Australian experience, American investigators observed the regional overlaps between the predominant tick species, such as the Lone Star tick, *Amblyomma americanum*, and red meat allergy cases, and between the cetuximab allergy cases and IgE antibodies specific for α-gal after tick bites (Figs. 14.1 and 14.2) (Van Nunen et al., 2009; Commins et al., 2011; Commins and Platts-Mills, 2013a).

Additional evidence in support of Lone Star tick bites as the cause of IgE antibody production specific for α-gal allergy to red meat in the United States was provided by a small case series of three patients (Carter et al., 2018). In this series, all three subjects reported tick bites in Lone Star tick-endemic regions of the United States, and two sub-jects were bitten by positively identified Lone Star ticks (Carter et al., 2018) In all 3 cases, IgE assays demonstrated statistically significant correlations between human IgE antibodies to α-gal and to salivary proteins derived from Lone Star ticks ($P < .001$) (Carter et al., 2018).

All ticks have three developmental stages with each stage requiring a different size host mammal to blood-feed on: (1) larvae feed on small rodents; (2) nymphs feed on larger rodents and small mammals; and (3) adults feed on the largest animals, such as deer, bears, and kangaroos. Ticks obtain α-gal sugars while blood-feeding on many nonprimate host animals during their lifetimes and inject small amounts of animal α-gal into the human circulation during human blood-feeding. The injected animal-derived α-gal sensitizes predisposed humans to an IgE-mediated allergic response on reexposures to α-gal anti-gens during cetuximab immunotherapy infusions for cancer or following ingestion of red meats, dairy products (milk and cheese), or gelatin-containing foods (Steinke et al., 2015). Although the exact incubation period for sensitization to red meat is unknown, it has been estimated to range from 1—3 months based on prior case reports (Steinke et al., 2015).

Recent investigations have now identified new immunological mechanisms of α-gal production in ticks and the α-gal syndrome in humans (Hilger et al., 2019; Cabezas-Cruz et al., 2019). Tick bite studies in mouse models have confirmed the link between tick bites and the IgE-mediated anti-α-gal response and have also demonstrated other unique immunological features of the α-gal response (Hilger et al., 2019). Both IgG and IgM anti-α-gal antibodies appear to confer protection against tick-transmitted pathogens, and only IgE anti-α-gal antibodies and not IgM or IgG antibodies trigger allergic responses to red meat and other α-gal containing products, such as gelatin and animal dander (Hilger et al., 2019). In another report, Cabezas-Cruz et al. proposed that tick salivary enzymes, particularly galactosyltransferases, and certain tick pathogenic gut bacteria, such as *Anaplasma phagocytophilum*, are involved in the synthesis of α-gal in ticks and in increasing the human risks of developing the α-gal syndrome following the bite of a pathogen-infected tick (Cabezas-Cruz et al., 2019).

Although the common denominator between tick bites and later cetuximab and red meat allergy was confirmed as IgE-mediated α-gal hypersensitivity, the cetuximab reactions were immediate in onset like other drug-induced allergies, and the red meat allergies were delayed by three or more hours in onset unlike other foodborne allergies (Carter et al., 2018; Steinke et al., 2015). Investigators have now attributed this delay in hypersensitivity reactions, including anaphylaxis, after red meat consumption to the time required for the intestinal absorption and lymphatic delivery of α-gal epitopes into the circulation in order to trigger IgE-mediated allergic reactions (Steinke et al., 2015).

In summary, the immunological connections between red meat allergy and tick bites require a prior sensitization to the nonprimate mammalian meat epitope α-gal by multiple, symptomatic tick bites from a single regional tick, such as the paralysis tick, *Ixodes holocyclus*, in Australia, the Lone Star tick, *Amblyomma americanum*, in the United States, the sheep tick, *Ixodes ricinus,* in Europe and Scandinavia, and the cayenne tick, *Amblyomma cajennense* in Latin America (Table 14.1).

Risk factors

In 2018, Carter et al. identified IgE antibodies to α-gal in six of 70 patients with idiopathic anaphylaxis, all of whom reported prior symptomatic tick bites and lived in Lone Star tick (*Amblyomma americanum*)-endemic American states (Fig. 14.2) (Carter et al., 2018). Unlike typical food allergies, which occur within minutes of ingestion, α-gal allergies following tick bites were delayed by 3—6 h and presented with combinations of urticarial reactions, angioedema, and anaphylaxis (Carter et al., 2018). In addition to having tick bite histories in Lone Star tick-endemic regions, all six patients in the study were male, and all had non-B blood types (Carter et al., 2018). Two of the six patients, who suffered more severe anaphylactic reactions, also had systemic mastocytosis, a hematological condition characterized by increased mast cell counts, high serum tryptase levels, and a predisposition to insect venom–induced allergic reactions (Carter et al., 2018). After adopting red meat-free diets that included chicken, turkey, and seafood, all six patients experienced no further episodes of unexplained anaphylaxis for follow-up periods ranging from 18 months to 3 years (Carter et al., 2018). The authors concluded that α-gal allergy should be excluded as a cause of unexplained, delayed anaphylaxis following red meat ingestion, especially in patients residing in Lone Star tick-endemic regions of the United States (Hamsten et al., 2013b; Carter et al., 2018). In addition, their study identified several risk factors for red meat allergy after tick bites including: (1) male gender due to increased occupational and recreational exposures to repeated tick bites in the United States and worldwide, (2) non-B blood type as the B-blood group antigen resembles α-gal stereochemically and probably provides some degree of cross-protection, and (3) a history of systemic mastocytosis (Carter et al., 2018).

Although asthma is not an established risk factor for red meat allergy after tick bites, preexisting atopic allergies to cat dander and to other furred animal dander are additional potential risk factors because the sensitizing epitope in animal dander or shed skin is α-gal which triggers the production of α-gal-specific IgE (Steinke et al., 2015).

More recently, another relatively common risk factor for red meat allergy after tick bites was described in patients with bovine or porcine prosthetic heart valves. The sensitizing epitope was once again confirmed as α-gal (Naso et al., 2013). In 2013, Naso and coinvestigators identified the α-gal epitope in glutaraldehyde-fixed bovine and porcine prosthetic heart valves and warned that histocompatibility or hypersensitivity reactions could result in patients with α-gal allergies (Naso et al., 2013). Most patients preferentially choose bioprosthetic heart valves over mechanical heart valves in order to avoid life-long anticoagulation (Naso et al., 2013; Mozzicato et al., 2014).

In 2014, Mozzicato et al. reported two patients with bioprosthetic heart valves who experienced postoperative or perioperative hypersensitivity reactions and were confirmed to have IgE-specific antibodies to α-gal (Mozzicato et al., 2014). In one case, a 53-year-old male with an extensive history of tick bites and a 3-year history of urticaria and flushing 2 h after eating beef or pork underwent a mitral valve replacement with a porcine valve for subacute bacterial endocarditis (Mozzicato et al., 2014). On postoperative day 1, he developed extensive urticaria on his chest and lower extremities that resolved after antihistamine treatment (Mozzicato et al., 2014). He continues to develop extensive urticaria after eating beef (Mozzicato et al., 2014).

In the other case, a 73-year-old male with an extensive history of tick bites and a 5-year history of delayed urticaria with and without syncope after eating red meat underwent aortic valve replacement with a bovine valve for aortic insufficiency (Mozzicato et al., 2014). At the end of the procedure, he developed a diffuse maculopapular rash, wheezing, and hypoxemia that resolved after fluid loading and treatment with epineph-rine, dexamethasone, and famotidine (Mozzicato et al., 2014). He continues to suffer allergic manifestations after consuming red meat, but not after consuming seafood and poultry (Mozzicato et al., 2014). The authors recommended that patients with preexist-ing IgE antibodies to α-gal following sensitization by repeated tick bites should be care-fully observed for hypersensitivity reactions including urticarial and anaphylaxis during and after heart valve replacements with either bovine or porcine bioprosthetic heart valves (Mozzicato et al., 2014).

Clinical manifestations

In most cases, patients with mammalian meat allergies will have a history of extensive local reactions to prior tick bites (van Nunen, 2015). If they cannot recall prior tick bites, there may give a history of a dark eschar with significant surrounding local reaction and edema or an excoriated scalp lesion providing indirect evidence of a prior tick bite in a tick endemic area (van Nunen, 2015). Patients will present with delayed allergic mani-festations from 2−10 h after ingesting cooked or raw mammalian meat, often at night-time (van Nunen, 2015). Anaphylaxis with syncope, hypotension, and stridor will characterize up to 60% of initial presentations with the remainder characterized by com-binations of pruritic urticarial reactions, angioedema, diarrhea, and abdominal pain (van Nunen, 2015). In some cases, a gelatin allergy may precede a mammalian meat allergy and may be immediate if the exposure is intravenous following gelatin-containing colloid infusions, or delayed if the exposure is to foodborne gelatin in desserts or in gelatin-containing medication capsules (van Nunen, 2015).

Diagnosis

The diagnosis of mammalian meat allergy and/or gelatin allergy associated with tick bites will require confirmation by both serological testing and skin testing. The most specific serological tests include blood antigen group typing, total serum IgE levels by chemilu-minescence assay (normal mean = 32 IU/mL), and specific IgE levels to beef, pork, and lamb extracts by fluoro-enzyme immunoassay (positive IgE reaction level to a-gal ≥0.35 IU/mL) (Commins and Platts-Mills, 2013c).

If such tests are unavailable, then cetuximab skin prick or intradermal skin testing will also confirm the diagnosis of α-gal sensitivity and IgE-mediated red meat allergy (Carter et al., 2018; van Nunen, 2015). Systemic mastocytosis should also be ruled out by measuring serum tryptase levels by fluoro-enzyme immunoassay (normal levels ≤11.5 ng/mL) (Commins and Platts-Mills, 2013c; van Nunen, 2015).

Skin prick or intradermal skin tests with extracts of beef, lamb, pork, chicken, turkey, fish, cat and dog dander are also recommended to establish the best meatless protein diets and to rule out co-existing dander allergy (Commins and Platts-Mills, 2013c; Carter et al., 2018; van Nunen, 2015). After the diagnosis is confirmed, a medical alert device, such as a medic-alert bracelet or neck chain, to be worn at all times, is highly recommended in order to alert medical providers of any coexisting anaphylaxis risks posed by oral or intravenous gelatin-containing colloid preparations, artificial bovine blood products, intravenous cancer chemotherapy with cetuximab, and bioprosthetic heart valve replacement (Commins and Platts-Mills, 2013c; van Nunen, 2015).

Treatment

The therapeutic management of mammalian meat allergic reactions is no different from the treatment of anaphylaxis, angioedema, and urticaria resulting from exposures to other foodborne allergens (van Nunen, 2014, 2015). The cornerstone of therapeutic management for acute anaphylaxis with syncope, shock, laryngeal edema, stridor, wheezing, and respiratory distress is with subcutaneous epinephrine to restore blood pressure and reverse bronchoconstriction (van Nunen, 2014, 2015). Oral or parenteral H-1 and H-2 blocking antihistamines are indicated for symptomatic relief from pruritic urticarial reactions (van Nunen, 2014, 2015). Oral or parenteral corticosteroids are indicated to reduce ongoing swelling from angioedema (van Nunen, 2014, 2015). Non-gelatin-containing intravenous fluids and electrolytes are indicated to reverse hypovolemia and restore circulatory volume in reactions with gastrointestinal involvement and severe diarrhea, usually without vomiting (van Nunen, 2014, 2015). All patients with confirmed mammalian meat allergies should be provided with and trained in the use of hand-held epinephrine auto-injectors to be carried on their person at all times (van Nunen, 2014, 2015).

Patients with α-gal sensitivity should avoid all red meat, including, beef, lamb, pork, goat, rabbit, horse, kangaroo, venison, and all animal organ meats (heart, kidney, sweatbreads [thymus gland and pancreas], tripe, etc.) and other game meats; all gelatin-containing foods; and cancer immunotherapy with intravenous cetuximab for life. Sensitivities may wane over a prolonged period of time during which red meat may be reintroduced gradually into one's diet.

Although the only treatment for red meat allergy is meat avoidance, patients should be encouraged to consult a dietician to supplement their diets with vitamins, such as vitamin B-12, iron, and protein from seafood and poultry, and to safely reintroduce meat protein into their diets. Skin testing will help to determine when certain meat products may be gradually reintroduced into the diet. Desensitization is unavailable.

Prevention and control

There are a number of strategies that can be used in the prevention and control of tick bites including personal protective measures, landscape management, and wildlife management. Personal protective measures to prevent tick bites include wearing appropriate clothing, using insect repellants, and performing regular tick checks. Wearing long pants tucked into socks, shoes not sandals, long-sleeved shirts, and light-colored clothing can aide in keeping ticks off the skin and in making them easier to spot on clothing. Impregnating clothing with permethrin, routinely performed by the military, is a highly effective repellant against ticks and other insects. The topical application of insect repellants containing 20%–50% formulations of N, N-diethyl-meta-toluamide (DEET) or 7%–20% picaridin directly on the skin is another effective and recommended measure.

Most patients will not recall tick-bites, especially bites by diminutive larval and nymphal ticks. Nevertheless, tick localization and removal as soon as possible, preferably within 24 h, remain recommended strategies to prevent tick transmitted infectious diseases and to reverse tick paralysis. Ticks should always be removed with forceps, tweezers, or specially designed tick removal devices, and not fingers as squishing ticks can transmit several tick borne diseases across dermal barriers or create infectious aerosols (Fig. 14.4). Ticks should always be removed in contiguity with their feeding mouthparts, rather than burning ticks with spent matches, or painting embedded ticks with adhesives or nail polishes (Fig. 14.4).

Landscape management strategies to prevent tick bites and tick borne diseases include widespread application of acaricides over tick-preferred, high grass ecosystems, removal of vegetation and leaf-litter near recreation sites, and creation of vegetation-free dry barriers of gravel, stone, or wood chips between forested areas and yards or playgrounds. Wildlife management strategies recommended to local authorities to prevent animal tick bites include applying acaricides actively to domestic animals and passively to deer, cattle, kangaroos, and other large mammals at baited feeding and watering stations, or salt licks; and setting out acaricide-baited rodent houses for rodents to occupy or acaricide-baited cotton balls for rodents to adopt as nesting materials, especially in crawl-spaces under wilderness cabins and houses, and near playgrounds and parks.

Conclusions

Humans are at risk of red meat allergy after tick bites in localized regions on every continent except Antarctica. Since 2007, over 200 cases of red meat allergy after tick bites have been reported. In most cases, one predominant tick species transmits the red meat-sensitizing antigen during blood feeding. The sensitizing antigen is a–gal, an oligosaccharide constituent of nonprimate blood and meat. The major risk factors for red meat allergy after tick bites include male gender, non-B blood type, systemic mastocytosis, a bioprosthetic (bovine or porcine) heart valve, and preexisting allergies to animal dander. Everyone should take personal protective measures to avoid tick bites and to reduce their risks of tick-transmitted infectious diseases and red meat allergies. In addition to meat avoidance, patients with red meat allergies should avoid all gelatin-containing foods and cancer immunotherapy with intravenous cetuximab, a monoclonal antibody

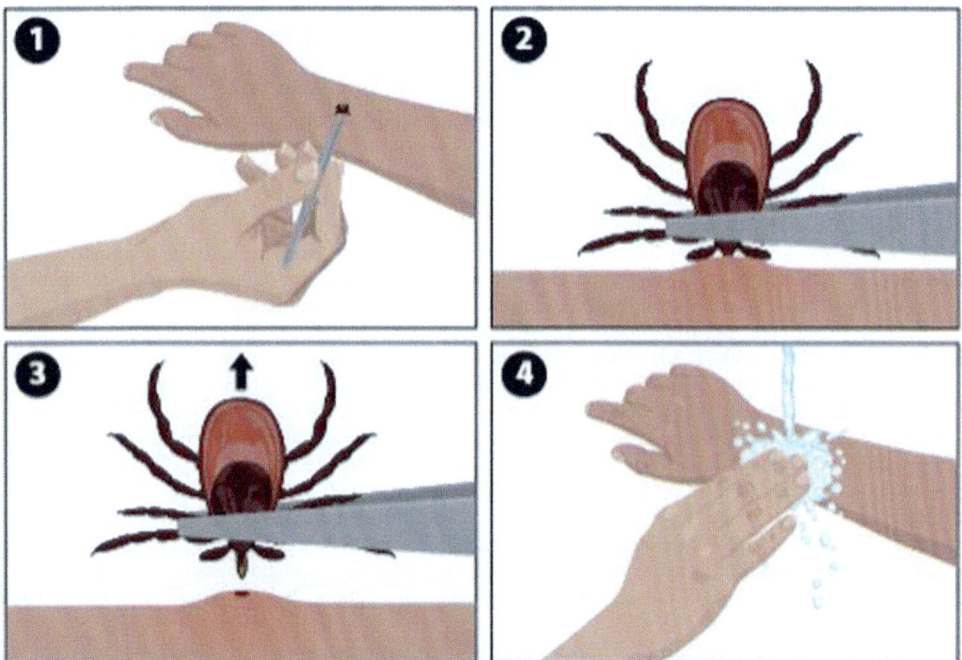

Figure 14.4 The proper techniques to remove embedded ticks include: (1) identifying the skin-embedded tick without dislodging it; (2) grasping the tick with tweezers, forceps, or other tick removal device across the thorax; (3) exerting a removal force straight upward and perpendicular to the skin in order to avoid splitting off the mouthparts that are injecting the salivary gland antigens and pathogens; and (4) washing the tick bite site with soap and water. *(United States Centers for Disease Control and Prevention, Atlanta, Georgia, USA. Public domain, no copyright permission required. Available at: https://www.google.com/search?q=cdc+proper+tick+removal+technique&rlz=1C1GCEU_enUS1012U S1012&oq=&gs_lcrp=EgZjaHJvbWUqCQgAECMYJxjqAjIJCAAQIxgnGOoCMgkIARAjGCcY6gIyCQgCECMY JxjqAjIJCAMQIxgnGOoCMgkIBBAjGCcY6gIyCQgFECMYJxjqAjIJCAYQIxgnGOoCMgkIBxAjGCcY6gLSAQszOD E5NTYzajBqN6gCCLACAQ&sourceid=chrome&ie=UTF-8#vhid=-FYDPNfjDbYgPM&vssid=I).*

produced in mouse cell lines, for life. Red meat allergy after tick bites represents another emerging threat from tick bites in addition to infectious diseases and tick paralysis. More cases of red meat allergy after tick bites will occur as persons with common risk factors spend more time outdoors in tick-endemic regions worldwide. Clinicians should advise their patients about their personal and regional health risks of tick-transmitted red meat allergy; now an established worldwide phenomenon.

References

Cabezas-Cruz, A., Hodžić, A., Román-Carrasco, P., Mateos-Hernández, L., Duscher, G.G., Sinha, D.K., Hemmer, W., Swoboda, I., Estrada-Peña, A., De La Fuente, J., 2019. Environmental and molecular drivers of the α-Gal syndrome. Frontiers in Immunology 10 (MAY), 1210. https://doi.org/10.3389/fimmu.2019.01210, 16643224.

Caponetto, P., Fischer, J., Biedermann, T., 2013. Gelatin-containing sweets can elicit anaphylaxis in a patient with sensitization to galactose-α-1,3-galactose. Journal of Allergy and Clinical Immunology: In Practice 1 (3), 302—303. https://doi.org/10.1016/j.jaip.2013.01.007, 22132198.

Carter, M.C., Ruiz-Esteves, K.N., Workman, L., Lieberman, P., Platts-Mills, T.A.E., Metcalfe, D.D., 2018. Identification of alpha-gal sensitivity in patients with a diagnosis of idiopathic anaphylaxis. Allergy 73 (5), 1131—1134. https://doi.org/10.1111/all.13366.

Chung, C.H., Mirakhur, B., Chan, E., Le, Q.-T., Berlin, J., Morse, M., Murphy, B.A., Satinover, S.M., Hosen, J., Mauro, D., Slebos, R.J., Zhou, Q., Gold, D., Hatley, T., Hicklin, D.J., Platts-Mills, T.A.E., 2008. Cetuximab-induced anaphylaxis and IgE specific for galactose-α-1,3-galactose. New England Journal of Medicine 358 (11), 1109—1117. https://doi.org/10.1056/nejmoa074943.

Commins, S.P., Platts-Mills, T.A.E., 2013a. Delayed anaphylaxis to red meat in patients with ige specific for galactose alpha-1,3-galactose (alpha-gal). Current Allergy and Asthma Reports 13 (1), 72—77. https://doi.org/10.1007/s11882-012-0315-y, 15346315.

Commins, S.P., Platts-Mills, T.A.E., 2013b. Tick bites and red meat allergy. Current Opinion in Allergy and Clinical Immunology 13 (4), 354—359. https://doi.org/10.1097/ACI.0b013e3283624560, 14736322.

Commins, S.P., Satinover, S.M., Hosen, J., Mozena, J., Borish, L., Lewis, B.D., Woodfolk, J.A., Platts-Mills, T.A.E., 2009. Delayed anaphylaxis, angioedema, or urticaria after consumption of red meat in patients with IgE antibodies specific for galactose-α-1,3-galactose. Journal of Allergy and Clinical Immunology 123 (2). https://doi.org/10.1016/j.jaci.2008.10.052. 426-e2.

Commins, S.P., James, H.R., Kelly, L.A., Pochan, S.L., Workman, L.J., Perzanowski, M.S., Kocan, K.M., Fahy, J.V., Nganga, L.W., Ronmark, E., Cooper, P.J., Platts-Mills, T.A.E., 2011. The relevance of tick bites to the production of IgE antibodies to the mammalian oligosaccharide galactose-α-1,3-galactose. Journal of Allergy and Clinical Immunology 127 (5), 1286—1293.e6. https://doi.org/10.1016/j.jaci.2011.02.019, 00916749.

Gauci, M., Loh, R.K.S., Stone, B.F., Thong, Y.H., 1989. Allergic reactions to the Australian paralysis tick, Ixodes holocyclus: diagnostic evaluation by skin test and radioimmunoassay. Clinical and Experimental Allergy 19 (3), 279—283. https://doi.org/10.1111/j.1365-2222.1989.tb02384.x, 13652222.

Hamsten, C., Starkhammar, M., Tran, T.A.T., Johansson, M., Bengtsson, U., Ahlén, G., Sällberg, M., Grönlund, H., van Hage, M., 2013a. Identification of galactose-α-1,3-galactose in the gastrointestinal tract of the tick Ixodes ricinus ; possible relationship with red meat allergy. Allergy 68 (4), 549—552. https://doi.org/10.1111/all.12128, 01054538.

Hamsten, C., Tran, T.A.T., Commins, S.P., et al., 2013b. Red meat allergy in Sweden: association with tick sensitization and B-negative blood groups. The Journal of Allergy and Clinical Immunology 132, 1431—1434.

Hilger, C., Fischer, J., Wolbing, F., 2019. Role and mechanism of galactose-alpha1,3-galactose in the elicitation of delayed anaphylactic reactions to red meat. Current Allergy and Asthma Reports 19 (1), 3. https://doi.org/10.1007/s11882-019-0385-9.

James, H.R., Commins, S.P., Kelly, L.A., Pochan, S.L., Workman, L.J., Mullins, R.J., Platts-Mills, T.A.E., 2011. Further evidence for tick bites as A cause of the IgE responses to alpha-gal that underlie A major increased in delayed anaphylaxis to meat. Journal of Allergy and Clinical Immunology 127 (2). https://doi.org/10.1016/j.jaci.2010.12.967. AB243-AB243.

Kwak, M., Somerville, C., van Nunen, S., 2018. A novel Australian tick Ixodes (Endopalpiger) australiensis inducing mammalian meat allergy after tick bite. Asia Pacific Allergy 8 (3), e31. https://doi.org/10.5415/apallergy.2018.8.e31.

Mariotte, D., Dupont, B., Gervais, R., Galais, M.P., Laroche, D., Tranchant, A., Comby, E., Bouhier-Leporrier, K., Reimund, J.M., Le Mauff, B., 2011. Anti-cetuximab IgE ELISA for identification of patients at a high risk of cetuximab-induced anaphylaxis. mAbs 3 (4), 396—401. https://doi.org/10.4161/mabs.3.4.16293, 19420870.

Morisset, M., Richard, C., Zanna, H., 2013. Allergy to cow's milk related to IgE antibodies specific for galactose-alpha-1,3-galactose, in Proceedings. In: European Academy of Allergology and Clinical Immunology Congress and World Allergy Organisation. Milan, Italy).

Mozzicato, S.M., Tripathi, A., Posthumus, J.B., Platts-Mills, T.A.E., Commins, S.P., 2014. Porcine or bovine valve replacement in 3 patients with IgE antibodies to the mammalian oligosaccharide galactose-alpha-1,3-galactose. Journal of Allergy and Clinical Immunology: In Practice 2 (5), 637—638. https://doi.org/10.1016/j.jaip.2014.04.016, 22132198.

Mullins, R.J., James, H., Platts-Mills, T.A.E., Commins, S., 2012. Relationship between red meat allergy and sensitization to gelatin and galactose-α-1,3-galactose. Journal of Allergy and Clinical Immunology 129 (5). https://doi.org/10.1016/j.jaci.2012.02.038. 1334-e1.

Naso, F., Gandaglia, A., Bottio, T., Tarzia, V., Nottle, M.B., d'Apice, A.J.F., Cowan, P.J., Cozzi, E., Galli, C., Lagutina, I., Lazzari, G., Iop, L., Spina, M., Gerosa, G., 2013. First quantification of alpha-G al epitope in current glutaraldehyde-fixed heart valve bioprostheses. Xenotransplantation 20 (4), 252—261. https://doi.org/10.1111/xen.12044.

van Nunen, S., 2014. Galactose-Alpha-1,3-Galactose, mammalian meat and anaphylaxis: a World-Wide phenomenon? Current Treatment Options in Allergy 1 (3), 262—277. https://doi.org/10.1007/s40521-014-0022-0.

van Nunen, S., 2015. Tick-induced allergies: mammalian meat allergy, tick anaphylaxis and their significance. Asia Pacific Allergy 5 (1), 3—16. https://doi.org/10.5415/apallergy.2015.5.1.3.

Nunen, S.A.V., Fernando, S.L., Clarke, L.R., 2007. The association between Ixodes holocyclus tick bite reactions and red meat allergy. Internal Medicine Journal 37 (5).

Van Nunen, S.A., O'Connor, K.S., Clarke, L.R., Boyle, R.X., Fernando, S.L., 2009. An association between tick bite reactions and red meat allergy in humans. Medical Journal of Australia 190 (9), 510—511. https://doi.org/10.5694/j.1326-5377.2009.tb02533.x, 13265377.

Nuñez, R., Carballada, F., Gonzalez-Quintela, A., Gomez-Rial, J., Boquete, M., Vidal, C., 2011. Delayed mammalian meat-induced anaphylaxis due to galactose-α-1,3- galactose in 5 European patients. Journal of Allergy and Clinical Immunology 128 (5), 1122—1124.e1. https://doi.org/10.1016/j.jaci.2011.07.020, 10976825.

O'Neil, B.H., Allen, R., Spigel, D.R., Stinchcombe, T.E., Moore, D.T., Berlin, J.D., Goldberg, R.M., 2007. High incidence of cetuximab-related infusion reactions in Tennessee and North Carolina and the association with atopic history. Journal of Clinical Oncology 25 (24), 3644—3648. https://doi.org/10.1200/JCO.2007.11.7812, 0732183X.

Rispens, T., Derksen, N.I.L., Commins, S.P., et al., 2013. IgE production to a-gal is accompanied by specific IgG1 antibodies and low amounts of IgE to blood group B. PLoS One 8, 1—6.

Sekiya, K., Fukutomi, Y., Nakazawa, T., Taniguchi, M., Akiyama, K., 2012. Delayed anaphylactic reaction to mammalian meat. Journal of Investigational Allergology and Clinical Immunology 22 (6), 446—447, 16980808. http://www.jiaci.org/issues/vol22issue6/8-19.pdf.

Steinke, J.W., Platts-Mills, T.A.E., Commins, S.P., 2015. The alpha-gal story: lessons learned from connecting the dots. Journal of Allergy and Clinical Immunology 135 (3), 589—596. https://doi.org/10.1016/j.jaci.2014.12.1947, 10976825.

Thompson, J.M., Carpenter, A., Kersh, G.J., Wachs, T., Commins, S.P., Salzer, J.S., 2023. Geographic distribution of suspected alpha-gal syndrome cases - United States, January 2017-December 2022. Morbidity and Mortality Weekly Report 72 (30), 815—820. https://doi.org/10.15585/MMWR.MM7230A2, 1545861X.

Wickner, P.G., Commins, S., 2014. The first Central American cases of delayed meat allergy with galactose-alpha-1,3-galactose positivity among field biologists in Panama. In: Proceedings. 2014 Meeting American Academy of Allergy and Immunology. San Diego, California USA).

CHAPTER 15

True bugs (Order Hemiptera) as ectoparasites: Bedbugs

Introduction and taxonomy

Bed bugs are small, flat, ectoparasitic arthropods that feed solely on the blood of humans and animals. They are considered "true bugs" belonging to the insect order Hemiptera (Phylum Arthropoda, Class Insecta, Order Hempitera, Family Cimicidae) (Parola and Izri, 2020; Goddard and DeShazo, 2009; Doggett et al., 2012). The sole genus of human bed bugs, *Cimex*, has only two species, *Cimex lectularius*, the common bedbug distributed worldwide, and *Cimex hemipterus*, the tropical bedbug, confined to the tropics and subtropics (Parola and Izri, 2020; Goddard and DeShazo, 2009; Doggett et al., 2012). Although unusual, humans may become the incidental hosts of nonhuman *Cimex* species of bed bugs that blood-feed on bats and birds (Doggett et al., 2012). Like other members of the Order Hemiptera, bed bugs have sharp, piercing, and sucking mouthparts (Parola and Izri, 2020; Goddard and DeShazo, 2009; Doggett et al., 2012).

Biology and life cycle

The sexually mature, adult bed bug is reddish-brown in color, oval in shape, and dorso-ventrally flattened. It averages 5.0 mm in length and 1.5—2.0 mm in width (Fig. 15.1) (Goddard and DeShazo, 2009). Since their hindwings are absent and their forewings are reduced to rudimentary buds, adult bed bugs cannot fly, but can crawl on three pairs of legs and can cover up to 100 feet at night to blood-feed (Goddard and DeShazo, 2009; Doggett et al., 2012). Juvenile bed bugs or nymphs resemble adults, but are smaller in size and paler in color (Fig. 15.1). A newly hatched nymph, the first of five developmental stages (instars), is the smallest life stage, and so pale and translucent that its initial blood meal can be visualized in its gastrointestinal tract (Fig. 15.1). Nymphs will enlarge and darken in color as they age and progress in life stage. During development, every life stage or instar requires a blood meal in order to progress to its next stage of development (Fig. 15.1) (Goddard and DeShazo, 2009; Doggett et al., 2012).

Eggs will hatch in about 4—12 days into first instar nymphs, which will require a blood meal to mature to the next instar life stage leading to adulthood (Fig. 15.2).

Ectoparasitic Diseases
ISBN 978-0-443-26724-6
https://doi.org/10.1016/B978-0-443-26724-6.00015-1

Figure 15.1 The developmental stages of *Cimex lectularius*, the most common species of bed bug. Juveniles (middle) are smaller and slightly paler versions of adults. A newly hatched nymph (right), the first stage of five life stages (instars), is translucent, and needs a blood meal to progress to its next stage of development. The black arrow points to blood in the nymph's gastrointestinal tract from a recent meal. *(United States Centers for Disease Control and Prevention (CDC). Public domain. No copyright permission required. Available at https://www.cdc.gov/dpdx/bedbugs.index.html)*

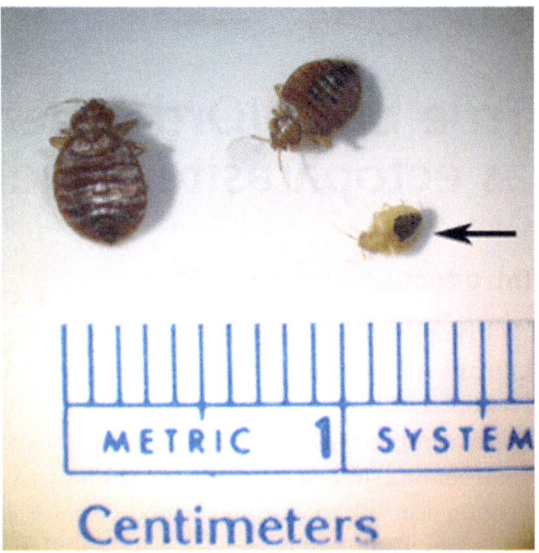

Mating between adult males and females occurs in the dark off of the host in a unique method of copulation known as traumatic insemination (Goddard and DeShazo, 2009; Doggett et al., 2012). In this performance, the male penetrates the female's ventral abdominal wall with his external genitalia and deposits sperm directly into the female's body cavity for fertilization. Adult bed bugs typically live from 6 to 12 months.

Bed bug behavior

Feeding behavior

Bed bugs will summon other bed bugs to feed on the same host by secreting potent airborne pheromones. Although bed bugs can crawl up to 100 feet to reach a host to feed upon at nighttime, they prefer to only travel up to about 8 feet from their colonies to a suitable, sleeping host (Goddard and DeShazo, 2009; Doggett et al., 2012).

Bed bugs secrete local anesthetics and anticoagulants in their saliva (Doggett et al., 2012). The salivary local anesthetics allow them to feed without awakening their hosts. The salivary anticoagulants assure constant blood flow while blood feeding (Parola and Izri, 2020; Goddard and DeShazo, 2009; Doggett et al., 2012).

Nesting behavior

After blood feeding for 5—10 min and obtaining a complete blood meal, bed bugs will return to their nearby colonies guided by pheromones. They will usually defecate on the

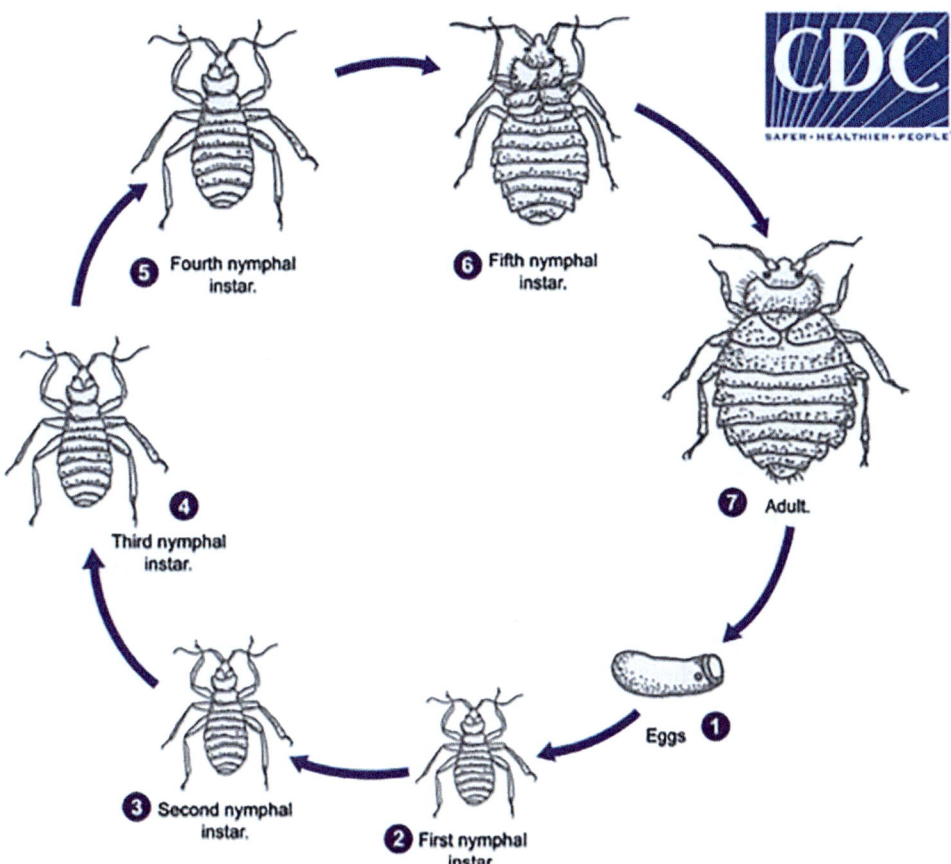

Figure 15.2 The life cycle of the common bed bug, *Cimex lectularius*, from egg to female adult through the five stages of instar development with each stage requiring a blood meal to progress to the next stage. Bed bugs prefer to ingest human blood, but will bite domestic pets, bats, and birds, especially chickens, for blood meals in the absence of humans. *(United States Centers for Disease Control and Prevention (CDC). Public domain. No copyright permission required. Available at https://www.cdc.gov/dpdx/bedbugs.index.html)*

way back leaving tell-tale reddish brown fecal streaks, which are important indicators of bed bug infestations (Parola and Izri, 2020).

Bed bug colonies are inhabited by all developmental forms from eggs to adults and are usually located within 8 feet or less of the host. Bed bugs nest together in tight, dark colonies within mattress seams, box springs, baseboards, headboards, carpets, bedroom dressers and other bedroom furniture, and even behind wall paper in order to conceal themselves from daylight and detection (Parola and Izri, 2020).

Epidemiology

Geographic distribution

Bed bugs are distributed worldwide. By the end of the 1950s, household bed bugs were nearly eradicated by the environmentally persistent organochlorine pesticide, dichlorodiphenyltrichloroethane (DDT) (See Chapter 16.) (Goddard and DeShazo, 2009; Doggett et al., 2012). The widespread use of DDT was directed at killing mosquitoes and eradicating malaria and other mosquito-borne infectious diseases. DDT also nearly eliminated other unwelcomed insect species, particularly cockroaches (Goddard and DeShazo, 2009). Unlike mosquitoes, cockroaches are not arthropod vectors of infectious diseases and consume bed bugs (Goddard and DeShazo, 2009). Only about 30% of households in the United States had bed bugs by the 1960s (Doggett et al., 2012; Parola and Izri, 2020). Modern vacuum cleaners and unupholstered, modern furniture designs also eliminated many household habitats for bed bugs.

Increasing infestations

With the banning of DDT in 1972 and increased immigration and international travel by the 1970s, the rates of household infestation with bed bugs soared worldwide (Doggett et al., 2012). The popularity of antique furniture and second-hand furnishings in home bedroom decoration further increased infestation rates by the 1980s (Doggett et al., 2012).

Pesticide resistance

Over time, bed bugs became increasingly resistant to pesticides and insect "bomb" foggers. (See Chapter 16) (Doggett et al., 2012; Parola and Izri, 2020). Today, most major cities have enacted bed bug control ordinances for hotel and motel chains, bed and breakfast establishments, furniture and mattress dealerships, public businesses, and public transportation in order to limit bed bug spread.

International travel

Bed bug spread is difficult to control because bed bug infestation is hard to detect and treat and rarely reported by embarrassed homeowners and hotel operators. They travel in the crevices of airline and train cushions and on the seats of public transit (Doggett et al., 2012). Bed bug colonies can be found in antique furniture and in second-hand furnishings, especially carpets and drapes. People often do not realize that they are transporting bed bugs as stow-away passengers on their belongings (Doggett et al., 2012; Parola and Izri, 2020).

Clinical manifestations

Bed bug bites may occur anywhere on the body and can range from no visible effects in 20%−30% of persons to a linear or scattered pattern of raised red spots to bullous blisters in 60%−70% of persons (Figs. 15.3 and Fig. 15.4) (Parola and Izri, 2020; Goddard and

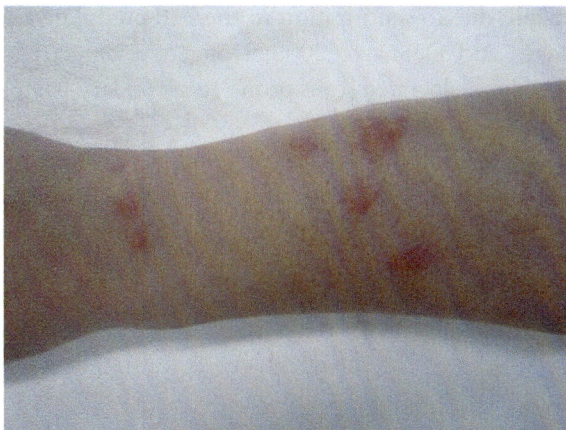

Figure 15.3 Bed bug bite complexes or cimicosis are usually present on exposed, uncovered skin on the face, neck, and extremities, and result in a linear or scattered pattern of intensely pruritic raised, erythematous, maculopapular lesions several days later. *(Wikipedia. Public domain. No copyright permission required. Available at https://en.wikipedia.org/wiki/Bed_bug)*

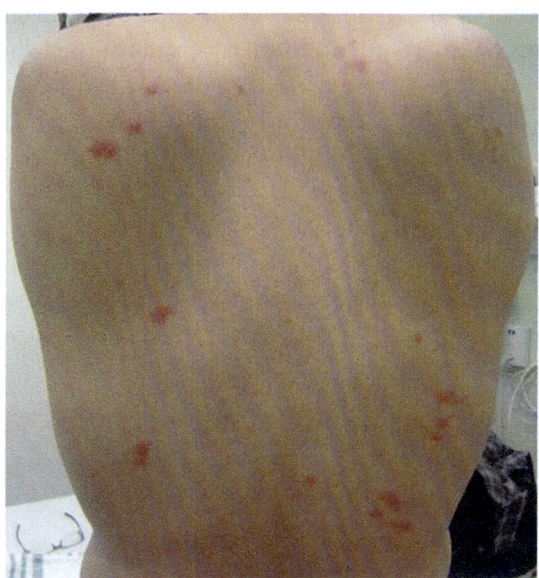

Figure 15.4 Bed bug bites in linear patterns are more frequently observed on the trunk, back, and legs with extended surface spaces for a solitary, blood-feeding bedbugs to traverse. Allergic manifestations, systemic reactions, and anaphylaxis are extremely rare. A central spot of bleeding may occur in the center of the lesion due to the injection of anticoagulants in the bedbug's saliva in order to maintain blood flow during feeding. *(Wikipedia. Public domain. No copyright permission required. Available at https://en.wikipedia.org/wiki/Bed_bug)*

DeShazo, 2009; Doggett et al., 2012). A central spot or punctum of bleeding may occur in the center of the bite lesion due to the injection of anticoagulants in the bedbug's saliva in order to maintain blood flow during feeding.

Complications of bed bug bites

Allergic manifestations, systemic effects, and anaphylaxis following bed bug bites can occur, but are extremely rare (Doggett et al., 2012; Goddard and DeShazo, 2009). However, bite inflammatory reactions with increased edema and erythema are often greater after multiple or recurrent bites most likely due to sensitization to the bed bug's salivary proteins (Parola and Izri, 2020; Goddard and DeShazo, 2009; Doggett et al., 2012). Scratching highly pruritic lesions can produce ulcerated sores prone to secondary bacterial infections, such as impetigo.

Recurrent bites over time in chronic infestations may lead to a microcytic, microchromic anemia of blood loss, loss of sleep, daytime sleepiness, and impaired daily work performance. Recovery from repeated attacks by bed bugs can be accompanied by anxiety, irritability, and insomnia and lead to delusions of parasitosis (See Chapter 17.) (Donabedian, 2007).

Detection and diagnosis

Many other skin conditions can produce cutaneous lesions similar to bed bug bites including other bug and mite bites, scabies, erythema nodosa, allergic reactions, hives, and viral and bacterial skin infections (Parola and Izri, 2020). Since bed bugs spend only 5—10 min blood feeding on humans before returning to their communal nests in mattresses, box springs, headboards, carpets, couches, and bedroom dressers and furniture, observation and detection studies of nests, usually within eight or more feet of sleeping spaces, are required for proof of infestation (Fig. 15.5) (Doggett et al., 2012).

Fecal spots

Bed bug fecal spots are reddish brown in color and can be found on mattress covers or in seams, on headboards, or inside a door or drawer of a bedroom dresser. Fecal streaks are reliable external indicators of bed bug infestations along with a sweet, fruity smell from

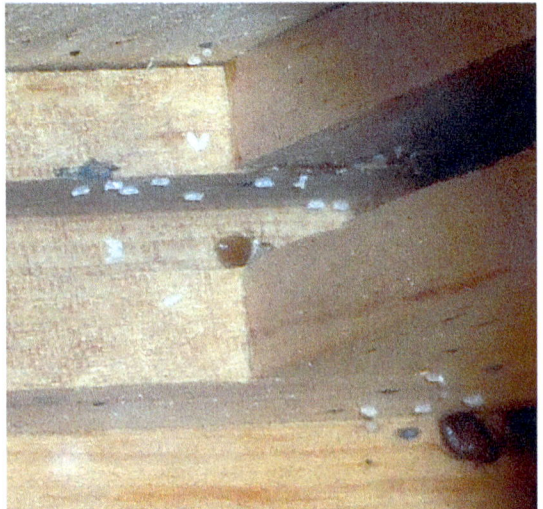

Figure 15.5 Bed bug eggs and two adults hiding inside a drawer of a bedroom dresser. Since bed bugs spend only 5—10 min blood feeding on humans before returning to their nests in carpets, mattresses, headboards, and bedroom furniture, observation with detection of nests, usually within 8 or more feet of sleeping spaces, is required for proof of infestation. *(Wikipedia. Public domain. No copyright permission required. Available at https://en.wikipedia.org/wiki/Bed_bug)*

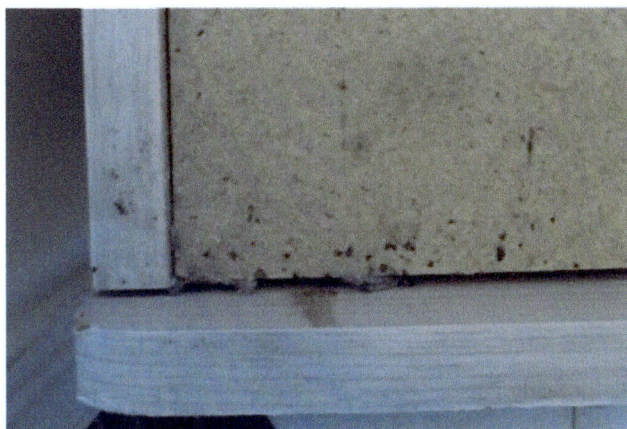

Figure 15.6 Bed bug reddish-brown fecal spots or streaks found inside a drawer of a bedroom dresser are another reliable indicator of bed bug infestation along with a sweet, fruity smell in the atmosphere from bedbug pheromones or dead bed bugs. *(Wikipedia. Public domain. No copyright permission required. Available at https://en.wikipedia.org/wiki/Bed_bug)*

bed bug pheromones in the infested rooms (Fig. 15.6). Since nymphs must molt and shed their exoskeletons in order to grow to the next stage toward adulthood, finding abandoned flat, oval exoskeletons are another positive indicator of bedbug infestation.

Dogs have been trained to detect bed bug infestations by sensing the odors released by living bed bugs and by dead bed bugs (Doggett et al., 2012). Bed bug detectors that release lactic acid or carbon dioxide can attract and trap bed bugs in small containers, but do not trap enough bed bugs for eradication.

Management

Avoiding repeated bites is the best management strategy for bed bugs and requires eradicating the bed bugs completely from the household or other occupied space.

Control and prevention

Chemical control

Insecticides and bug bomb-foggers are ineffective for bedbug infestations as bed bugs are now resistant to most pesticides (Parola and Izri, 2020). The only pesticide that remains highly effective for bed bugs is the carbamate, propoxur, which is not approved for indoor use due to its toxicity (See Chapter 16.) (Parola and Izri, 2020; Doggett et al., 2012). Although effective for control of cockroaches, boric acid tablets are also ineffective against bed bugs. Starving bed bugs in closed bags or containers filled with contaminated bedding and other soft items is also ineffective as bedbugs can survive up to 300 days without blood meals (Doggett et al., 2012).

Mechanical control

Bed bugs are killed by exposures to temperatures of 45°C (113°F) and above for 1 h, or exposures to temperatures of −17°C (1°F) and below for 2 h (Parola and Izri, 2020). Although consumer-grade freezers cannot reach temperatures low enough to kill bed bugs, domestic clothes driers can reach temperatures high enough to kill bed bugs during hot water washing for one or more hours (Parola and Izri, 2020). Whole household high temperature treatments are effective, but have caused fires, and are not recommended.

Preventive strategies

Preventive strategies for bed bugs are all directed at keeping bed bugs out of households and other occupied spaces and include the following measures (Parola and Izri, 2020)

1. Check office chairs, airplane, train, and public transit seats, cushions, and headrests, hotel mattresses, headboards, and bedroom furniture for bed bugs.
2. Do not sit down on public transportation.
3. Monitor and vacuum all home beds once a month.
4. Put suitcases and backpacks on raised stands and not on beds when traveling.
5. Hang up your clothes or leave them in your suitcase when traveling and never leave them on the floor.
6. Check the bottom of your shoes for crushed bed bugs or empty exoskeletons whenever leaving new lodgings or checking luggage.
7. Decontaminate your clothes and luggage upon returning home.

Conclusions

The differential diagnosis of bed bug bites requires detection and confirmation of bed bug infestation. Bed bugs may harbor pathogens obtained in blood meals, but cannot transmit them. Bed bug bites will resolve with or without medications within days as long as recurrent bites are prevented. Beg bugs are resistant to most pesticides. Mechanical control methods are more effective than chemical control methods for bed bug eradication.

References

Doggett, S.L., Dwyer, D.E., Peñas, P.F., Russell, R.C., 2012. Bed bugs: clinical relevance and control options. Clinical Microbiology Reviews 25 (1), 164–192. https://doi.org/10.1128/CMR.05015-11.

Donabedian, H., 2007. Delusions of parasitosis. Clinical Infectious Diseases 45 (11), e131–e134. https://doi.org/10.1086/523004.

Goddard, J., DeShazo, R., 2009. Bed bugs (cimex lectularius) and clinical consequences of their bites. JAMA 301 (13), 1358–1366. https://doi.org/10.1001/jama.2009.405.

Parola, P., Izri, A., 2020. Bedbugs. New England Journal of Medicine 382 (23), 2230–2237. https://doi.org/10.1056/NEJMcp1905840.

CHAPTER 16

Insect repellents, insecticides, and vector control

Introduction

Since insect repellents offer important topical barriers of personal protection from mite-borne infectious diseases and all other arthropod-borne infestations and infectious diseases, this chapter will define the differences between insect repellents and insecticides; compare the efficacies and toxicities of chemical versus plant-derived insect repellents and insecticides; recommend the best combinations of insect repellents and insecticides for personal protection; and describe the most effective nonchemical methods of personal protection from insect bites.

Definitions

An insect repellent is a chemical or organic agent that makes the atmosphere within 4 centimeters of human skin so noxious to insects as to discourage contact, biting, and blood or tissue juice feeding (Debboun and Strickman, 2013). On the other hand, an insecticide is a chemical or organic agent, originally plant-derived, that kills insects on contact, most commonly with a paralyzing neurotoxin (Debboun and Strickman, 2013). Some insect repellents are also insecticides, such as permethrin and all other synthetic pyrethroids (Debboun and Strickman, 2013).

In the United States (US), the Food and Drug Administration (FDA) tests and approves topical insect repellents, such as N, N-diethyl-3-methylbenzamide (formerly N, N-diethyl-m-toluamide or DEET) for human use and safety during pregnancy. The Environmental Protection Agency (EPA) approves insecticides for use by applicators under the Federal Insecticide, Fungicide, and Rodenticide Act. Many insecticides are EPA-approved only for outdoor application, such as the carbamates and organophosphates, but not for indoor use. The only insecticides approved for indoor use in the United States are the pyrethroids, which are two classes of synthetic extracts originally derived from crushed, dried *Chrysanthemum* flowers.

Why use insect repellents?

The three major reasons to use insect repellents are: (1) the new threats to human health posed by emerging and imported arthropod-borne infectious diseases, such as West Nile

Ectoparasitic Diseases
ISBN 978-0-443-26724-6
https://doi.org/10.1016/B978-0-443-26724-6.00016-3

and Zika viruses; (2) the dominance of new competent insect vectors of infectious diseases, such as *Aedes albopictus*; and (3) the inability to primarily prevent the transmission of most arthropod-borne infectious diseases by vaccinations with the exceptions of yellow fever vaccine in South America and Africa; the Japanese encephalitis vaccine in Southeast Asia, and several regional tick-borne encephalitis virus vaccines in the Scandinavian countries, Eastern Europe, and Asia. Dengue and malaria vaccines are now in development with the dengue vaccine soon to be released and malaria vaccines in field testing.

The history of insect repellents

The first effective insect repellents included smoke and flames from burning tar and cooking fires; and a variety of grasses and flowers hung in homes or porches, or rubbed on the skin, including chrysanthemum, geranium, and lantana (Brown and Hebert, 1997). Many plant oils were extracted from these and other plants, such as citronella, clove, geranium, mint, nutmeg, pennyroyal, and soybean oils, and molded into wax candles or applied topically as soaps or ointments. These plant oils would repel insects for short periods, but their high volatility limited their duration of effectiveness when burned in candles or applied topically (Brown and Hebert, 1997).

Prior to World War II, there were only four insect repellents: (1) oil of citronella discovered in 1901; (2) the dialkyl phthalates (dibutyl and dimethyl phthalate) discovered in 1929; (3) indalone, a contact repellent, effective against ticks, introduced in 1937; and (4) Rutgers 612 introduced in 1939 (Brown and Hebert, 1997). Rutgers 612, or just 612, became very popular until DEET, developed by the US Armed Forces, was first marketed in 1956 (Brown and Hebert, 1997).

Selecting the best insect repellents

Insect repellents must be effective, safe, and pleasant to apply in children and adults, and during pregnancy, without damaging skin or clothing. Table 16.1 presents the most desired characteristics of an ideal insect repellent. Table 16.2 describes the range of insect repellents and insecticides available worldwide as stratified by their active ingredients, formulations, strengths (in %), efficacies against various arthropods, precautions, and most common adverse effects.

Chemical versus plant-based insect repellents: Which are the best?

Insect repellents may be divided into two basic chemical classes: (1) the synthetic chemicals, such as DEET, picaridin, and IR3535 (*Avon Skin So Soft*); and (2) the plant-derived oils and synthetics extracted from plants, such as oil of lemon eucalyptus, oil of citronella, and pyrethrin (Table 16.1).

Table 16.1 The characteristics of an ideal insect repellent.

1. Effective against broad range or arthropods including fleas, flies, mosquitoes, biting midges (*no-see-ums*), mites, and ticks.
2. No damage to clothing (i.e., staining, bleaching, or thinning).
3. Can be applied with sunscreen (no such product is available).
4. No odor or has pleasing odor.
5. No oily residues are left on skin.
6. Difficult to remove by light washing, wiping, or sweating.
7. No effect on plastics (i.e., glasses, watches, and upholstery).
8. Chemically stable.
9. Reasonably priced for broad range of people.
10. No adverse effects on the skin: nontoxic, nonallergenic, and noncomedogenic.
11. Safe to use during pregnancy and breastfeeding.

In 1942, the US Department of Agriculture and the US Army began clinical trials with many chemical compounds in order to replace the dialkyl phthalates with less toxic and less oily and messy topical insect repellents effective against a broader variety of insects with a longer duration of action (Brown and Hebert, 1997; Katz et al., 2008). By 1946, N, N-diethyl-3-methylbenzamide (previously N, N-diethyl-m-toluamide or DEET) was in use by US Armed Forces and later marketed to the public in 1956 (Brown and Hebert, 1997; Katz et al., 2008).

DEET remains available worldwide today in a variety of formulations including aerosols, lotions, sprays, gels, sticks, and wipes (*towelettes*) at concentrations ranging from 5% to 100%. Most products contain concentrations of 30%—40% DEET or less, and human studies have now confirmed a plateau insect repellent effect as the concentration of DEET applied topically exceeds 50% (Rutledge et al., 1985). In addition, volunteers who have applied concentrations of 50%—75% DEET have developed erythema with vesiculobullous skin necrosis and residual scarring (McKinlay et al., 1998). DEET concentrations in the range of 10%—35% will provide adequate insect bite protection with concentrations below 30% recommended for children 2 years of age and older (Insect Bites. The Medical Letter, 2015). The American Academy of Pediatrics does not recommend the topical application of DEET in children less than 2 years of age (Insect bites, 2015).

Field testing of topical DEET has demonstrated a longer duration of protection against the Culicine species of mosquitoes that can transmit arboviruses and filarial parasites than against the Anopheline species of mosquitoes that can transmit malaria (Frances et al., 2004). Higher levels of DEET up to 33% may be required to provide better protection against ticks for up to 12 hours (Carroll et al., 2008).

DEET will not damage cotton, wool, or nylon clothing; but can damage rayon, spandex, and leather, and dissolve plastic and vinyl upholstery (Brown and Hebert,

Table 16.2 Available insect repellents: formulations, efficacy, safety, and toxicity.

Insect repellents (Chemical names)	Formulations (Strength %)	Efficacy against anopheline (malaria) mosquitoes	Efficacy against culicine (arbovirus) mosquitoes	Efficacy against ticks	Efficacy against flies and biting midges (no-see-ums)	Safety in children and pregnancy	Toxicity and other adverse effects
Chemical-based repellents							
DEET (N, N-diethyl-3-methyl-benzamide. Formerly N, N-diethyl-*m*-toluamide)	Aerosols Lotions Pump sprays Wipes (5%–100%)	+ +	+ + +	+	+ +	FDA: do not use in children under age 2 years. Potential neuro-toxicity in children if ingested or if over-applied. American Academy Pediatrics recommends maximum strength of 30%. DEET crosses the placenta. FDA pregnancy category N.	Potential neuro-toxicity if applied under sunscreen. May damage plastic and some synthetic fabric clothing. Safe for cotton, wool, and nylon.
Picaridin (US) and Icaridin (EU) (2-(2-hydroxyethyl)-1-piperidine-carboxylic acid 1-methylpropyl-ester)	Lotions Pump sprays Wipes (7%–20%)	+ +	+ + +	+ +	+ + + High levels of protection up to 12 h against *Amblyomma americanum*	No studies in children, but manufacturers do not recomb-mend use in children younger than 2 years of age. No develop-mental toxicity in animals. FDA pregnancy category N.	Possible skin irritation. No damage to plastics or clothing.

IR3535 (3-[N-butyl-N-acetyl]-amino-propionic acid ethyl ester)	Aerosols Lotions Pump sprays Wipes (7.5%–19.7%)	++	+++ EPA: up to 2 h protection time for mosquitoes.	++ EPA: up to 3 h protection time for ticks.	+++	FDA pregnancy category B.	Causes eye irritation. Potential toxicity if ingested or inhaled. May damage plastic and clothing.

Plant-Based repellents

Oil of lemon eucalyptus (p-menthane-3, 8-diol)	Pump sprays (10%–40%)	+++	+++ EPA: up to 2 h protection time for mosquitoes.	+++ EPA: up to 3 h protection time for ticks.	+++	May cause seizures or death if ingested. FDA: do not use under age 3 years. FDA pregnancy category N.	Potential skin irritation in atopic individuals.
Citronella (3, 7-dimethyloct-6-en–1-al) natural plant oil obtained from *Cymbopogon* spp. grasses.	Bath oils Candles Lotions (0.5%–20%)	+	+	0	0	Potential neuro-toxicity if ingested or inhaled. FDA pregnancy category N.	May damage clothing. Potential eye irritation and skin irritation and allergies.

Continued

Table 16.2 Available insect repellents: formulations, efficacy, safety, and toxicity.—cont'd

Insect repellents (Chemical names)	Formulations (Strength %)	Efficacy against anopheline (malaria) mosquitoes	Efficacy against culicine (arbovirus) mosquitoes	Efficacy against ticks	Efficacy against flies and biting midges (no-see-ums)	Safety in children and pregnancy	Toxicity and other adverse effects
Permethrin (3-phenoxybenzyl (1RS)-cis, trans-3-(2, 2-dichlorovinyl)-2, 2-dimethyl-cyclo-propane-carboxylate) Pyrethroid derived from dried, crushed flowers of *Chrysanthemum* spp.	Sprays for clothes, insect nets, sleeping bags, boots (0.5%)	+++	+++	+++	+++	Potential neuro-toxicity if ingested or inhaled. FDA: do not use under age 2 years. FDA pregnancy category B.	Not useful on skin. Possible skin irritation. Pyrethroid resistance is now developing in mosquitoes. No damage to plastics or clothing.

Protective efficacy scale: 0: No protection provided. +: minimal level of protection. ++: moderate level of protection. +++: maximal level of protection.
FDA pregnancy categories: A: Human studies have demonstrated no evidence of risk to the fetus. B: Animal studies have demonstrated no evidence of risk to the fetus. C: Animal studies have demonstrated adverse effects on the fetus. D: Investigational or marketing experiences or human studies have demonstrated adverse effects on the fetus, but potential benefits may warrant use of the drug in pregnancy despite the risks. X: Studies in animals or humans have demonstrated fetal abnormalities. N: FDA has not classified the drug.

1997). Although DEET does cross the placenta, developmental toxicity has not been reported in animals or humans in over 50 years of testing and use by over 30% of the US population (McGready et al., 2001). With proper application, the safety record of DEET has proven to be excellent over decades with most cases of toxicity confined to children following overapplications and accidental or suicidal ingestions (Briassoulis et al., 2001; Snyder et al., 1986; Heick et al., 1988; Lietman et al., 1980; Leo et al., 2001; Pronczuk de Garbino et al., 1983; Zadikoff, 1979; Osimitz and Grothaus, 1995; Osimitz and Murphy, 1997; Lipscomb et al., 1992; Gryboski et al., 1961; Roland et al., 1985; Seizures temporarily associated with the use of DEET insect repellent—New York and Connecticut, 1989; Edwards and Johnson, 1987; Hampers et al., 1999; Veltri et al., 1994; Tenenbein, 1987; Petrucci and Sardini, 2000).

Between 1956 and 2008, there were 43 confirmed case reports of DEET toxicity; 25 with central nervous system (CNS) involvement, 1 with cardiovascular effects, and 17 with allergic or cutaneous manifestations (Briassoulis et al., 2001; Snyder et al., 1986; Heick et al., 1988; Lietman et al., 1980; Leo et al., 2001; Pronczuk de Garbino et al., 1983; Zadikoff, 1979; Osimitz and Grothaus, 1995; Osimitz and Murphy, 1997; Lipscomb et al., 1992; Gryboski et al., 1961; Roland et al., 1985; Seizures temporarily associated with the use of DEET insect repellent—New York and Connecticut, 1989; Edwards and Johnson, 1987; Hampers et al., 1999; Veltri et al., 1994; Tenenbein, 1987; Petrucci and Sardini, 2000). The CNS manifestations of DEET toxicity included lethargy, headache, confusion, disorientation, ataxia, tremors, seizures, and acute encephalopathy with psychosis (Briassoulis et al., 2001; Snyder et al., 1986; Heick et al., 1988; Lietman et al., 1980; Leo et al., 2001; Pronczuk de Garbino et al., 1983; Zadikoff, 1979; Osimitz and Grothaus, 1995; Osimitz and Murphy, 1997; Lipscomb et al., 1992; Gryboski et al., 1961; Roland et al., 1985; Seizures temporarily associated with the use of DEET insect repellent—New York and Connecticut, 1989; Edwards and Johnson, 1987; Hampers et al., 1999; Veltri et al., 1994; Tenenbein, 1987; Petrucci and Sardini, 2000). Cutaneous manifestations were mostly urticarial reactions and hemorrhagic vesiculobullous erosions following topical applications of 50% and stronger preparations (McKinlay et al., 1998).

A 61-year-old woman presented with orthostatic hypotension and bradycardia after topical overapplication of DEET and stabilized within hours of supportive treatment (Clem et al., 1993). Of the six reported deaths attributed to DEET poisoning, three followed intentional ingestion; one occurred in a child with ornithine transcarbamylase deficiency; and two cases occurred in children with convulsive CNS reactions after repeated overapplications (Heick et al., 1988; Lietman et al., 1980; Leo et al., 2001; Pronczuk de Garbino et al., 1983; Zadikoff, 1979; Tenenbein, 1987; Petrucci and Sardini, 2000).

The newest insect repellent, picaridin or icaridin (KBR 3023, 2-(2-hydroxyethyl)-1-piperidinecarboxylic acid-1-methylpropyl ester), was developed in Europe in the 1990s;

released in the US more than 10 years ago; and offered several immediate advantages over DEET.

Picaridin's advantages over DEET included no chemical odor, nonsticky or greasy on application, and no damage to clothing or plastics (Katz et al., 2008). Like DEET, the exact mechanism of action of picaridin is unknown, but its vapor barrier is so noxious to insects' taste and olfactory senses that it discourages insect contact and biting (Katz et al., 2008). Picaridin is effective against mosquitoes, flies, chiggers (larval trombiculid mites), and ticks; and is available as lotions, sprays, and wipes in strengths of 7%—20% (Katz et al., 2008). Like DEET, picaridin appears to offer greater protection against Culicine than Anopheline mosquitoes, and may offer a longer duration of action and greater protection than DEET against ticks in 20% preparations (Frances et al., 2004).

In human field trials, Carroll and coinvestigators demonstrated that 10% and 20% concentrations of picaridin provided very high levels of protection for up to 12 hours against lone star ticks (*Amblyomma americanum*), the newly recognized insect vectors of heartland virus disease and tickborne red meat allergy (Carroll et al., 2008). Human field and animal investigations in Australia and Europe have demonstrated no dermal, solid organ, or reproductive toxicity from picaridin (Brown and Hebert, 1997; Katz et al., 2008). The manufacturers do not recommend using picaridin in children under 2 years of age (Brown and Hebert, 1997; Katz et al., 2008).

IR3535 or ethyl butylacetylaminoproprionate (3-N-butyl-N-acetyl aminopropionic acid) was initially marketed in the US as a skin emollient and moisturizer (*Avon Skin So Soft*) and was quickly recognized and adopted for use by hunters because of its greater efficacy against bothersome biting midges, or *no-see-ums*, than DEET. In addition, IR3535 demonstrated greater efficacy against onchocerciasis-transmitting blackflies and leishmaniasis-transmitting sandflies in endemic areas than DEET; and was shown to provide a longer duration of protection (mean 10.4 hours) against leishmaniasis-transmitting phlebotomine sand-fly bites than DEET (mean 8.8 hours) (Naucke et al., 2006). Like DEET and picaridin, IR3535 is more effective at repelling Culicine mosquitoes than Anopheline mosquitoes (Goodyer et al., 2010). Although IR3535 has been used in Europe for over 20 years and animal studies have not demonstrated developmental toxicity, there are no specific recommendations for its use or avoidance in children or during pregnancy (FDA Pregnancy Category B).

Oil of lemon eucalyptus or p-menthane-3, 8-diol (PMD) is an extract of the leaves of lemon eucalyptus, *Corymbia citriodora*, or a synthetic version of its major repellent component, PMD (Fig. 16.1) (Carroll and Loye, 2006).

PMD is available in pump sprays in concentrations of 10%—40%. PMD has a mosquito repellent efficacy and duration equal to that of DEET, and, like picaridin, may offer better protection against ticks than DEET (Carroll and Loye, 2006). PMD reduced successful attachment and blood-feeding by 77% against the tick vectors of Lyme disease (*Ixodes scapularis*, *Ixodes pacificus*) and Rocky Mountain spotted fever (*Dermacentor*

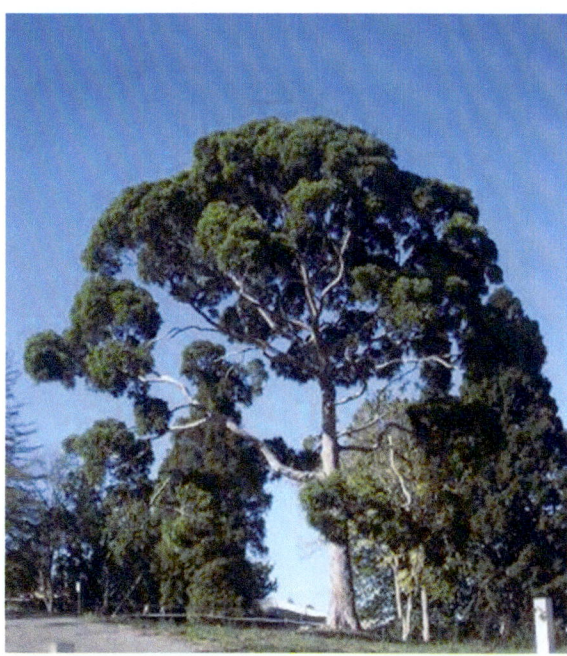

Figure 16.1 The lemon eucalyptus tree, *Corymbia citriodora,* is the source of the insect repellent chemical, p-menthane-3, 8-diol (PMD). PMD has a mosquito repellent efficacy and duration equal to that of DEET, and, like picaridin, may offer better protection against ticks than DEET. *(Wikepedia. Public domain.)*

andersoni), and is also effective against some species of biting midges (Trigg and Hill, 1996). The FDA has recommended that PMD not be used in children under 3 years of age.

Citronella (3, 7-dimethyloct-6-en-1-aL) is a natural plant oil obtained from several species of *Cymbopogon* lemongrasses (Fig. 16.2).

Citronella is available as a lotion, oil, or solid wax impregnated into candles and flame pots in strengths ranging from 0.5% to 20%. Due to its high volatility, citronella has a short duration of action; but can deter nuisance biting by mosquitoes for up to 2 hours (Tawatsin et al., 2001). It is ineffective against flies, fleas, biting midges, mites, and ticks (Tawatsin et al., 2001).

Permethrin, first marketed in 1973, is a synthetic pyrethroid insect repellent and contact insecticide that was originally derived from the crushed dried flowers of *Chrysanthemum cinerarifolium* (Fig. 16.3).

Permethrin is not absorbed topically and requires direct insect contact to be effective (Katz et al., 2008). Its mechanism of action is via initial excitation of the insect's nervous system by sodium channel blockade followed by acetylcholinesterase inhibition and fatal paralysis (Katz et al., 2008; Goodyer et al., 2010). Clothing and other products treated with pyrethroids should be retreated after five to up to 70 washings as indicated on the product label to provide continued insect bite protection (Chapter 2. The Pre-Travel Consultation. Protection against mosquitoes, ticks, and

Figure 16.2 *Cymbopogon citratus,* or lemongrass, is the source of citronella (3, 7-dimethyloct-6-en-1-al), a natural plant oil with insect repellent properties. *(Wikepedia. Public domain.)*

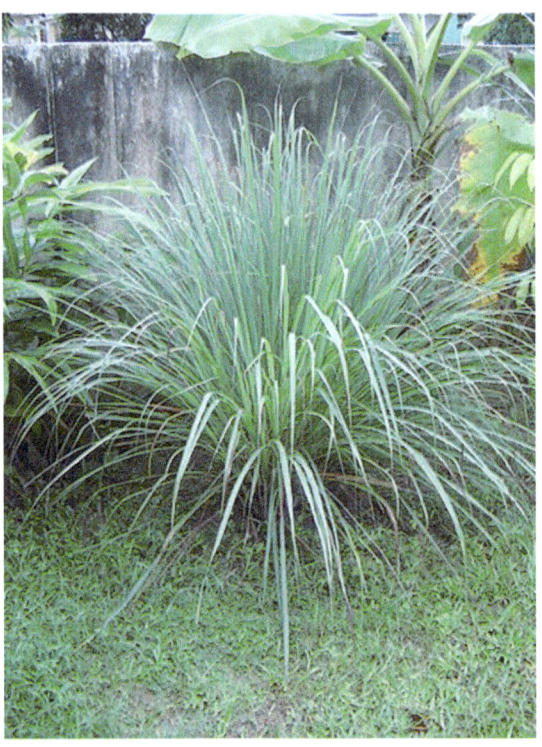

Figure 16.3 Crushed dried flowers of *Chrysanthemum cinerarifolium,* the chrysanthemum, contain pyrethrins with natural insect repellent properties. When applied to clothing, bed nets, tents, and sleeping bags, permethrin and other newer, synthetic pyrethroids (allethrin, alpha-cypermethrin, cyfluthrin, deltamethrin, etofenprox, lambda-cyhalothrin, and metofluthrin) all provide very high-level protection against mosquitoes, flies, biting midges, chiggers, fleas, sandflies, mites, and ticks, especially when combined with topically applied insect repellents (Goodyer et al., 2010). *(Wikepedia. Public domain.)*

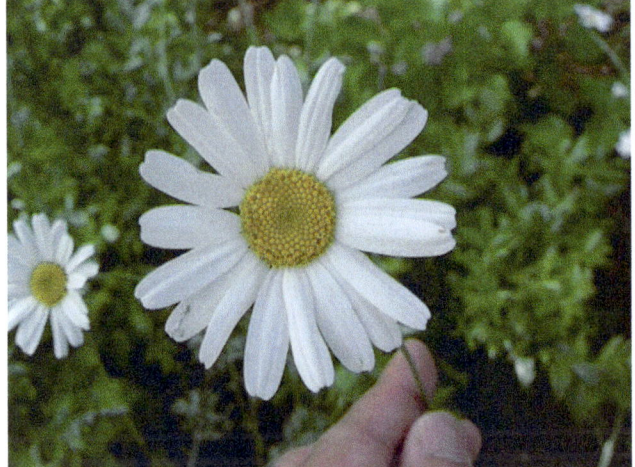

other insects and arthropods, 2015). Long-duration, pyrethroid-treated mosquito bed nets are now available that maintain effective insecticide levels for 3 years (Insect bites, 2015).

Permethrin can kill ticks on contact and provides better tick protection than DEET and picaridin (Solberg et al., 1995). Permethrin-impregnated bed nets have provided improved protection of long duration against all Anopheline malaria mosquito vectors (Insect bites, 2015).

Human neurotoxicity with ataxia, hyperactivity, hyperthermia, seizures, and paralysis has been reported after massive ingestions of liquid preparations or inhalations of permethrin-containing sprays (Brown and Hebert, 1997; Katz et al., 2008). Animal studies conducted by the FDA have demonstrated no developmental toxicity from permethrin exposures (FDA Pregnancy Category B) (Pesticides and Toxic Substances (7508P). Permethrin Facts. EPA 738-F-09-001, 2009).

Although some plant-derived insect repellents are highly effective, such as PMD and permethrin, others only discourage nuisance biting, such as citronella; and others are completely ineffective. Garlic consumption has continued to be recommended as natural insect repellent; but a double-blinded, placebo-controlled trial of garlic consumption to prevent mosquito bites has confirmed garlic's ineffectiveness as a mosquito repellent (Rajan et al., 2005).

In summary, the most effective uses of insect repellents are to combine a topically applied repellent, such as DEET or picaridin, with wearing permethrin or other synthetic pyrethroid-impregnated clothing that act as contact insecticides and provide better and longer lasting protection against malaria-transmitting mosquitoes and ticks.

Compared to studies with ticks, few studies have investigated the use of insect repellents or insecticides to prevent mite bites. Since ticks and mites are related phylogenetically (Order Acarina, Class Arachnida), it is assumed that acaricides effective against ticks will also be effective against mites.

In special cases, where exposures to ticks, biting midges, sandflies, or blackflies are anticipated, topical insect repellents containing IR3535, picaridin, or PMD may offer better protection than topical DEET alone, especially when exposed skin is covered by permethrin-impregnated clothing.

Insect repellent use in children and during pregnancy

Table 16.2 compares available insect repellents and their safe use in children and during pregnancy. The use of DEET is relatively contraindicated in all persons diagnosed with ornithine transcarbamylase deficiency due to the potential risks of hyperammonemia with hepatic encephalopathy (Lietman et al., 1980). As noted, of the six reported deaths attributed to DEET poisoning, one occurred in a child with ornithine transcarbamylase deficiency; and two cases occurred in children with convulsive CNS reactions after repeated overapplication (Heick et al., 1988; Lietman et al., 1980; Leo et al., 2001; Pronczuk de Garbino et al., 1983; Zadikoff, 1979; Tenenbein, 1987; Petrucci and Sardini, 2000).

Insect repellents and sunscreens

Insect repellents should not be applied under sunscreens because sunscreens are applied more frequently after sweating, swimming, bathing, and drying. In addition, the FDA has recommended against using products that combine insect repellents with sunscreens because sunscreens have to be reapplied more frequently than insect repellents (Hexsel et al., 2008). In 2004, Ross and coinvestigators demonstrated increased absorption of DEET applied under sunscreen in a mouse model which resulted in a CDC recommendation to always apply sunscreen prior to DEET application (Goodyer et al., 2010; Ross et al., 2004).

Area and barrier chemical insect repellents

In addition to topically applied insect repellents and pyrethroid-impregnated clothing, there are a number of area and barrier methods used to repel insects including permethrin-impregnated curtains, screens, and bed nets; insecticide vaporizers; mosquito or bug coils; knockdown insecticide aerosol sprays; and a variety of plant-oil burning candles. Some of these measures are effective; others are not.

Permethrin and other synthetic pyrethroid-treated fabrics have proven highly effective as adjuncts to topical repellents and provide both contact insecticidal and repellent activity. Electric insecticide vaporizers can be set to release pyrethroid insecticides and will inhibit nuisance biting by mosquitoes, but there is no evidence that they will prevent the transmission of arthropod-borne infectious diseases (Goodyer et al., 2010). Knockdown insecticide aerosol sprays are designed to kill flying insects indoors, but there is also no evidence to support their use over arthropod avoidance and topical insect repellents (Goodyer et al., 2010).

Mosquito coils are made from compacted pastes or powders containing pyrethroids and other volatile chemicals, including formaldehyde (Chen et al., 2008; Liu et al., 2003). When lit, the coils will smolder and produce smoke for hours, discouraging nuisance biting by mosquitoes; but contaminating the atmosphere with particulates and volatile chemicals from combustion, especially in enclosed spaces (Chen et al., 2008; Liu et al., 2003). Repeated exposures to mosquito coil smoke may pose significant risk factors for lung disease, including lung cancer (Chen et al., 2008; Liu et al., 2003). Burning a variety of plant oil—based candles will also discourage nuisance biting by mosquitoes and flies for a couple of hours, but, like aerosol sprays and insecticide vaporizers, there is no evidence to support their use over arthropod avoidance and topical insect repellents (Goodyer et al., 2010).

Nonchemical measures for the management, control, and prevention of arthropod-borne infectious diseases

In order to minimize insect bites outdoors, individuals should wear light-colored clothing, long-sleeved shirts, long pants, socks, and covered shoes. They should sleep indoors in screened or air-conditioned areas. The Anopheline mosquitoes that transmit malaria typically bite at dawn and dusk, which are prime times to avoid their exposures. However, the Culicine mosquitoes that transmit dengue, Chikungunya, West Nile virus, yellow fever, and Zika virus are container breeders residing nearby that bite aggressively throughout the day, providing good reasons to apply insect repellents throughout the day when outdoors.

Most people do not recall painless tick and mite bites, especially bites by diminutive larvae and nymphs, and attachment sites may be unseen or hidden by hair or underclothing. Nevertheless, tick localization and removal for expert identification as soon as possible, preferably within 24 hours, remain recommended initial management strategies.

Ticks should be removed with forceps or fine-tipped tweezers gripped close to the point of skin attachment with gentle, steady traction applied to avoid decapitating ticks and leaving imbedded mouthparts with pathogen-filled salivary glands. Ticks should always be removed with forceps (or tweezers) and not fingers as squishing ticks can transmit several tick-borne microbial diseases across dermal barriers or create infectious aerosols. Ticks should be removed in contiguity with their feeding mouthparts, rather than burning ticks with spent matches, or painting embedded ticks with adhesives, solvents, nail polishes, or nail polish removers.

Personal protective measures to prevent tick-borne infectious diseases include wearing long pants tucked into socks, long-sleeved shirts, and light-colored clothing to aide in keeping ticks off of the skin and in making them easier to spot on clothing. Other recommended measures include applying pyrethroid-containing insect repellents to clothing and picaridin, IR3535, or PMD to exposed skin, and performing regular whole-body and scalp tick-checks.

Conclusions

With few exceptions, there are no vaccines to prevent mosquito and tick-borne infectious diseases; and disease transmission to humans can only be prevented by arthropod avoidance, insect repellents, and insecticides. The most effective use of insect repellents is to combine topically applied repellents, such as DEET or picaridin, with synthetic pyrethroid-impregnated clothing that act as contact insecticides and provide better and longer duration protection against mosquitoes, mites, and ticks. In special cases, where regional exposures to ticks, biting midges, sandflies, or blackflies are anticipated, topical insect repellents containing IR3535, picaridin, or PMD offer better protection than DEET alone.

References

Briassoulis, G., Narlioglou, M., Hatzis, T., 2001. Toxic encephalopathy associated with use of DEET insect repellents: a case analysis of its toxicity in children. Human & Experimental Toxicology 20 (1), 8–14. https://doi.org/10.1191/096032701676731093.

Brown, M., Hebert, A.A., 1997. Insect repellents: an overview. Journal of the American Academy of Dermatology 36 (2), 243–249. https://doi.org/10.1016/S0190-9622(97)70289-5.

Carroll, S.P., Loye, J., 2006. PMD, a registered botanical mosquito repellent with deet-like efficacy. Journal of the American Mosquito Control Association 22 (3), 507–514. https://doi.org/10.2987/8756-971X(2006)22[507:PARBMR]2.0.CO;2.

Carroll, J.F., Benante, J.P., Klun, J.A., White, C.E., Debboun, M., Pound, J.M., Dheranetra, W., 2008. Twelve-hour duration testing of cream formulations of three repellents against *Amblyomma americanum*. Medical and Veterinary Entomology 22 (2), 144–151. https://doi.org/10.1111/j.1365-2915.2008.00721.x.

Chen, S.C., Wong, R.H., Shiu, L.J., Chiou, M.C., Lee, H., 2008. Exposure to mosquito coil smoke may be a risk factor for lung cancer in Taiwan. Journal of Epidemiology 18 (1), 19–25. https://doi.org/10.2188/jea.18.19.

Clem, J.R., Havemann, D.F., Raebel, M.A., 1993. Insect repellent (N,N-Diethyl-m-Toluamide) cardiovascular toxicity in an adult. The Annals of Pharmacotherapy 27 (3), 289–293. https://doi.org/10.1177/106002809302700305.

Debboun, M., Strickman, D., 2013. Insect repellents and associated personal protection for a reduction in human disease. Medical and Veterinary Entomology 27 (1), 1–9. https://doi.org/10.1111/j.1365-2915.2012.01020.x.

Edwards, D.L., Johnson, C.E., 1987. Insect-repellent-induced toxic encephalopathy in a child. Clinical Pharmacy 6 (6), 496–498.

Frances, S.P., Waterson, D.G.E., Beebe, N.W., Cooper, R.D., 2004. Field evaluation of repellent formulations containing deet and picaridin against mosquitoes in Northern Territory, Australia. Journal of Medical Entomology 41 (3), 414–417. https://doi.org/10.1603/0022-2585-41.3.414.

Goodyer, L.I., Croft, A.M., Frances, S.P., Hill, N., Moore, S.J., Onyango, S.P., Debboun, M., 2010. Expert review of the evidence base for arthropod bite avoidance. Journal of Travel Medicine 17 (3), 182–192. https://doi.org/10.1111/j.1708-8305.2010.00402.x.

Gryboski, J., Weinstein, D., Ordway, N.K., 1961. Toxic encephalopathy apparently related to the use of an insect repellent. New England Journal of Medicine 264 (6), 289–291. https://doi.org/10.1056/NEJM196102092640608.

Hampers, L.C., Oker, E., Leikin, J.B., 1999. Topical use of DEET insect repellent as a cause of severe encephalopathy in a healthy adult male. Academic Emergency Medicine 6 (12), 1295–1297. https://doi.org/10.1111/j.1553-2712.1999.tb00147.x.

Heick, H.M.C., Peterson, R.G., Dalpe-Scott, M., Qureshi, I.A., 1988. Insect repellent, N,N-diethyl-m-toluamide, effect on ammonia metabolism. Pediatrics 82 (3), 373–376.

Hexsel, C.L., Bangert, S.D., Hebert, A.A., Lim, H.W., 2008. Current sunscreen issues: 2007 Food and Drug Administration sunscreen labelling recommendations and combination sunscreen/insect repellent products. Journal of the American Academy of Dermatology 59 (2), 316–323. https://doi.org/10.1016/j.jaad.2008.03.038.

Insect bites. Medical Letter 57, 2015, 53–58.

Katz, T.M., Miller, J.H., Hebert, A.A., 2008. Insect repellents: Historical perspectives and new developments. Journal of the American Academy of Dermatology 58 (5), 865–871. https://doi.org/10.1016/j.jaad.2007.10.005.

Leo, R.J., Del Regno, P.A., Gregory, C., Clark, K.L., 2001. Insect repellant toxicity associated with psychosis. Psychosomatics 42 (1), 78–80. https://doi.org/10.1176/appi.psy.42.1.78.

Lietman, P.S., Heick, H.M.C., Shipman, R.T., Norman, M.G., James, W., 1980. Reye-like syndrome associated with use of insect repellent in a presumed heterozygote for ornithine carbamoyl transferase deficiency. The Journal of Pediatrics 97 (3), 471–473. https://doi.org/10.1016/s0022-3476(80)80209-5.

Lipscomb, J.W., Kramer, J.E., Leikin, J.B., 1992. Seizure following brief exposure to the insect repellent N,N-Diethyl-m-toluamide. Annals of Emergency Medicine 21 (3), 315–317. https://doi.org/10.1016/S0196-0644(05)80896-0.

Liu, W., Zhang, J., Hashim, J.H., Jalaludin, J., Hashim, Z., Goldstein, B.D., 2003. Mosquito coil emissions and health implications. Environmental Health Perspectives 111 (12), 1454–1460. https://doi.org/10.1289/ehp.6286.

McGready, R., Hamilton, K.A., Simpson, J.A., Cho, T., Luxemburger, C., Edwards, R., Looareesuwan, S., White, N.J., Nosten, F., Lindsay, S.W., 2001. Safety of the insect repellent N, N-diethyl-m-toluamide (DEET) in pregnancy. The American Journal of Tropical Medicine and Hygiene 65 (4), 285–289. https://doi.org/10.4269/ajtmh.2001.65.285.

McKinlay, J.R., Ross, E.V., Barrett, T.L., 1998. Vesicobullous reaction to diethyltoluamide revisited. Cutis 62, 44.

Naucke, T.J., Lorentz, S., Grünewald, H.W., 2006. Laboratory testing of the insect repellents IR3535® and DEET against Phlebotomus mascittii and P. duboscqi (Diptera: psychodidae). International Journal of Medical Microbiology 296 (1), 230–232. https://doi.org/10.1016/j.ijmm.2006.01.003.

Osimitz, T.G., Grothaus, R.H., 1995. The present safety assessment of deet. Journal of the American Mosquito Control Association 11 (2), 274–278.

Osimitz, T.G., Murphy, J.V., 1997. Neurological effects associated with use of the insect repellent N,N-diethyl-m-toluamide (DEET). Journal of Toxicology - Clinical Toxicology 35 (5), 435–441. https://doi.org/10.3109/15563659709001224.

Petrucci, N., Sardini, S., 2000. Severe neurotoxic reaction associated with oral ingestion of low-dose diethyltoluamide-containing insect repellent in a child. Pediatric Emergency Care 16 (5), 341–342. https://doi.org/10.1097/00006565-200010000-00009.

Pronczuk de Garbino, J., Laborde, A., Fogel de Korc, E., 1983. Toxicity of an insect repellent: N-N-diethyltoluamide. Veterinary & Human Toxicology 25 (6), 422–423.

Rajan, T.V., Hein, M., Porte, P., Wikel, S., 2005. A double-blinded, placebo-controlled trial of garlic as a mosquito repellant: a preliminary study. Medical and Veterinary Entomology 19 (1), 84–89. https://doi.org/10.1111/j.0269-283X.2005.00544.x.

Roland, E.H., Jan, J.E., Rigg, J.M., 1985. Toxic encephalopathy in a child after brief exposure to insect repellents. Canadian Medical Association Journal 132 (2), 155–156.

Ross, E.A., Savage, K.A., Utley, L.J., Tebbett, I.R., 2004. Insect repellant interactions: sunscreens enhance deet (N,N-diethyl-M- toluamide) absorption. Drug Metabolism and Disposition 32 (8), 783–785. https://doi.org/10.1124/dmd.32.8.783.

Rutledge, L.C., Wirtz, R.A., Buescher, M.D., Mehr, Z.A., 1985. Mathematical models of the effectiveness and persistence of mosquito repellents. Journal of the American Mosquito Control Association 1 (1), 56–62.

Seizures temporarily associated with the use of DEET insect repellent—New York and Connecticut. Morbidity & Mortality Weekly Report 38, 1989, 678–680.

Snyder, J.W., Poe, R.O., Stubbins, J.F., Garrettson, L.K., 1986. Acute manic psychosis following the dermal application of n,n-diethyl-m-toluamide (deet) in an adult. Clinical Toxicology 24 (5), 429–439. https://doi.org/10.3109/15563658608992605.

Solberg, V.B., Klein, T.A., McPherson, K.R., Bradford, B.A., Burge, J.R., Wirtz, R.A., 1995. Field evaluation of deet and a piperidine repellent (AI3-37220) against Amblyomma americanum (Acari: Ixodidae). Journal of Medical Entomology 32 (6), 870–875. https://doi.org/10.1093/jmedent/32.6.870.

Tawatsin, A., Wratten, S.D., Scott, R.R., Thavara, U., Techadamrongsin, Y., 2001. Repellency of volatile oils from plants against three mosquito vectors. Journal of Vector Ecology 26 (1), 76–82.

Tenenbein, M., 1987. Severe toxic reactions and death following the ingestion of diethyltoluamide-containing insect repellents. JAMA, the Journal of the American Medical Association 258 (11), 1509–1511. https://doi.org/10.1001/jama.258.11.1509.

Chapter 2. The Pre-travel Consultation. Protection against Mosquitoes, Ticks, and Other Insects and Arthropods, 2015. Centers for Disease Control and Prevention.

Trigg, J.K., Hill, N., 1996. Laboratory evaluation of a eucalyptus-based repellent against four biting arthropods. Phytotherapy Research 10 (4), 313—316. https://doi.org/10.1002/(SICI)1099-1573(199606)10:4<313::AID-PTR854>3.0.CO;2-O.

US Environmental Protection Agency, 2009. Pesticides and Toxic Substances (7508P). Permethrin Facts. EPA 738-F-09-001, pp. 1—11.

Veltri, J.C., Osimitz, T.G., Bradford, D.C., Page, B.C., 1994. Retrospective analysis of calls to poison control centers resulting from exposure to the insect repellent n, n-diethyl-m-toluamide (DEET) from 1985-1989. Clinical Toxicology 32 (1), 1—16. https://doi.org/10.3109/15563659409000426.

Zadikoff, C.M., 1979. Toxic encephalopathy associated with use of insect repellant. The Journal of Pediatrics 95 (1), 140—142. https://doi.org/10.1016/S0022-3476(79)80109-2.

Further reading

Centers for Disease Control and Prevention, Lyme disease. Available at: http://www.cdc.gov/lyme/stats/index/html. (Accessed 8 August 2015).

Centers for Disease Control and Prevention, Chikungunya hits US Mainland. Available at: http://www.cdc.gov/ncezid/dvbd/. (Accessed 8 August 2015).

Hahn, M.B., Monaghan, A.J., Hayden, M.H., et al., 2015. Meteorological conditions associated with increased activity of West Nile virus disease in the United States, 2004-2012. The American Journal of Tropical Medicine and Hygiene 92, 1013—1022.

Kosoy, O.I., Lambert, A.J., Hawkinson, D.J., et al., 2015. Novel thogotovirus associated with febrile illness and death, United States, 2014. Emerging Infectious Diseases 21, 760—764.

Krause, P.J., Fish, D., Narasimhan, S., Barbour, A.G., 2015. Borrelia miyamotoi infection in nature and in humans. Clinical Microbiology and Infections 21, 631—639.

Lindsey, N.P., Lehman, J.A., Staples, J.E., Fischer, M., 2014. West Nile virus and other arboviral diseases—United States, 2013. Morbidity & Mortality Weekly Report 63, 521—526.

Lindsey, N.P., Prince, H.E., Kosoy, O., et al., 2015. Chikungunya virus infections among travelers—United States, 2010-2013. The American Journal of Tropical Medicine and Hygiene 92, 82—87.

Muehlenbachs, A., Fata, C.R., Lambert, A.J., et al., 2014. Heartland virus associated death in Tennessee. Clinical Infectious Diseases 59, 845—850.

Shapiro, M.R., Fritz, C.L., Tait, K., et al., 2010. Rickettsia 364D: a newly recognized cause of eschar-associated illness in California. Clinical Infectious Diseases 50, 541—548.

Wagemakers, A., Staarink, P.J., Sprong, H., Hovius, J.W., 2015. Borrelia miyamotoi: a widespread tick-borne relapsing fever spirochete. Trends in Parasitology 31, 260—269.

Weatherhead, J.E., Miller, V.E., Garcia, M.N., et al., 2015. Long-term neurological outcomes in West Nile virus infected-patients: an observational study. The American Journal of Tropical Medicine and Hygiene 92, 1006—1012.

CHAPTER 17

Delusional ectoparasitosis (Morgellons disease)

Introduction

A case series of delusional infestations in patients convinced of infestations with microscopic arthropods that demonstrated the most common behavioral and clinical manifestations of the condition is presented with a review of the current literature.

Case series

Report of cases

Case 1 (Adapted from Meehan et al. (2006))

A 56-year-old female with a history of depression presented with a 2-month history of intensely pruritic sensations of "*bugs that were crawling*" on her posterior neck at her hairline. These sensations were resistant to topical therapy with antihistamines and corticosteroids. Physical examination demonstrated a localized plaque of self-excoriated nodules and papules. Microscopic examination of skin scrapings was negative for scabies mites or eggs; and a potassium hydroxide mount was negative for any organisms or fungi. Intralesional triamcinolone was injected into the largest nodule; and the patient was instructed to apply a topical steroid cream twice daily to the affected area and to complete a 10-day course of oral cephalexin before returning for follow-up. At follow-up, the patient was tearful and distraught and produced a specimen of a "*bug*" from her hairline; later identified as a dried pea. The patient was started on oral atypical antipsychotic therapy with olanzapine, 5 mg/day, and demonstrated dramatic improvement and resolution of all symptoms at her 1-month follow-up appointment.

Case 2 (Author's case)

A physician and his wife experienced episodic crawling sensations on their faces, chests, and backs especially at night and developed an increasing number of pruritic, papular lesions in the same locations that became excoriated from scratching. Dermatoscopic examination of the lesions and microscopic examination of skin scrapings from the lesions revealed no evidence of scabies or mite infestations. A pest extermination company examined the premises and found no evidence of animal or arthropod infestation, and a veterinarian found no evidence of ectoparasitic infection on examination of the family's dog. Later, the episodes of pruritic crawling sensations in similar locations causing self-excoriations occurred in other family members in other areas of the residence. The

Ectoparasitic Diseases
ISBN 978-0-443-26724-6
https://doi.org/10.1016/B978-0-443-26724-6.00017-5

physician treated his family with oral ivermectin and topical permethrin. He treated the family's dog with topical permethrin. The family then spent two nights in a hotel while their house was being professionally fumigated with a pyrethroid pesticide. On return to the household, the pruritic crawling sensations had improved but persisted. There was no further follow-up.

Case 3 (Author's case)

A 45-year-old nurse, who lived with two cats in an apartment whose carpets had been treated for carpet beetles, developed pruritic bite-like lesions with scratch marks on the anterior abdominal wall and breasts. Microscopic examination of skin scrapings and potassium hydroxide mounts demonstrated no evidence of scabies mites or eggs, or other arthropods, or fungi. Repeated examination of the two cats by a veterinarian demonstrated no evidence of ectoparasitic infections. After moving to another apartment in an old home with a basement, the patient reported fewer episodes of itching with topical antihistamine therapy until mice were discovered and trapped in the basement; and moths were observed in her bedroom. Following control of the mice and moths by an exterminator, the itching and scratch marks improved again. Finally, the patient reported excessively vacuuming all of the carpets in her apartment and was later lost to follow-up.

Case 4 (Adapted from Donabedian (2007))

A 51-year-old dog breeder whose dogs had been treated for ectoparasites several months earlier reported to an infectious disease specialist that she had "*worms crawling under her skin*" that occasionally exited her skin, jumped into her nose and eyes, and then traveled to her brain causing severe headaches. The physical examination and all laboratory tests were negative including a serologic test for leptospirosis. Later, the patient produced a sealed plastic bag containing round "*worms*" rolled in tissue paper. Microscopic examination demonstrated the "worms" to be inanimate, fiber-like matter. When a recommendation was made for psychiatric consultation and possible treatment with antipsychotic medications, the patient accused her physician of being totally uncaring of her suffering and completely ignorant of her disabling condition. The patient dismissed her physician and was lost to further follow-up.

Discussion

The cases reported have all demonstrated several common, pathognomonic, behavioral features, and clinical manifestations of delusional infestations including: (1) onset in well-educated, middle-aged females who are pet owners; (2) sharing symptoms with a close relative or spouse; (3) pesticide overtreatment of themselves, their households, and their pets with insecticides; (4) excessive cleaning or vacuuming of their entire households; and (5) display of the purported ectoparasite in a box or other container.

Some cases were characterized by a unique variation of delusional infestation, now known as Morgellons disease or syndrome, by producing "*round worms*" or other parasites in cardboard or plastic boxes or rolled up in paper tissues (Middelveen et al., 2018). Morgellons syndrome is defined as an unrecognized medical and neuro-psychiatric disorder in which embedded fibers of cellulose or cotton from clothing or paper can be demonstrated microscopically in self-excoriated, intensely pruritic skin lesions in patients suffering from delusional infestations (Fig. 17.1) (Middelveen et al., 2018).

History and disease definitions

An unusual skin disease in rural French children with hairs or worms protruding from the skin on the back, arms, or legs was first identified and referred to as "*the Morgellons*" by English physicians in the late 17th century (Middelveen et al., 2018). The earliest reports of delusions of infestations were published in the late 19th century and attributed to Thibierge, who reported cases of "*acarophobia*", or fear of spiders (Middelveen et al., 2018; Wilson and Miller, 1946). In 1938, Karl Ekbom, a Swedish neurologist, described "*delusions of animals on the skin*", but his long German description was so cumbersome (*Dermatozoenwahn*), that the condition was simply called Ekbom's syndrome (Middelveen et al., 2018; Wilson and Miller, 1946). In 1946, Wilson and Miller coined a new name for the condition, "*delusion of parasitosis*" (Wilson and Miller, 1946). More recently, Freudenmann and Lepping have recommended a broader term "*delusional infestation*" (Freudenmann and Lepping, 2009).

In a 2012 case series, investigators from the United States Centers for Disease Control and Prevention (CDC) described 115 patients with delusional infestations and established a case definition for Morgellons disease (Pearson et al., 2012). According to the CDC, Morgellons disease is an unexplained dermopathy characterized by self-reported skin lesions with emerging fibers and disturbing skin sensations (Pearson et al., 2012). The designation, Morgellons disease, gradually replaced the older term, delusional infestation, for the unexplained dermopathy.

Epidemiology

In 1995, Trabert reported the results of his comprehensive metaanalysis of 193 reports of delusional infestations over a study period of 100 years that included 1123 case-patients (Trabert, 1995). The incidence in Germany was 1.6 cases per million cases per year with a mean age of case-patients of 57 years (Trabert, 1995). The ratio of female-to-male cases was 1.4:1.0 for those under age 50 years and 2.5:1.0 for those 50 years of age and older (Trabert, 1995). The later CDC study confirmed similar demographic characteristics (Pearson et al., 2012).

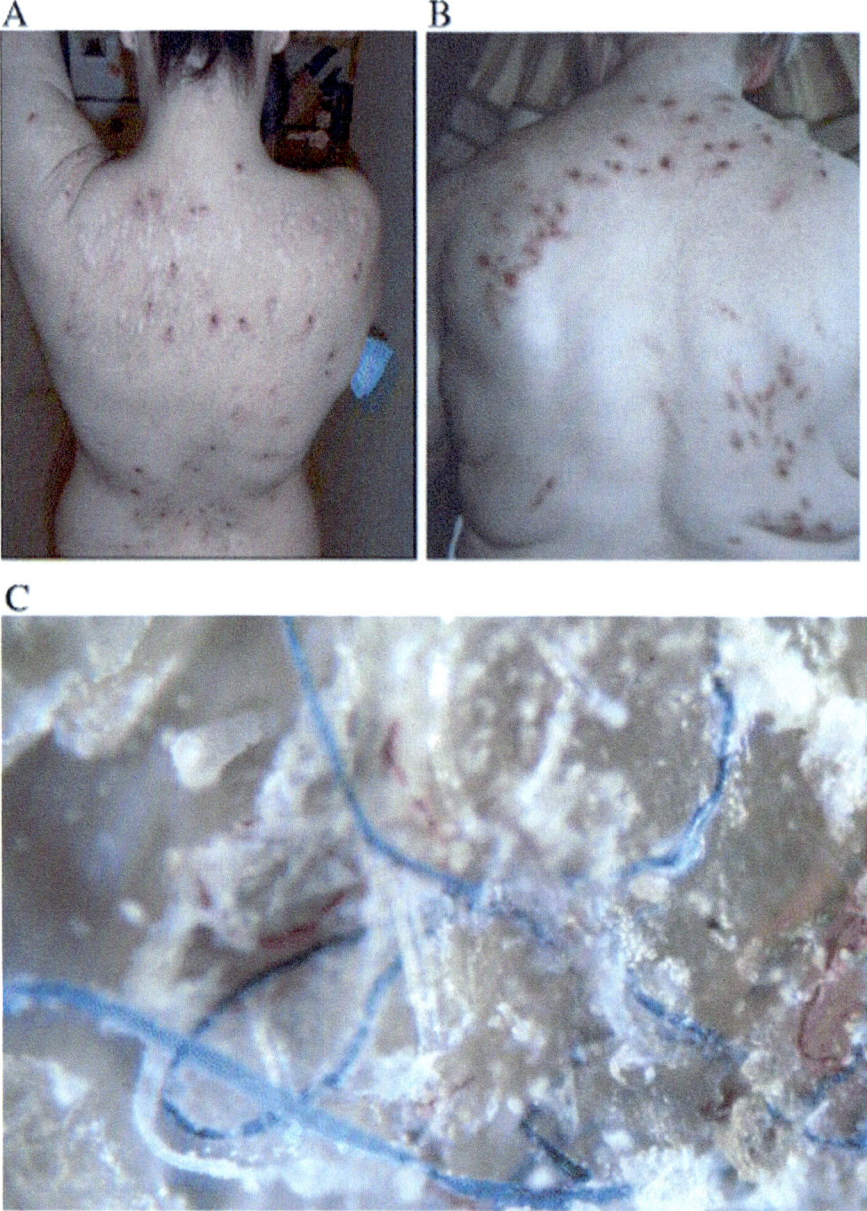

Figure 17.1 A study of Morgellons syndrome: (A) Self-excoriated and other lesions of the patient's back including those outside of the patient's reach. (B) Distribution of self-excoriated back lesions within the patient's reach. (C) Microscopic examination of lesion skin biopsy demonstrating multicolored cloth fibers and no pathogenic microorganisms. *(Wikipedia. Public domain. No copyright permission required.)*

In the CDC study, 115 case-patients meeting the definition of Morgellons disease were identified in a 13-county catchment area of Northern California (Pearson et al., 2012). The prevalence rate was 3.65 per 100,000 persons (95% Confidence Interval = 2.98—4.40) without case clustering (Pearson et al., 2012). Case-patients had a mean age of 52 years (range = 17—93 years) and were primarily female (77%) and Caucasian (77%) (Pearson et al., 2012). No parasites or mycobacteria were detected in skin biopsies (Pearson et al., 2012). Most materials obtained in skin biopsies and in suspected samples were composed of cellulose, most likely of cotton origin (Pearson et al., 2012).

Subsequent descriptive and analytical epidemiological investigations have confirmed similar demographic characteristics over time (Reilly and Batchelor, 1986). When Reilly and Batchlor surveyed 386 dermatologists in the United Kingdom, 66% reported seeing at least one patient with delusional infestation within the past 5 years (Reilly and Batchelor, 1986).

Clinical behavioral manifestations

Approximately 5%—15% of patients with delusional infestations will exhibit delusions shared with a spouse or relative (a behavioral symptom also known in French as *folie à deux*) or shared with more than one family member or close friend (a behavioral symptom also known as *folie partagé*) (Bourgeois et al., 1992). The most common shared delusions are between husband and wife, between siblings, especially twins; or between a parent, usually the mother, and a son, or daughter (Bourgeois et al., 1992).

(Bourgeois et al., 1992) Patients with delusional infestations will dismiss their initial providers quickly to seek other medical opinions from a variety of specialists ranging from dermatologists to internists, infectious disease specialists, and nurses (Bourgeois et al., 1992). In 1992, Bourgeois and coauthors reported a case of shared delusional infestations between husband and wife (*folie à deux*) in which a 58-year-old woman was institutionalized for attempting to kill her primary care provider who refused to confirm her delusions (Bourgeois et al., 1992). In some cases, patients with delusional infestations have killed their pets to rid themselves of their perceived delusions (Bourgeois et al., 1992).

Differential diagnosis

These conditions must be ruled out initially by careful recreational, occupational, and travel histories, and microscopic, microbiological, and molecular tests.

Ectoparasitic infections, such as scabies and other mite infestations, may occur in large seasonal clusters, such as in Pittsburg, Kansas, in August 2004, when 300 residents sought immediate medical care for intensely pruritic, erythematous, papular rashes, which were subsequently determined to because by multiple bites from oak tree gall mites, *Peymotes herfsi* (See Chapter 7) ("United States Centers for Disease Control and Prevention. Outbreak of pruritic rashes associated with mites—Kansas," 2004). These insect mites are ectoparasites of leaf-rolling fly larvae that fall from oak trees or get carried by the wind and land on people outdoors causing summertime community outbreaks of pruritic rashes (See Chapter 7.) ("United States Centers for Disease Control and Prevention. Outbreak of pruritic rashes associated with mites—Kansas," 2004).

Another common cause of seasonal clusters of pruritic rashes may be caused by aquatic exposures to the infective stage cercariae of several avian or rodent schistosomes or flatworms that are released into freshwater lakes and rivers in the tens of thousands by infected aquatic snail intermediate hosts in a complicated life cycle (Fig. 17.2) (Diaz, 2021). Cercarial dermatitis, also known as duck hunter's itch or swimmer's itch, is an

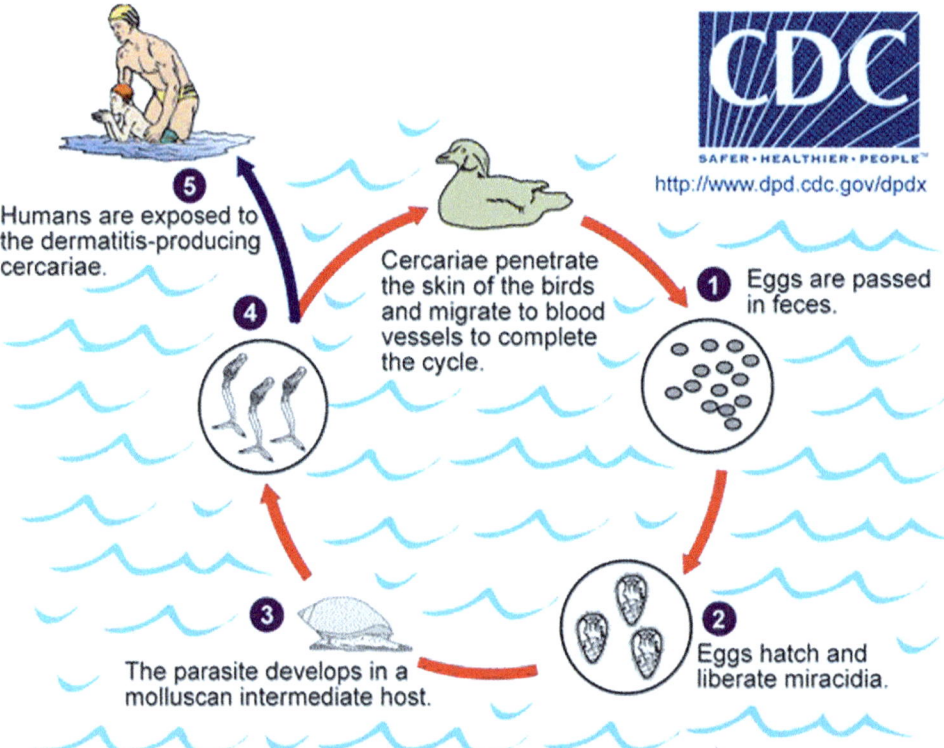

Figure 17.2 The life cycle of several species of avian schistosomes of resident and migratory waterfowl whose eggs are passed in bird feces and hatch into ciliated miricidia that penetrate aquatic snail intermediate hosts. Infected snails later release infective cercariae into freshwater sources to penetrate the skin of definitive bird hosts or inadvertent or dead-end hosts, such as humans, causing self-limited, intensely pruritic cercarial dermatitis. *(United States Centers for Disease Control and Prevention, DpDx Image Library. No copyright permission required. Available at http://www.dpd.cdc.gov/dpdx/HTML/CercarialDermatitis.htm. Source: CDC. Public domain. No copyright permission required.)*

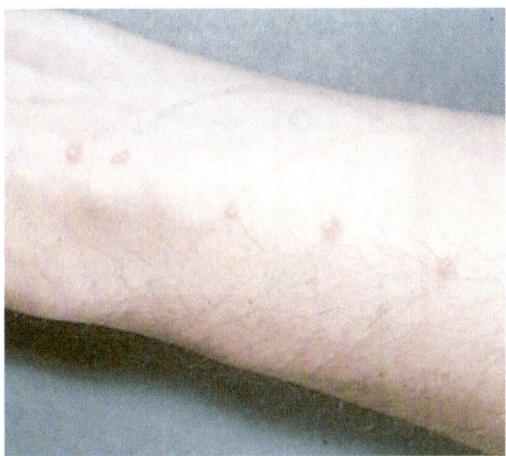

Figure 17.3 This image presents the typical, self-limited, intensely pruritic, papulovesicular rash of cercarial dermatitis or swimmer's (duck hunter's) itch caused by penetration of the skin by the cercariae of avian (waterfowl) schistosomes. *(United States Centers for Disease Control and Prevention, DpDx Image Library. No copyright permission required. Available at http://www.dpd.cdc.gov/dpdx/ HTML/CercarialDermatitis.htm. CDC. Public domain. No copyright permission required.)*

intensely pruritic maculopapular dermatitis caused by migratory cercariae that penetrate the dermis, die in the subcutaneous tissues after failing to complete their life cycles in human dead-end hosts, and incite local inflammatory reactions (Fig. 17.3) (Diaz, 2021).

Cercarial dermatitis typically occurs during the summers after freshwater exposures in inland lakes in the United States, but can also occur year-round and after coastal marine exposures worldwide (Diaz, 2021). Periodic outbreaks of cercarial dermatitis often recur in persons wading or swimming in the same bodies of water in the United States and worldwide as a result of high schistosome prevalence rates in local mammals, shorebirds, and waterfowl (Diaz, 2021).

Cutaneous larva migrans (CLM) is a parasitic skin infection typically caused by hookworm larvae that usually infest stray cats and dogs and other animals. Humans can be infected with the larvae by walking barefoot or lying naked on sandy beaches in contact with sand that has been contaminated with animal feces (Figs. 17.4 and 17.5). CLM is also known as creeping eruption as once infected, the larvae migrate under the skin's surface and cause intensely itchy red, movable lines, or tracks (Figs. 17.4 and 17.5). The larvae do not mature to adulthood to mate and complete their life cycles in human or "dead end" hosts.

Lastly, several drugs; metabolic disorder-associated peripheral neuropathies, especially diabetic neuropathy; and some neurodegenerative diseases, especially Parkinson's and Alzheimer's diseases, can cause dysesthesias with bug-crawling skin sensations that mimic ectoparasite infestations (Meehan et al., 2006; Donabedian, 2007; Fleury et al., 2008; Bhatia et al., 2013).

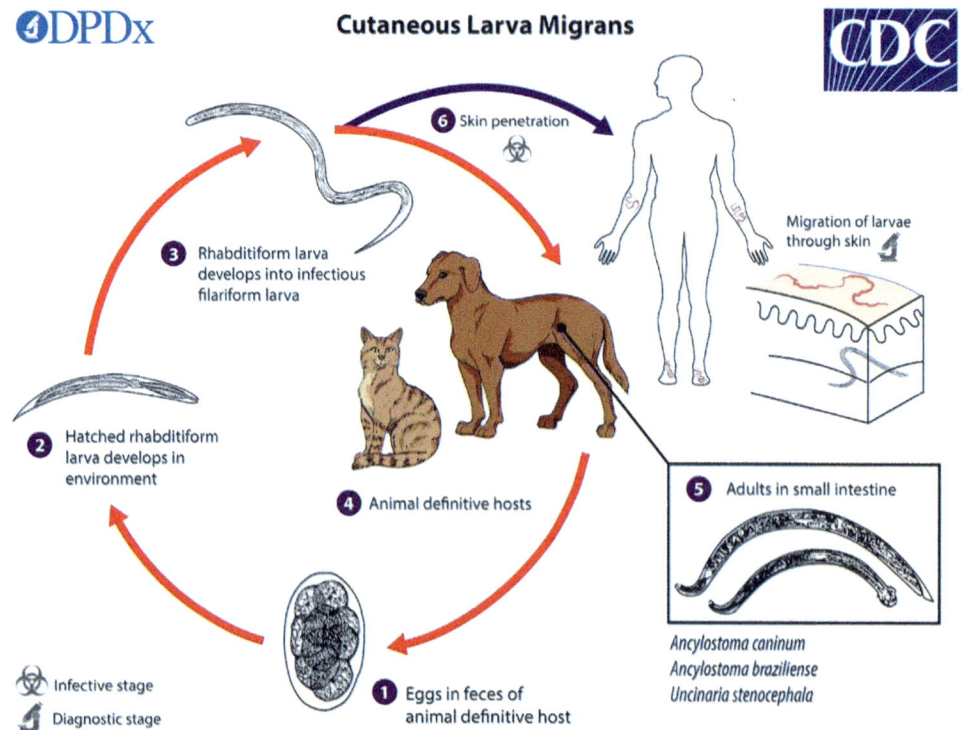

Figure 17.4 This image depicts the life cycle of cutaneous larva migrans caused by migrating hookworm larvae. Cutaneous larva migrans (CLM) is a parasitic skin infection typically caused by hookworm larvae that usually infest stray cats and dogs and other animals. Humans can be infected with the larvae by walking barefoot or lying naked on sandy beaches in contact with sand that has been contaminated with animal feces. *(United States Centers for Disease Control and Prevention. Available at https://www.cdc.gov/dpdx/zoonotichookworm/modules/CLM_LifeCycle_lg.jpg.CDC. Public domain. No copyright permission required.)*

Treatment

Before the discovery of antipsychotic medications, Wilson and Miller reported a poor prognosis for patients with delusional infestations with 82% of 51 reported patients having no change in their illnesses (Wilson and Miller, 1946). However, by the 1990s and with the use of the first generation of antipsychotics in managing delusional infestations, especially pimozide, Trabert reported nearly 70% improvement in patients with pharmacotherapy (Trabert, 1995; Bhatia et al., 2013; Reilly et al., 1978; Gowda et al., 2002; Narumoto et al., 2006; Meehan et al., 2006; Donabedian, 2007; Reilly, Jopling and Beard, 1978; Gowda et al., 2002; Narumoto et al., 2006). Unlike pimozide and all other first-generation antipsychotics, the second-generation antipsychotics carry less risk of precipitating extrapyramidal syndromes, tardive dyskinesias, and cardiac arrhythmias,

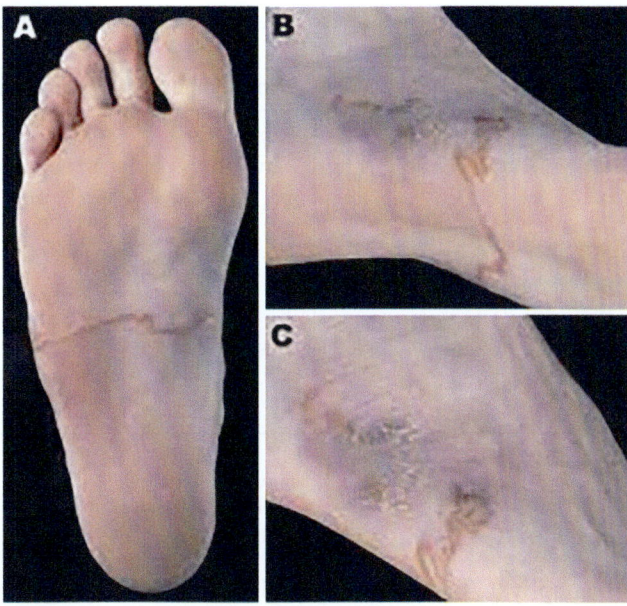

Figure 17.5 Cutaneous larva migrans on the right foot (a) and ankle (b, c) acquired from walking on a beach barefooted in Brittany, France. Nienke Tamminga, Wouter *(F.W. Bierman, and Peter J. de Vries Cutaneous larva migrans acquired in Brittany, France. Letter. Emerging Infectious Disease. 2009;15 (11). CDC Publication. Public Domain.)*

such as prolonged QT intervals and *torsades de pointes*(Meehan et al., 2006; Donabedian, 2007; Reilly, Jopling and Beard, 1978; Gowda et al., 2002; Narumoto et al., 2006).

Several reports have now confirmed that relatively small daily doses of these antipsychotics or neuroleptics are dramatically effective in reducing the delusions of infestation (Meehan et al., 2006; Donabedian, 2007; Reilly, Jopling and Beard, 1978; Gowda et al., 2002; Narumoto et al., 2006). Some of the second generation antipsychotics are associated with sedation, weight gain, anticholinergic symptoms, and hyperglycemia, especially olanzapine; but all have significantly lower potentials for causing cardiac arrhythmias, prolonged QT syndromes, *torsades de pointes,* extrapyramidal syndromes, and tardive dyskinesias than the first generation antipsychotics. Table 17.1 compares the adverse effects of the second generation antipsychotics recommended for the management of delusional infestations and their dosing schedules.

In 2006, Narumoto and coinvestigators reported a case that has now provided more convincing scientific evidence for a physiochemical mechanism of dopaminergic and serotonergic neurotransmitter dysfunction in delusional infestation and for the continued use of second generation antipsychotics in treating the disorder (Narumoto et al., 2006). In their case, a patient developed delusional infestation following an acute, ischemic stroke in the right temporoparietal region and was treated with risperidone with rapid, dramatic improvement (Narumoto et al., 2006). A pretreatment single-photon emission

Table 17.1 Second-generation antipsychotics recommended for delusional infestation: Comparison of dosing schedules and adverse effects.

Medications: Generic names	Olanzapine	Risperidone	Ziprasidone
Medications: Trade names	*Zyprexa*	*Risperdal*	*Geodon*
Daily dosing schedules	5 mg po q d hs	2 mg po q d hs	Advance over 2 d from 20 mg bid to 40 mg tid (120 mg.day^{-1})
Weight gain	+++	++	0/+
Hyperglycemia	+	0	0
Dyslipidemias	+	0	0
Sedation	++	++	+
Hypotension	+	+	0
Anticholinergic effects	+++	+	+

+++: High effect; ++: Moderate effect; +: Minimal effect; 0.
Adapted from Diaz JH. Delusional infestations by mites and other parasites. Chapter 12. In Diaz JH *Mite-Human Encounters: Nuisances, Vectors, Parasites, Allergens, and Commensals*, Elsevier, Philadelphia, 2023. Elsevier publication.

computerized tomography (CT) scan showed a global decrease in regional cerebral blood flow (rCBF), but a posttreatment CT scan showed marked increase in rCBF in the region of the infarct and in the basal ganglia bilaterally (Narumoto et al., 2006). This report was the first objective confirmation using sensitive neuroimaging techniques of the utility of second-generation antipsychotics in the management of the disorder by increasing rCBF in specific brain regions (Narumoto et al., 2006). In addition, the neuroimaging study demonstrated an association between reduced rCBF and the dysesthesias of delusional infestation and the reversal of dysesthesias with the restoration of rCBF with antipsychotic treatment, suggesting an underlying vascular mechanism for the disorder (Narumoto et al., 2006).

Conclusions

Although some reports have suggested that cases of Morgellons disease are increasing today, especially in arid and tropical regions where arthropod-borne infestations and infectious diseases are hyperendemic, most studies have now confirmed a stable incidence rate over time and similar disease demographics worldwide (Meehan et al., 2006; Donabedian, 2007; Freudenmann and Lepping, 2009; Sabry et al., 2012). The management strategies for Morgellons disease have, however, changed significantly over time with second generation antipsychotics offering safer adverse effect profiles and better prognoses than earlier therapies with behavior modification or first generation antipsychotics. The most effective current management strategies for delusional infestations include: (1) empathetic history-taking and active listening to the patient; (2) careful exclusion of spirochetal infections, such as Lyme disease, and true parasitoses, such as schistosomal, cercarial dermatitis and cutaneous larva migrans; (3) exclusion of cerebrovascular, neurodegenerative and metabolic disorders; and (4) a therapeutic regimen that includes a second generation antipsychotic agent.

References

Bhatia, M.S., Jhanjee, A., Srivastava, S., 2013. Delusional infestation: a clinical profile. Asian Journal of Psychiatry 6 (2), 124–127. https://doi.org/10.1016/j.ajp.2012.09.008.

Bourgeois, M.L., Duhamel, P., Verdoux, H., 1992. Delusional Parasitosis: Folie à Deux and Attempted Murder of a Family Doctor. British Journal of Psychiatry 161 (5), 709–711. https://doi.org/10.1192/bjp.161.5.709.

Diaz, J.H., 2021. What's the diagnosis? Dermal distress (cercarial dermatitis). Infect Dis Clin Prac 29 (5), 324–327.

Donabedian, H., 2007. Delusions of parasitosis. Clinical Infectious Diseases 45 (11), e131–e134. https://doi.org/10.1086/523004.

Fleury, V., Wayte, J., Kiley, M., 2008. Topiramate-induced delusional parasitosis. Journal of Clinical Neuroscience 15 (5), 597–599. https://doi.org/10.1016/j.jocn.2006.12.017.

Freudenmann, R.W., Lepping, P., 2009. Delusional infestation. Clinical Microbiology Reviews 22 (4), 690–732. https://doi.org/10.1128/cmr.00018-09.

Gowda, B.S.N., Heebar, S., Sathyanarayana, M.T., 2002. Delusional parasitosis responding to risperidone. Indian Journal of Psychiatry 44 (4), 382–383.

Meehan, W.J., Badreshia, S., Mackley, C.L., 2006. Successful treatment of delusions of parasitosis with olanzapine. Archives of Dermatology 142 (3), 352–355. https://doi.org/10.1001/archderm.142.3.352.

Middelveen, M.J., Fesler, M.C., Stricker, R.B., 2018. History of Morgellons disease: from delusion to definition. Clinical, Cosmetic and Investigational Dermatology 11, 71–90. https://doi.org/10.2147/CCID.S152343.

Narumoto, J., Ueda, H., Tsuchida, H., Yamashita, T., Kitabayashi, Y., Fukui, K., 2006. Regional cerebral blood flow changes in a patient with delusional parasitosis before and after successful treatment with risperidone: a case report. Progress in Neuro-Psychopharmacology and Biological Psychiatry 30 (4), 737–740. https://doi.org/10.1016/j.pnpbp.2005.11.029.

Pearson, M.L., Selby, J.V., Katz, K.A., Cantrell, V., Braden, C.R., Parise, M.E., Paddock, C.D., Lewin-Smith, M.R., Kalasinsky, V.F., Goldstein, F.C., Hightower, A.W., Papier, A., Lewis, B., Motipara, S., Eberhard, M.L., 2012. Clinical, epidemiologic, histopathologic and molecular features of an unexplained dermopathy. PLoS One 7 (1). https://doi.org/10.1371/journal.pone.0029908.

Reilly, T.M., Batchelor, D.H., 1986. The presentation and treatment of delusional parasitosis: a dermatological perspective. International Clinical Psychopharmacology 1 (4), 340–353. https://doi.org/10.1097/00004850-198610000-00009.

Reilly, T.M., Jopling, W.H., Beard, A.W., 1978. Successful treatment with pimozide of delusional parasitosis. British Journal of Dermatology 98 (4), 457–459. https://doi.org/10.1111/j.1365-2133.1978.tb06541.x.

Sabry, A.H.A.T., Fouad, M.A.H., Morsy, A.T.A., 2012. Entomophobia, acarophobia, parasitic dermatophobia or delusional parasitosis. Journal of the Egyptian Society of Parasitology 42 (2), 417–430. https://doi.org/10.12816/0006328.

Trabert, W., 1995. 100 Years of delusional parasitosis. Psychopathology 28 (5), 238–246. https://doi.org/10.1159/000284934.

United States Centers for Disease Control and Prevention, 2004. Outbreak of pruritic rashes associated with mites—Kansas. Morb Mort Week Rep 54 (38), 952–955.

Wilson, J.W., Miller, H.E., 1946. Delusion of parasitosis (acarophobia). Archives of Dermatology and Syphilology 54 (1), 39–56. https://doi.org/10.1001/archderm.1946.01510360043006.

CHAPTER 18

Conclusions

Introduction

Recent epidemiologic evidence now supports the endemicity of several emerging ecto-parasitic diseases and their arthropod vectors and human and animal reservoir hosts throughout the developing world and in many parts of the developed world, including Europe and the United States. Historic ectoparasitic diseases, such as pediculosis and scabies, have reemerged in regions where they were once effectively controlled. Ectopar-asitic diseases will continue to persist throughout the world for several reasons. Among these reasons are (1) the globalization of trade and commerce with ectoparasites and their human and animal hosts traveling worldwide on modern transportation; (2) mass move-ments of populations from rural to urban areas and from developing to developed na-tions; (3) the worldwide legitimate and illegal trade of domestic and exotic animals; (3) the accidental and intentional introduction of exotic animal species into new regions with supportive ecosystems; (4) the increasing frequency of pyrethroid-resistant strains of ectoparasites, such as head lice and trombiculid mites; (5) an expanding population of host animal reservoirs for arthropod-borne diseases, especially ungulates and rodents; and (6) a growing worldwide populations of naïve, and often immunocompromised, human hosts (Demma et al., 2005).

Bartonella quintana — A reemerging pathogen

The isolation of the trench-fever pathogen, *Bartonella quintana,* in head lice from home-less persons in the United States illustrates how socioeconomic factors, human behavioral trends, and vector adaptations can support ectoparasite persistence with public health consequences (Bonilla et al., 2009). The new clade of African body and head lice infected by both *Bartonella quintana* and *Yersinia pestis* demonstrated that body and head lice could possibly represent new arthropod vectors for trench fever, *Bartonella* endocarditis, and plague (Drali et al., 2015).

Babesiosis — Increasing regional prevalence

The incidence of babesiosis has now increased five times in some New England states with Connecticut reporting an incidence of two cases per 100,000 persons in 2011 and nine cases per 100,000 persons in 2019 (Demma et al., 2005).

Ectoparasitic Diseases
ISBN 978-0-443-26724-6
https://doi.org/10.1016/B978-0-443-26724-6.00018-7

Rhipicephalus sanguineus — **A new and unanticipated vector**

In a seemingly unending era of discoveries of tick-transmitted diseases, another new and unanticipated vector for Rocky Mountain spotted fever (RMSF), the brown dog tick, *Rhipicephalus sanguineus*, was identified in the US Southwest and rapidly expanded its range of distribution into southern Arizona, California, and Texas and northern Mexico (Gray and Herwaldt, 2011). New strains of encephalitis and coagulopathy-causing Alongshan flaviviruses are now circulating in ixodid tick vectors in China and throughout Western Europe, adding to an expanding list of emerging, unanticipated tickborne infectious diseases.

Haemaphysalis longicornis — **A highly competent introduced vector**

According to the US Centers for Disease Control and Prevention (CDC), the Asian long-horned tick, *Haemaphysalis longicornis,* represents the most dangerous introduced species of foreign tick in the USA today. The Asian long-horned tick poses a significant threat of transmission of several tickborne disease to humans and domestic animals (Beard et al., 2018).

Native to eastern China, Japan, Korea, and the Russian Far East, the Asian long-horned tick was first detected on a domestic animal (goat) in the United States in New Jersey in 2017. By 2018, the tick had extended its range from New Jersey to seven other states in the eastern United States and as far south as Arkansas (Beard et al., 2018). Animal host reservoirs for the introduced tick are abundant and include six species of domestic animals, six species of wildlife, and humans (Beard et al., 2018). Although there is no evidence that *H. longicornis* has transmitted any pathogens to animals or humans in the US to date, *H. longicornis* is capable of transmitting several pathogens including bacteria (*Rickettsia, Borrelia, Ehrlichia, Anaplasma,* and *Theileria* spp), viruses (Bourbon, Heartland, severe fever with thrombocytopenia syndrome virus), and, probably, the protozoan, *Babesia*.

Ectoparasitic Diseases — **meeting its objectives**

Ectoparasitic Diseases has identified emerging ectoparasitic diseases, differentiated between infections transmitted by ectoparasites from ectoparasitic infestations and allergies caused by ectoparasites, and provided clinicians with recommendations for diagnoses, treatments, prevention, and control strategies. The text has also examined the psychological and socioeconomic impacts of infections, infestations, health disparities, ectoparasite-induced allergies, and predisposing risk factors for ectoparasitic diseases. Several featured topics of *Ectoparasitic Diseases* have not been addressed in other current texts on parasitic diseases, including the tick sialome, tick-transmitted coinfections, tick paralysis, the alpha-gal-syndrome, and Morgellons disease.

Conclusions

Ectoparasitic diseases are no longer exotic diseases afflicting barefoot children, the displaced, and the socioeconomically disadvantaged in the tropics. Human ectoparasitic diseases, such as myiasis, scabies, tungiasis, and scrub typhus, have reemerged as unusual and often misdiagnosed, diseases of tourists, executives, missionaries, and soldiers from industrialized nations returning from vacations or job-related assignments in locations throughout developed and developing nations, including popular resort destinations.

Ectoparasitic diseases are significant sources of morbidity in humans and should not be neglected as international outbreaks will continue to occur with pesticide-resistant strains that are difficult to control. Clinicians should be aware of new and reemerging ectoparasitic diseases in order to make timely diagnoses and institute proper therapies. In addition, public health officials should be informed of regional ectoparasitic disease outbreaks in order to institute investigation, prevention, and control strategies to protect vulnerable populations.

References

Beard, C.B., Occi, J., Bonilla, D.L., Egizi, A.M., Fonseca, D.M., Mertins, J.W., Backenson, B.P., Bajwa, W.I., Barbarin, A.M., Bertone, M.A., Brown, J., Connally, N.P., Connell, N.D., Eisen, R.J., Falco, R.C., James, A.M., Krell, R.K., Lahmers, K., Lewis, N., Little, S.E., Neault, M., de León, A.A.P., Randall, A.R., Ruder, M.G., Saleh, M.N., Schappach, B.L., Schroeder, B.A., Seraphin, L.L., Wehtje, M., Wormser, G.P., Yabsley, M.J., Halperin, W., 2018. Multistate infestation with the exotic disease—vector tick haemaphysalis longicornis — United States, August 2017—September 2018. Morbidity and Mortality Weekly Report 67 (47), 1310—1313. https://doi.org/10.15585/MMWR.MM6747A3, 1545861X.

Bonilla, D.L., Kabeya, H., Henn, J., Kramer, V.L., Kosoy, M.Y., 2009. Bartonella quintana in body lice and head lice from homeless persons, San Francisco, California, USA. Emerging Infectious Diseases 15 (6), 912—915. https://doi.org/10.3201/eid1506.090054, 10806059.

Demma, L.J., Traeger, M.S., Nicholson, W.L., Paddock, C.D., Blau, D.M., Eremeeva, M.E., Dasch, G.A., Levin, M.L., Singleton, J., Zaki, S.R., Cheek, J.E., Swerdlow, D.L., McQuiston, J.H., 2005. Rocky Mountain spotted fever from an unexpected tick vector in Arizona. New England Journal of Medicine 353 (6), 587—594. https://doi.org/10.1056/NEJMoa050043.

Drali, R., Shako, J.C., Davoust, B., Diatta, G., Raoult, D., 2015. A new clade of african body and head lice infected by bartonella quintana and yersinia pestis-democratic republic of the Congo. The American Journal of Tropical Medicine and Hygiene 93 (5), 990—993. https://doi.org/10.4269/ajtmh.14-0686, 00029637.

Gray, E.B., Herwaldt, B.L., 2011. Babesiosis surveillance—United States. Morbidity & Mortality Weekly Report 68 (6), 1—11.

Index

'*Note:* Page numbers followed by "f"indicate figures and "t" indicate tables.'

A

Alongshan virus (ALSV), 179
Amblyomma americanum, 130, 130f, 198f
Anaplasmosis, 157—158
Animal (zoonotic) mites, 72t—73t
  domestic animal-transmitted cheyletiellosis, 71—75
  rat, bat, and snake mite bites, 79—81
  scabietic mange, 75—76
  zoonotic acariasis, 77—78
Anticoagulant proteins, 185—186
Antipruritics, chigger mites, 32
Argasid ticks, 128—129
Arthropod ectoparasites, 5t—6t
  infectious diseases transmission, 3, 6t—7t
  socioeconomic and behavioral factors, 7—8
Arthropod vectors, 35—36
Atrophic rhinitis, 107
Autoimmune hemolytic anemia, 169
Avian bites and infestations
  clinical manifestations, 77—78
  definitions, 77—78
  prevention and control, 78
  treatment, 78

B

Babesia divergens, 165—166
Babesia duncani, 165—166
Babesia microti, 165—166
Babesiosis
  autoimmune hemolytic anemia, 169
  causal agents, 167t—168t
  clinical manifestations, 167t—168t, 169—170
  epidemiology, 166—169
  history, 165
  incidence, 166, 249
  laboratory diagnosis, 170
  microbiology, 165—166
  neurologic effects, 169—170
  prevention and control, 171—172
  regional distributions, 165
  reservoirs, 165
  risk factors, 166—169

  therapy, 171
  vectors, 165
Bartonella quintana, 13, 249
Bat mite, 79, 81
Bed bugs
  biology and life cycle, 213—214, 215f
  Cimex species, 213
  clinical manifestations, 216—218, 217f
  complications, 217—218
  control and prevention, 219—220
  detection and diagnosis, 218—219
  epidemiology, 216
  feeding behavior, 214
  geographic distribution, 216
  International travel, 216
  management, 219
  nesting behavior, 214—215
  pesticide resistance, 216
  taxonomy, 213
Body lice
  Bartonella quintana, 13
  clinical manifestations and differential diagnosis, 19
  diagnosis, 14
  epidemiological analysis, 12
  life cycles, pathogenesis, and clinical manifestations, 15t—17t
  prevalence, 12
  preventive interventions, 25
  Rickettsia prowazekii, 13
  risk factors, 12
  therapy, 24
Borrelia burgdorferi, 129f
Borrelial lymphocytoma, 138
Borrelia miyamotoi, 130
Borrelioses, 133—143
  Lyme borreliosis (LB), 136—140
  Southern tick-associated rash illness (STARI), 140
  tickborne relapsing fevers (TBRFs), 141—143
Bubonic plague, 121, 121f
Bullous scabies, 51
Burrow ink test (BIT), 55—56

C

California tick fever virus of rabbits (CTFV-Ca), 181–182
Canadian tick paralysis, 191–194
Cardiac vasculitis, 148–149
Carpoglyphuslactis, 87–91
Cavitary myiasis, 103–104, 107
Cercarial dermatitis, 242–243
Cetuximab-mediated allergic reactions, 202–203
Cheese mites, 91, 92f
Cheyletiella yasguri, 74, 74f
Cheyletiellosis
  clinical manifestations, 75, 75f
  domestic animal-transmitted
    with alopecia, 74f
    clinical manifestations, 75
    definition, 71–74
    life cycle, 74, 74f
    treatment, 75
Chigger mites
  clinical manifestations, 31–32, 31f
  complications, 33
  ecology, 29
  feeding behavior, 30–31, 30f
  immune responses, 32
  larval trombiculid mites, 28t
  life cycle, 27f, 28–29
  prevention and control, 33
  regional distribution, 29
  taxonomy, 27–28
  treatment, 32
Chiroptonyssus robustipes, 79
Chloramphenicol, rickettsialpox, 69
Cimex lectularius, 214f
Citronella, 229, 230f
Classic scabies, 50f, 51, 53t–54t
  clinical manifestations, 50
  immune responses, 55t
  skin eruptions, 51
CNS Q fever, 151
Cochliomyia hominivorax, 106t
Coconut mite, 87–91, 90f
Colorado tick fever virus (CTFV), 181–182
Copra itch, 87–91, 90f
Corticosteroids, chigger mites, 32
Crab lice, 14, 19–20. *See also* Pubic lice
Crimean-Congo hemorrhagic fever (CCHF) virus, 180

Crusted scabies, 47–49, 48f
  immune responses, 55t
  immunosuppressive conditions, 54
  porcine models, 54–55
Cutaneous larva migrans (CLM), 243, 244f

D

Deer tick virus, 178
Delusional ectoparasitosis
  avian schistosomes life cycle, 242f
  case series, 237–238
  clinical behavioral manifestations, 241
  definition, 239
  differential diagnosis, 241–243
  epidemiology, 239–241
  history, 239
  management, 246t
  treatment, 244–246
Demodex blepharitis, 99–100
Demodex brevis, 97
Demodex folliculorum follicle mite, 97f
Demodicidosis gravis, 99
Dermacentor andersoni, 128f
Dermacentor occidentalis, 132f
Dermacentor tick paralysis
  neurotoxic paralysis, 187–190
  treatment, 194
Dermanyssus americanus, 77–78
Dermatobia hominis, 106–107, 106t
Dermatophagoides pteronyssinus, 93f
DNA-dependent protein kinase (DNA-PK) activation, house dust mite-induced asthma, 94, 95f
Doxycycline
  murine typhus, 113
  rickettsialpox, 69
  srub typhus, 43–44
Dust mites
  definitions and taxonomy, 92
  feeding behavior and life cycle, 92–93
  immune response, 93–94
  prevention and control, 95–96
  treatment, 95–96

E

Ehrlichioses, 155–159
Ekbom's syndrome, 239
Electric insecticide vaporizers, 232
Epiluminescence dermatoscopes, 56

Erythema migrans, 137f
Eschar phase, rickettsialpox, 67
Ethyl butylacetylaminoproprionate, 228
European Eyach virus (EYAV), 181—182
European house dust mite, 93f
Eutrombicula alfreddugesi, 27—28, 29f

F

Facial leprosy, 107
Facultative myiasis, 103
Fecal spots, bed bugs, 218—219
Flea-transmitted infectious diseases, 110t—111t
    murine typhus, 112—113
    plague, 117—124
    tungiasis, 113—116
Follicle mites
    clinical manifestations, 99—100
    as commensals, 96—97
    immune responses, 98
    life cycle, 98
    treatment, 100
Francisella tularensis, 153
Furuncular myiasis, 103—104, 107, 109

G

Genitourinary myiasis, 103—104
Glyciphagus domesticus, 87—91
Guillain-Barré syndrome, 191—194

H

Haemaphysalis longicornis, 181, 250
Hay/grain itch mite, 82f
Head lice
    clinical manifestations, 19
    definition, 10
    diagnosis, 14
    differential diagnosis, 19
    epidemiology, 12
    life cycles, pathogenesis, and clinical
        manifestations, 15t—17t
    preventive interventions, 25
Hemorrhagic fever viruses, 180—181
Human cheyletiellosis, 75f
Human immunodeficiency virus (HIV) infection,
    12—13
Human T-cell lymphotropic virus type 1
    (HTLV-1) infection, 47—49

I

Immune response
    dust mite allergens, 93—94
    follicle mites, 98
Immunization strategies, 160
Impetigo, scabies, 61
Infectious disease transmission, 3
Insect (itch) mites, 81—86
Insect repellents
    chemical *vs.* plant-based, 222—231
    children and pregnancy, 231—232
    definition, 221
    efficacy, 223t
    formulations, 223t
    history, 222
    reasons to use, 221—222
    safety and toxicity, 223t
    and sunscreens, 232
Intestinal myiasis, 103—104
IR3535, 228
Ivermectin, scabies, 59
Ixodes pacificus, 130—131, 132f
Ixodes scapularis, 130—131, 131f, 186, 187f
Ixodid ticks, 127—128

J

Japanese spotted fever (JSF), 150
Jarisch-Herxheimer reaction (JHR), 140, 143

K

Knock-down insecticide aerosol sprays, 232

L

Landscape management strategies, 208
Leptotrombidium species chigger arvae, 36f
Life cycles, human ectoparasites, 3, 4t
Liponyssoides sanguineus, 65f
Lone Star tick, 130, 203
Lyme borreliosis (LB), 129, 134t—135t, 136—140
    Borrelial lymphocytoma, 138
    Borrelia organisms, 136
    diagnosis and treatment, 138
    erythema migrans, 136
    incidence, 136—137, 139—140
    neurologic manifestation, 138
    United States and Europe, 136—138
Lyme disease, 129

M

Mechanical control, bed bugs, 220
Mediterranean Spotted Fever (MSF), 149
Morgellons syndrome, 240f. *See also* Delusional
    ectoparasitosis
Mosquito coils, 232
Murine typhus
    clinical manifestations, 113
    differential diagnosis, 113
    flea vectors, 112, 112f
    laboratory diagnostic strategies, 113
    prevention and control strategies, 113
    treatment, 113
Myiasis
    causing flies, 105t
    clinical manifestations, 107–108
    epidemiology, 104–107
    facultative, 103
    management strategies, 109
    obligatory, 103
    prevention and control, 109
    types, 103–104

N

N, N-diethyl-m-toluamide (DEET)
    field testing, 223
    formulations, 223
    safety record, 223–227
    toxicity, 227
Nodular scabies, 51–52, 52f, 53t–54t
Nonchemical measures, 233

O

Oak leaf gall mites, 82–83, 82f
Ophionyssus natricis, 79, 80f
Orientia tsutsugamushi infection, 40f. *See also* Srub
    typhus
    clinical manifestations, 41
    geographic distribution, 38
    immunoglobin responses, 38
    larval feeding, 37
    treatment, 43
Ornithonyssus bursa, 77–78, 78f

P

Pediculosis (lice)
    body lice. *See* Body lice
    definition, 9–11
    head lice. *See* Head lice
    pubic lice. *See* Pubic lice
Pediculosis capitis, 15t–17t, 21–24, 22t–23t.
    See also Head lice
Pediculosis corporis. *See* Body lice
Pediculosis (phthiriasis) pubis, 19–20. *See also*
    Pubic lice
Pediculus humanus, 9
Pediculus humanus var. *capitis*, 10f
Periungual lesion, tungiasis, 115, 116f
Permethrin, 229–231
Personal protective measures, 233
    babesiosis, 171–172
    red meat allergies after tick bites, 207–208
    tick-transmitted diseases, 160–161
Phthirus pubis, 11f
Picaridin, 228
Pityriasis folliculorum, 99
Plague
    clinical manifestations, 121–123
    diagnosis, 123, 123f
    ecology, 117, 118f
    epidemiology, 118–120
    history, 117
    pathophysiology, 120
    prevention and control strategies, 124
    therapy, 124
Plant, food, and food storage mites
    clinical manifestations, 87–91
    definitions and taxonomy, 87
    host reservoirs, 88t–89t
    prevention and control, 91
    treatment, 91
p-menthane-3, 8-diol (PMD), 228–229, 229f
pneumonia, Q fever, 151
Pneumonic plague, 122
Powassan encephalitis, 177–178
Powassan virus (POWV) disease, 178
Pubic lice
    diagnosis, 14
    differential diagnosis, 19–20
    epidemiology, 12
    life cycles, pathogenesis, and clinical
        manifestations, 15t–17t
    preventive interventions, 25
Pyemotes herfsi, 82–83, 82f
Pyemotes tritici, 81–82, 82f
Pyemotes ventricosus mite bite, 83–85, 84f
Pyemotid mite bites
    clinical manifestations, 85

definitions and taxonomy, 81–85
prevention and control, 86
treatment, 85

Q

Q (Query) fever
  diagnosis, 151–152
  human illness, 151
  pregnancy, 151
  therapy, 152
  transmission, 150–151
  US military personnel, 151
Quinine, babesiosis, 171

R

Rash phase, rickettsialpox, 67
Rat mite bite. *See also* Rickettsialpox
  clinical manifestations, 79
  prevention and control, 81
  treatment, 81
Red meat allergies
  alpha-gal, 197
  blood group antigens, 201
  cetuximab, 202–203
  clinical manifestations, 206
  diagnosis, 206–207
  epidemiology, 197–198
  gelatin, 202
  geographic distribution, 198–199
  global reports, 200t–201t
  immunoglobulin E (IgE)-mediated allergic
    reactions, 197
  immunology, 199–204
  prevalence, 197–198
  prevention and control, 207–208
  radioallergosorbent testing (RAST), 203
  risk factors, 204–206
  treatment, 207
Rhipicephalus sanguineus, 130, 131f, 250
Rickettsia, taxonomy, 35
Rickettsia 364D eschar, 133, 133f
Rickettsialpox, 45, 150–152
  clinical manifestations, 66–67
  differential diagnosis, 68
  epidemiology, 66
  feeding behavior, 65
  laboratory diagnosis, 68
  life cycle, 65
  prevention and control, 69

reservoirs and vectors, 65
  therapy, 69
Rickettsia parkeri rickettsiosis, 146, 147f
Rickettsia prowazekii, 13
Rickettsioses
  Rickettsialpox, 150–152
  spotted fever, 144–150
Rocky mountain spotted fever (RMSF), 145t
  CNS complications, 148–149
  digital ischemia with gangrene, 149f
  fatal cases, 146–148
  incidence rate, 146
  spotty rashes, 146
Rocky Mountain wood tick, 191
Rosacea-like demodicidosis, 99, 99f

S

Salmon River virus (SRV), 181–182
Scabies, 48f
  atypical forms, 51–52
  clinical manifestations, 49–55, 50f
  crusted scabies, 48f
  diagnosis, 55–56
  drug resistance, 60
  epidemiology, 47–49
  immune responses, 52–55
  impetigo, 61
  molecular mechanisms, 54
  prevalence, 47
  prevention and control strategies, 60–61
  therapy, 56–60, 57t–58t
  transmission, 49
Scabietic mange, 75–76, 76f
Scalp scabies, 53t–54t
Second-generation antipsychotics, 246t
Septicemic plague, 122, 122f
Snake mite bites, 79, 80f
  prevention and control, 81
  treatment, 81
Southern tick-associated rash illness (STARI), 130,
    130f, 134t–135t, 140
Spotted fevers rickettsioses
  distal maculopapular-petechial rash, 148f
  Japanese spotted fever (JSF), 150
  Mediterranean Spotted Fever (MSF), 149
  Rickettsia parkeri, 146
  Rickettsia rickettsii, 144f
  Rocky mountain spotted fever (RMSF). *See*
    Rocky mountain spotted fever (RMSF)

Srub typhus
    clinical manifestations, 41–42, 42f
    disease transmission, 35–36
    ecology, 36–37
    epidemiology, 37–39
    geographic distribution, 38, 45
    immune responses, 37–38
    laboratory diagnosis, 42–43
    larval feeding, 37
    noninfectious chigger bites, 37
    prevention and control, 44–45
    risk factors, 39
    seasonal transmission, 38–39
    treatment, 43
Summer penile syndrome, 32
Sunscreens, 232

T

Taxonomy, 1, 2t
Tickborne diseases
    anaplasmosis, 157–158
    borrelioses, 133–143
    ehrlichioses, 158–159
    epidemiology, 129–133
    prevention and control, 160–161
    Rickettsioses, 143–152
    tularemia, 152–155
    vector behavior, 127
Tickborne encephalitis viruses (TBVE)
    New World, 177–178
    Old World, 177–179
    representative, 174t–175t
    risk factors, 173
    wild animal reservoirs, 177
Tickborne hemorrhagic fever (TBHF) viruses,
        180–181
Tickborne relapsing fever (TBRFs), 134t–135t,
        141–143
    Borrelia hermsii, 142
    Borrelia turicatae, 142
    clinical manifestations, 142–143
    laboratory diagnostics, 143
    Ornithodoros species bites, 141–142, 141f
    transovarian transmission, 141
    treatment strategies, 143
Tick paralysis
    differential diagnosis, 191–194,
        192t–193t
    marsupial ixodid tick, 191
    Rocky Mountain wood tick, 191
    ticks species, 187–190

Ticks
    advantages, 127
    biology and taxonomy, 127–129
    life cycle, 128–129
Tick sialome
    chemical constituents, 185–186
    immunomodulatory compounds, 185
    nonproteinaceous compounds, 186
    proteinaceous compounds, 185–186
Ticks removal
    babesiosis, 172
    red meat allergies after tick bites, 209f
Tick-transmitted coinfections
    decision tree models, 187, 188f
    geographic areas, 186
    immunologic confirmation, 186
Tick-transmitted viral diseases
    coltiviruses, 181–182
    emerging flaviviruses, 179
    epidemiology, 173–177
    hemorrhagic fever viruses, 180–181
Trombidiosis. *See* Chigger mites
Tsutsugamushi triangle, 39f
Tularemia, 152–155
    clinical classification, 154t
    diagnosis, 153–155
    Francisella tularensis, 153
    transmission, 152–153
    treatment strategies, 155
Tungiasis
    clinical manifestations, 114–115, 115f
    differential diagnosis, 115
    epidemiology, 114
    management strategies, 115–116
    prevention and control, 116
Tyrophagus casei, 87–91
Tyrophagus longior, 87–91, 90f
Tyrophagus putrescentiae, 87–91

V

Vesiculopapular dermatitis, 79

W

Walking dandruff. *See* Cheyletiellosis
Wildlife management strategies, 208

Y

Yersinia pestis, 13–14

Z

Zoonotic acariasis, 77–78

Printed and bound by CPI Group (UK) Ltd, Croydon, CR0 4YY

06/09/2024

01032554-0002